Application of Nursing Process and Nursing Diagnosis

An Interactive Text for Diagnostic Reasoning

Application of Nursing Process and Nursing Diagnosis

An Interactive Text for Diagnostic Reasoning

FOURTH EDITION

Marilynn E. Doenges, RN, BSN, MA
Adult Psychiatric/Mental Health Nurse, retired
Adjunct Faculty
Beth-El College of Nursing & Health Science,
CU-Springs
Colorado Springs, Colorado

Mary Frances Moorhouse, RN, BSN, CRRN, CLNC
Nurse Consultant
TNT-RN Enterprises
Clinical Instructor
Pikes Peak Community College
Colorado Springs, Colorado

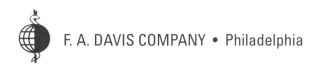

F. A. DAVIS COMPANY • Philadelphia

F. A. Davis Company
1915 Arch Street
Philadelphia, PA 19103

Printed in the United States of America

Last digit indicates print number: 10 9 8 7 6 5 4 3 2 1

Publisher: Robert Martone
Cover Designer: Louis J. Forgione

As new scientific information becomes available through basic and clinical research, recommended treatments and drug therapies undergo changes. The author(s) and publisher have done everything possible to make this book accurate, up to date, and in accord with accepted standards at the time of publication. The authors, editors, and publisher are not responsible for errors or omissions or for consequences from application of the book, and make no warranty, expressed or implied, in regard to the contents of the book. Any practice described in this book should be applied by the reader in accordance with professional standards of care used in regard to the unique circumstances that may apply in each situation. The reader is advised always to check product information (package inserts) for changes and new information regarding dose and contraindications before administering any drug. Caution is especially urged when using new or infrequently ordered drugs.

ISBN 0-8036-1066-1

To our families, who support us in all we do and who continue to support our dreams, fantasies, and obsessions.

With special thanks to:

The Doenges family: the late Dean, whose support and encouragement are sorely missed; Jim; Barbara and Bob Lanza; David, Monita, Matthew, and Tyler; John, Holly, Nicole, and Kelsey; and the Daigle family: Nancy, Jim, Jennifer, and Brandon Smith-Daigle, and Jonathan and Kim.

The Moorhouse family: Jan, Paul; Jason, Alexa, and Mary Isabella.

Alice Geissler-Murr, for being available when we need help.

The staff at Memorial Hospital library, for cheerfully filling in all the blanks and by helping us find those elusive references.

To the students of Beth-El College of Nursing and the nursing students of the Pikes Peak Community College, who continue to challenge us to make the nursing process and nursing diagnosis understandable.

To our colleagues, who continue to provide a sounding board and feedback for our professional beliefs and expectations. We hope this interactive text will help you and your students at all stages to clarify and apply these concepts.

To our F. A. Davis family, especially our publisher and friend, Robert (Bob) Martone;

Bob Butler, Jessica Howie Martin, and all who facilitated the revision process to get this project completed in a timely fashion.

To NANDA and the international nurses who are developing and using nursing diagnoses. And to the nurses who have patiently awaited this revision, we hope it will help in applying theory to practice and will enhance the delivery and effectiveness of your care.

Notes to the Educator

The nursing process has been used for over 25 years as a systematic approach to nursing practice. The process is an efficient and effective method for organizing nursing knowledge and clinical decision making in providing planned client care. Although it has been undergoing constant re-evaluation and revision, the concepts within the process still remain central to nursing practice.

Healthcare accrediting agencies and nursing organizations have developed standards of nursing practice that focus on the tenets of the nursing process, that is, assessing, diagnosing, planning, implementing, evaluating, and documenting client care. Although the formats used to document the plan of care may change with the interpretation and evaluation of standards, the nursing responsibilities and interventions required for planned client care still need to be learned, shared, performed, evaluated, and documented.

The nursing process is by its nature an interactive method of practicing nursing. This text mirrors that interactive focus by presenting a step-by-step problem-solving design to help students develop an understanding of the meaning and language of nursing. We have included definitions and professional standards that will serve as a solid foundation for your students to understand and apply the nursing process. The vignettes, practice activities, work pages, and case studies provide an opportunity to examine and scrutinize client situations and dilemmas in practice, consider alternatives, and evaluate outcomes. The worksheets serve as graphic summaries that provide students with criteria to evaluate their decisions and demonstrate their understanding of the concepts and integration of the material presented. Tear-out pages for independent learning provide an opportunity for practical application and beginning mastery of the nursing process. These pages can be taken to the clinical area to reinforce selected aspects of the nursing process. Finally, review of client situations and the Code for Nurses can serve as a catalyst for philosophical and ethical discussions. All these activities encourage the student to actively seek solutions rather than passively assimilate knowledge, thus stimulating the student's critical thinking ability.

Chapter 1, The Nursing Process: Delivering Quality Care

This introductory chapter presents an overview of the nursing process. Students are introduced to the definitions of nursing and nursing diagnosis and the American Nurses Association's Standards of Clinical Nursing Practice.

Chapter 2, The Assessment Step: Developing the Client Database

This chapter introduces students to the first step of the nursing process. Organizational formats for constructing nursing assessment tools are discussed, and both the physical and psychosocial aspects of assessment are blended into the interview process. Examples of client data assist students to identify categories of nursing diagnostic labels.

Chapter 3, The Diagnosis or Need Identification Step: Analyzing the Data

The definition and concepts of nursing diagnosis are presented in this chapter. We use the term *Client Diagnostic Statement* to describe the combination of the NANDA-approved label, the client's related factors (etiology), and associated defining characteristics (signs/symptoms). A six-step diagnostic reasoning process is presented to assist students in their beginning efforts to accurately analyze the client's assessment data. The remainder of this chapter focuses on ruling out, synthesizing, evaluating, and constructing the client diagnostic statement.

Chapter 4, The Planning Step: Creating the Plan of Care

Information on developing the individualized outcomes for the client is provided in this chapter. A focus on correctly writing measurable outcomes is initially presented. In addition, examples from the standardized nursing language for outcomes, Nursing Outcomes Classification (NOC), are also presented. Nursing interventions are defined and acknowledgment of the work by the Iowa Intervention Project's Nursing Interventions Classification (NIC) is included. The topics, priorities of interventions, discharge planning, and selecting appropriate nursing interventions are discussed along with examples of a fourth standardized language, the Omaha System. A practice activity for recording the steps of the nursing process learned thus far is included to provide the student with a realistic application. An interactive plan of care worksheet is used to present examples and guidelines for developing the client's outcome statement, selecting nursing interventions, and providing rationales for nursing interventions. Finally, information about the use of mind mapping to stimulate right brain activity to facilitate the planning process is presented along with a sample plan of care.

Chapter 5, The Implementation Step: Putting the Plan of Care into Action

Information is presented about the validation and implementation of the plan of care. Concerns regarding the day-to-day organization of the nurse's work is creatively used in a practice activity in which students use time management to plan the day's client care interventions. Change-of-shift reporting principles are also discussed and practiced.

Chapter 6, The Evaluation Step: Determining Whether Desired Outcomes Have Been Met

The crucial step of evaluation and its accompanying reassessment and revision processes are presented in this chapter on the last step of the nursing process. A practice activity is provided to help students evaluate the plan of care partially constructed in Chapter 4. Revisions to the plan of care are necessary, and the activity provides a realistic exercise for this final step. The interactive plan of care worksheet is designed to ask your students questions about their client's progress and the effectiveness of their implemented nursing interventions.

Chapter 7, Documenting the Nursing Process

This chapter introduces students to ways of successfully documenting their use of the nursing process. Communication, legal responsibilities, and reimbursement are a few of the topics introduced in this chapter. The documentation systems of SOAP and FOCUS CHARTING™ are presented to depict two possible methods of documenting the nursing process. The last section of the interactive worksheet focuses the students' attention on three important aspects of documentation: the reassessment data, interventions implemented, and the client's response.

Chapter 8, Interactive Care Planning: from Assessment to Client Response

This final chapter provides an evaluation checklist that can be used to evaluate your students' progress in all aspects of the nursing process. The checklist is designed to include the criteria listed on the Interactive Care Plan Worksheets, ANA Standards of Clinical Nursing Practice, and the JCAHO nursing standards. The chapter ends with a case study that gives your students an opportunity to apply all the steps of the nursing process. The evaluation checklist along with the TIME OUTS included in the plan of care worksheets provide the students with the required guidance when constructing their first complete plan of care.

Appendices

A listing of the NANDA (formerly the North American Nursing Diagnosis Association) nursing diagnoses are included in Appendix A. Each nursing diagnosis' definition, related/risk factors, and defining characteristics are provided to assist the student in accurately selecting the appropriate nursing diagnosis.

Appendix B defines the seven axes of the new NANDA Taxonomy II.

Appendix C provides an adult medical-surgical nursing assessment tool as referenced in Chapter 2, along with excerpts from assessment tools developed for the psychiatric and obstetric settings. The tools are helpful to students in their assessment of the client's response to health problems as well as the gathering of physical assessment data.

Appendix D organizes the NANDA diagnostic labels within Maslow's hierarchy of needs to aid in visualizing and determining priorities for providing client care.

Appendix E, ANA's Code of Ethics for Nurses, was included for your use both in the classroom and during clinical rounds to share with your students the values that guide nursing practice today. A reference to the Code and the introduction of a discussion of beliefs that affect nursing practice are contained in Chapter 1, and an ethical activity is presented in Chapter 5.

Appendices F and G provide tools for the student to measure the accuracy of their choice of nursing diagnosis labels. The Ordinal Scale of Accuracy of a Nursing Diagnosis assigns a point value to a diagnosis that is consistent with the number of cues and disconfirming cues identified. This tool aids students in validating their analysis of the collected data and choice of nursing diagnosis. The Integrated Model for Self-Monitoring of the Diagnostic Process provides direct feedback to students but can also be shared with you to demonstrate the students' progress in data analysis and diagnosis.

Appendix H is a sample of a Clinical (Critical) Pathway, providing you with the opportunity to address alternate forms for planning and evaluating care.

Appendix I presents some commonly accepted charting abbreviations, which may be useful in your discussion of the documentation process.

Appendix J provides a glossary of common terms.

Appendix K outlines the 17 Likert scales used to measure the variability in the client's state, behavior, or perception as depicted in NOC outcomes.

Finally, Appendices K and L are the Keys to the Learning Activities provided in the text.

The National League for Nursing emphasizes the need for graduates of nursing programs to think critically, make decisions, and formulate independent judgments. To achieve this outcome, you as an instructor are encouraged to use teaching strategies that will "stimulate higher-order critical thinking in both theory and practice situations" (Klaassens, 1988). These strategies include: questioning, analysis, synthesis, application, writing, problem-solving games, and philosophical discussions.

It is our hope that the interactive features of this text will provide the strategies to assist you in successfully sharing with your students the meaning and language of the nursing process and in making a smooth and effective transition from the classroom to any clinical setting.

Marilynn E. Doenges

Mary Frances Moorhouse

Notes to the Student

The nursing process will be described by your instructors as a systematic approach to the practice of nursing. Shortly, you will find that this process is an efficient and effective method for organizing both nursing knowledge and practice. The process will also assist you in accurately performing clinical decision-making activities in planning your client's care. The process has been continually refined since its inception in the 1960s. However, to date, the concepts within the process still remain central to nursing practice. Through the use of this text, your instructors will share the meaning of the concepts and this evolving nursing practice language with you.

The nursing process is an interactive method of practicing nursing, with the components fitting together in a continuous cycle of thought and action. This interactive focus was used in developing and writing this text for you. The text focuses on the steps of the nursing process and provides information and exercises to aid your understanding and application of the process. Included are practice activities, ongoing reference to simulated clinical experiences through the use of vignettes, and end-of-chapter work pages to promote your understanding. Definitions of both nursing and the nursing process, along with the American Nurses Association's (ANA) Standards of Clinical Nursing Practice, are presented to provide a solid foundation for you to build an understanding of the language and knowledge of nursing and application of the nursing process.

In addition, a six-step diagnostic reasoning/critical thinking process is presented for accurately analyzing the client's assessment data. It will assist you in ruling out, synthesizing, evaluating, and constructing the client diagnostic statement, which is pivotal for developing individualized plans of care for your clients. A practice activity for writing a nursing plan of care was developed to provide a realistic application of your newly learned knowledge. An example of a typical day's work requirements is used in a practice activity in which you are given the opportunity to use time management principles and skills to plan your client's care within an 8-hour shift. A third practice activity is provided to give you a chance to choose client information you would include in a change-of-shift report to communicate the outcomes of your use of the nursing process.

Next, you are given an opportunity to test your beginning skills in developing a complete plan of care. A set of step-by-step forms is provided for you to document your clinical judgment by selecting client diagnostic statements, developing the goals/outcomes, and identifying the nursing interventions. Finally, an evaluation checklist is provided to serve as a valuable self-assessment of the appropriateness and accuracy of your comprehension of the planning exercise and future plans of care that you will design for your clients.

At the end of the chapters, a bibliography and list of suggested readings are included to guide you in further and future reading and understanding of both nursing knowledge and nursing process. In Chapter 1, a suggested reading list provides a listing of publications from a historical perspective. The listing should be helpful to you in searching out the meaning of nursing and the nursing process. The list may also prove valuable in writing varied required papers on similar topics. Use and enjoy. The second section gives you the most current listing of publications at the time of the printing of this edition. Once again, the selected publications are provided to assist you in this learning process.

The perforated tear-out pages for the end-of-chapter work pages, interactive care plan worksheets, and the evaluation checklist were especially designed for your independent learning. These tear-out pages can be taken to the clinical area to reinforce selected aspects of the nursing process. It is our hope that the interactive features of this text will assist you in making the successful and effective transition from the classroom to your assigned clinical setting. We wish you well in this beginning phase of your new profession.

Marilynn E. Doenges

Mary Frances Moorhouse

Acknowledgments

To Joe Burley, RN, MNED
College of Nursing
University of Florida
Gainesville, Florida

To Jean Jenny, MS, MEd, BScNEd, RN
Former Professor
Faculty of Health Sciences
University of Ottawa
School of Nursing
Ottawa, Ontario
Canada

To Alice C. Geissler-Murr, RN, BSN
Triage Nurse
Legal Nurse Consultant
Colorado Springs, Colorado

To Paladin Productions,
whose computer talents clarified
our ideas and made them visible

Contents

Practice Activities and Work Pages

Chapter 1

The Nursing Process: Delivering Quality Care

The Nursing Profession

Nursing is both a science and an art concerned with the physical, psychological, sociological, cultural, and spiritual concerns of the individual. The science of nursing is based on a broad theoretical framework; its art depends on the caring skills and abilities of the individual nurse. The importance of the nurse within the healthcare system is being recognized in many positive ways, and the profession of nursing is itself acknowledging the need for its practitioners to be professional and accountable.

In its early developmental years, nursing did not seek or have the means to control its own practice. Florence Nightingale, in discussing the nature of nursing, observed that "nursing has been limited to signify little more than the administration of medicines and the application of poultices" (Nightingale, 1859). Although this attitude still persists in some cases, the nursing profession has defined what makes nursing unique and has identified a body of professional knowledge.

Thus, barely a century after Miss Nightingale noted that "the very elements of nursing are all but unknown" (Nightingale, 1859), the American Nurses' Association (ANA) developed the first Social Policy Statement (1980) defining nursing as "the diagnosis and treatment of human responses to actual or potential health problems." Recently the statement was revisited, updated, and entitled *Nursing's Social Policy Statement* (1995). The new policy statement acknowledges that since the release of the original statement, nursing has been influenced by many social and professional

Definition of Nursing
Nursing is the diagnosis and treatment of human responses to health and illness (ANA, 1995).

changes, as well as by the science of caring. Nursing has integrated these changes with the 1980 definition to include treatment of human responses to health and illness.

The new statement provides four essential features of today's contemporary nursing practice:

1. Attention to the full range of human experiences and responses to health and illness without restriction to a problem-focused orientation
2. Integration of objective data with knowledge gained from an understanding of the client's or group's subjective experience
3. Application of scientific knowledge to the processes of diagnosis and treatment
4. Provision of a caring relationship that facilitates health and healing (ANA, 1995, pp 3–4)

In the modern world of nursing, therefore, human responses, defined as people's experiences with and responses to health and illness, are the phenomena of concern for nurses. Thus, nursing's role includes health promotion as well as activities that contribute to recovery from or adjustment to illness. Also, nurses support the right of clients to define their own health-related goals and engage in care that reflects their values.

Keep in mind there are other well-known nursing resources (some included in the "Suggested Readings" section) that offer additional definitions of nursing. As your knowledge and experience develop, your definition of nursing may change to reflect your focus on a particular care setting or population, or your specific role. For example, although the definition of nursing developed by Erickson, Tomlin, and Swain (1983) is 20 years old, it remains viable and timely as it incorporates the concepts noted previously with today's holistic approach to care. Their definition includes what nursing is, how it is accomplished, and the goals of nursing: "Nursing is the holistic helping of persons with their self-care activities in relation to their health. This is an interactive, interpersonal process that nurtures strengths to enable development, release, and channeling of resources for coping with one's circumstances and environment. The goal is to achieve a state of perceived optimum health and contentment."

In your journey to discover, understand, and apply this body of knowledge, each chapter guides and presents the knowledge of nursing diagnoses, nursing interventions, and client outcomes. These three components of nursing knowledge are applied in practice activities and end-of-chapter work pages to further your understanding and correct application of this knowledge.

You will soon be introduced to the language described in the nursing process. This introduction includes the classification of nursing diagnoses put forth by NANDA International Inc (formerly the North American Nursing Diagnosis Association), the Iowa Intervention and Outcome Projects: Nursing Intervention Classification (NIC) (2000) and the Nursing Outcomes Classification (NOC) (2000), and the Omaha Classification System (Martin & Scheet, 1992). NANDA, NIC, and NOC have combined their classification systems (NNN Alliance); the Omaha Classification System also combines all three aspects of the language, to provide comprehensive nursing languages. The four client scenarios presented in the text use examples from NANDA, NIC, NOC, and the Omaha Classification to provide you with differing ways of seeing the nursing process in action.

Now, let's move on and describe the nursing process.

The nursing process provides an orderly, logical problem-solving approach for administering nursing care so that the client's needs for such care are met comprehensively and effectively.

The Nursing Process

Nursing leaders have identified a process that "combines the most desirable elements of the art of nursing with the most relevant elements of systems theory, using the scientific method" (Shore, 1988). This process incorporates an interactive/interpersonal approach with a problem-solving and decision-making process (Peplau, 1952; King, 1971; Yura & Walsh, 1988).

The nursing process was first introduced in the 1950s as a three-step process of assessment, planning, and evaluation based on the scientific method of observing, measuring, gathering data, and analyzing the findings. Years of study, use, and refinement have led nurses to expand the nursing process to five distinct steps that provide an efficient method of organizing thought processes for clinical decision making, problem solving, and delivery of higher quality, individualized client care. The nursing process consists of the following steps:

> *Assessment,* or the systematic collection of data relating to clients
> *Diagnosis/need identification,* involving the analysis of collected data to identify the client's needs or problems
> *Planning,* which is a two-part process of identifying goals and the client's desired outcomes to address the assessed health and wellness needs, and selecting appropriate nursing interventions to assist the client in attaining the outcomes
> *Implementation,* or putting the plan of care into action, and
> *Evaluation,* which is done by determining the client's progress toward attaining the identified outcomes and by monitoring the client's response to and the effectiveness of the selected nursing interventions, for the purpose of altering the plan as indicated

Because these five steps are central to nursing actions in any setting, the nursing process is now included in the conceptual framework of nursing curricula and is accepted as part of the legal definition of nursing in the Nurse Practice Acts of most states.

When a client enters the healthcare system, whether as an acute care, clinic, or home care client, the steps of the nursing process are set into motion. The nurse collects data, identifies client needs (nursing diagnoses), establishes goals, identifies outcomes, and selects nursing interventions to assist the client in achieving these outcomes and goals. Finally, after these interventions have been implemented, the nurse evaluates the client's responses and the effectiveness of the plan of care in reaching the desired outcomes and goals to determine whether or not the needs or problems have been resolved and the client is ready to be discharged from the care setting. If the identified needs or problems remain unresolved, further assessment, additional need identification, alteration of outcomes and goals, and/or changes in interventions are required.

Definition of Nursing Process
The nursing process consists of five steps:
1. Assessment
2. Diagnosis/Need Identification/ Analysis
3. Planning
4. Implementation
5. Evaluation

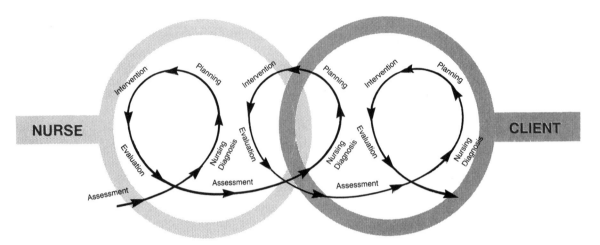

FIGURE 1–1. Diagram of the nursing process. The steps of the nursing process are interrelated, forming a continuous circle of thought and action that is both dynamic and cyclic.

Although we use the terms *assessment, need identification, planning, implementation,* and *evaluation* as separate, progressive steps, in reality they are interrelated. Together, these steps form a continuous circle of thought and action, which recycles throughout the client's contact with the healthcare system. Figure 1–1 shows a model of how this cycling process can be visualized. You can see that the nursing process uses the nursing diagnosis (the clinical judgment product of critical thinking). Based on this judgment, nursing interventions are selected and implemented. These two products of critical thinking—clinical judgment and implementation of selected nursing interventions—are reviewed in upcoming chapters.

Figure 1–1 further shows how the progressive steps of the nursing process create an understandable model of both the products and processes of critical thinking contained within the nursing process. The model graphically emphasizes both the dynamic and cyclic characteristics of the nursing process.

How the Nursing Process Works

The scientific method of problem solving introduced in the previous section is used almost instinctively by most people, without conscious awareness.

FOR EXAMPLE: You have celebrated completion of your semester finals with a very spicy, late-evening dinner. You awaken during the night with a burning sensation in the center of your chest. You are young and in good health and note no other symptoms (**ASSESSMENT**). You decide that your pain is the result of the spicy food you have eaten (**DIAGNOSIS**). You then determine that you need to relieve the discomfort with an over-the-counter preparation before you will be able to return to sleep (**PLANNING**). You take a liquid antacid for your discomfort (**IMPLEMENTATION**). Within a few minutes, you note the burning sensation is relieved, and you return to bed without further concern (**EVALUATION**).

As you see, this is a process you routinely use to solve problems in your own life that can be readily applied to client-care situations. You only need to learn the new terms describing the nursing process, rather than having to think about each step (ASSESSMENT, DIAGNOSIS/NEED IDENTIFICATION, PLANNING, IMPLEMENTATION, and EVALUATION) in an entirely new way.

To effectively use the nursing process, the nurse must possess and be able to apply some basic abilities. Particularly important is a thorough knowledge of science and theory, as applied not only in nursing, but also in other related disciplines such as medicine and psychology. Creativity is needed in the application of nursing knowledge, as well as adaptability in handling change and the many unexpected happenings that occur. As a nurse, you must make a commitment to practice your profession in the best possible way, trusting in yourself and your ability to do your job well and displaying the necessary leadership to organize and supervise as your position requires. In addition, intelligence, well-developed interpersonal skills, and competent technical skills are essential.

> **FOR EXAMPLE:** A client's irritable behavior could be a sign of anger or it could arise from a sense of helplessness regarding life events. However, it could also be the result of low serum glucose or the effect of excessive caffeine intake. A single behavior may have varied causes. It is important that your nursing assessment skills identify the underlying etiology so that you can provide appropriate care.

In addition to these abilities, several fundamental beliefs (Box 1–1) provide guidance for the application of the nursing process and enhance the quality of nursing care. To further increase your knowledge and clinical decision-making skills, Appendix E contains the nine statements of the ANA Code of Ethics for Nurses (ANA, 2001). We suggest you take the time to read, think about, and incorporate these nine statements into your professional practice and refer to the complete work for interpretation of the code statements.

The practice responsibilities presented in the definitions of nursing and the nursing process are explained in detail in the publication *Standards of Clinical Nursing Practice* (ANA, 1991). The standards provide workable guidelines to ensure that the practice of nursing can be carried out by each individual nurse. Box 1–2 presents an abbreviated description of the standards of clinical practice. With the ultimate goal of quality health care, the effective use of the nursing process will result in a viable nursing-care system that is recognized and accepted as nursing's body of knowledge and that can be shared with other healthcare professionals.

Practice Advantages of the Nursing Process

The use of the nursing process has many advantages:

- The nursing process provides a framework for meeting the individual needs of the client, the client's family/significant other(s), and the community.
- The steps of the nursing process focus the nurse's attention on the "individual" human responses of a client/group to a given health situation, resulting in a holistic plan of care addressing their specific needs.
- The nursing process provides an organized, systematic method of problem solving, which may minimize dangerous errors or omissions in caregiving and avoid time-consuming repetition in care and documentation.

Practice Advantages of the Nursing Process:

Organizing framework

Human response focus

Structured decision making

Client involvement

Common language

Economic contributions

BOX 1-1

Fundamental Philosophical Beliefs in Nursing

Several fundamental philosophical beliefs are essential to the practice of nursing and need to be kept in mind when using the nursing process. The recent update of the ANA's Nursing's Social Policy Statement includes several values and assumptions that are included in the following list:

- The client is a human being who has worth and dignity.
- Humans manifest an essential unity of mind/body/spirit (ANA, 1995).
- There are basic human needs that must be met (see Chapter 4, Maslow's Hierarchy).
- When these needs are not met, problems arise that may require intervention by another person until the individuals can resume responsibility for themselves.
- Human experience is contextually and culturally defined (ANA, 1995).
- Health and illness are human experiences (ANA, 1995).
- Clients have a right to quality health and nursing care delivered with interest, compassion, and competence, with a focus on wellness and prevention.
- The presence of illness does not preclude health nor does optimal health preclude illness (ANA, 1995).
- The therapeutic nurse-client relationship is important in the nursing process.

- The use of the nursing process promotes the active involvement of the client in his or her own health care, enhancing consumer satisfaction. Such participation increases the client's sense of control over what is happening to him or her, stimulates problem solving, and promotes personal responsibility, all of which strengthen the client's commitment to achieving identified goals.
- The use of the nursing process enables you as a nurse to have more control over your own practice. This enhances the opportunity for you to use your knowledge, expertise, and intuition constructively and dynamically to increase the likelihood of a successful client outcome. This, in turn, promotes greater job satisfaction and professional growth.
- The use of the nursing process provides a common language for practice, unifying the nursing profession. Using a system that clearly communicates the plan of care to coworkers and clients enhances continuity of care, promotes achievement of client goals, provides a vehicle for evaluation, and aids in the development of nursing standards. In addition, the structure of the process provides a format for documenting the client's response to all aspects of the planned care.
- The use of the nursing process provides a means of assessing nursing's economic contribution to client care. The nursing process supplies a vehicle for the quantitative and qualitative measurement of nursing care that meets the goal of cost effectiveness and still promotes holistic care.

BOX 1–2

ANA Standards of Clinical Nursing Practice

Standards of Care

Describes a competent level of nursing care as demonstrated by the nursing process that encompasses all significant actions taken by the nurse in providing care, and forms the foundation of clinical decision making.

1. **Assessment:** the nurse collects client health data.
2. **Diagnosis:** the nurse analyzes the assessment data in determining diagnoses.
3. **Outcome Identification:** the nurse identifies expected outcomes individualized to the client.
4. **Planning:** the nurse develops a plan of care that prescribes interventions to attain expected outcomes.
5. **Implementation:** the nurse implements the interventions identified in the plan of care.
6. **Evaluation:** the nurse evaluates the client's progress toward attainment of outcomes.

Standards of Professional Performance

Describes roles expected of all professional nurses appropriate to their education, position, and practice setting.

1. **Quality of Care:** the nurse systematically evaluates the quality and effectiveness of nursing practice.
2. **Performance Appraisal:** the nurse evaluates his/her own nursing practice in relation to professional practice standards and relevant statutes and regulations.
3. **Education:** the nurse acquires and maintains current knowledge in nursing practice.
4. **Collegiality:** the nurse contributes to the professional development of peers, colleagues, and others.
5. **Ethics:** the nurse's decisions and actions on behalf of clients are determined in an ethical manner.
6. **Collaboration:** the nurse collaborates with the client, significant others, and healthcare providers in providing client care.
7. **Research:** the nurse uses research findings in practice.
8. **Resource Utilization:** the nurse considers factors related to safety, effectiveness, and cost in planning and delivering client care.

Summary

In using the nursing process to administer nursing care to clients, the nursing profession has identified a body of knowledge that contributes to the prevention of illness, as well as to the maintenance and/or restoration of the client's health (or relief of pain/discomfort and provision of support when a return to health is not possible). The nursing process is the basis of all nursing actions and is the essence of nursing. It can be applied in any healthcare or educational setting, in any theoretical or conceptual framework, and within the context of any nursing philosophy. The process is flexible and yet sufficiently structured to provide a base for nursing actions.

The following chapters identify, discuss, and clarify each step of the nursing process. As noted, each step of the process builds on and interacts with the other steps, ensuring an effective practice model. Inclusion of the standards of clinical nursing practice in the appropriate chapters provides additional information to reinforce your understanding and opportunities to apply your knowledge by means of Practice Activities and a Work Page at the end of each chapter. Four clients help you in your learning process by sharing their personal experiences. Please note, the term *client* is used here rather than *patient* to reflect the philosophy that the individuals or groups you work with are legitimate members of the decision-making process with some degree of control over the planned regimen, and are able, active participants in the planning and implementation of their own care (Erickson, Tomlin, & Swain, 1983).

- Robert is a 72-year-old African-American male admitted to a medical acute care unit for a recurrence of bilateral lower lobe pneumonia. He is a retired truck driver, living alone since his wife's death 5 years ago. He is concerned about his future and about losing control of his life, which presents you with ethical concerns and challenges in dealing with family dynamics.
- Sally is a 30-year-old female who is pregnant and experiencing beginning labor. This is her third pregnancy. Sally completed her evening shift as a respiratory therapist, although she noted early signs of labor at 8:00 PM. You will follow Sally through labor, delivery, and home visits by a public health nurse to enhance your understanding of the continuity of care.
- Michelle, a 14-year-old female, has suffered multiple injuries in a mountain bike accident. She is a ninth grader at the local high school and lives with her parents (who immigrated from Vietnam 16 years ago), an older brother, and a younger sister. You will find pain management a major aspect of your nursing interventions for Michelle along with several cultural concerns.
- Donald, a 46-year-old male, is being treated for depression after the loss of his position as a loan banker because of his chronic absenteeism and poor job performance related to alcohol abuse. He has been drinking heavily recently and is suffering alcohol withdrawal since his admission. You will follow Donald through his other assessed healthcare needs of nutrition, coping, and changes in his role expectations.

The use of these vignettes provides many clinical examples throughout the text, offering a simulated practice environment and a touch of reality in planning the required continuity of client care.

Two suggested reading lists are included at the end of this first chapter to assist you in your journey of understanding the historical development of the nursing process and becoming knowledgeable about current publications describing these topics. We suggest that sometime during your busy program you take the time to read and reflect on these early authors' meaning and the language of nursing and the nursing process.

1. The ANA has defined nursing as: _____
   _____
   _____

2. My own definition of nursing is: _____
   _____
   _____

3. How has the information in this chapter affected your definition? _____
   _____

4. The ANA Social Policy Statement defines the phenomena of concern for nurses as: _____
   _____

5. The definition of *nursing process* is: _____
   _____
   _____
   _____

6. Name and define the five steps of the nursing process and provide an example of each step:

Step	Definition	Example
a. _____	_____	_____
b. _____	_____	_____
c. _____	_____	_____
d. _____	_____	_____
e. _____	_____	_____

7. List three advantages of using the nursing process:
   a. _____
   b. _____
   c. _____

8. List two of the fundamental philosophical beliefs that you believe are basic to decision making within the nursing process:
   a. _____
   b. _____

9. Identify the steps of the nursing process by placing the appropriate number of the activity in the space following the data presented in the following vignette: 1 = ASSESSMENT; 2 = DIAGNOSIS/NEED IDENTIFICATION; 3 = PLANNING; 4 = IMPLEMENTATION; 5 = EVALUATION.

VIGNETTE: Robert, a 72-year-old African-American male, is admitted with recurrent bilateral lower lobe pneumonia.

He reports this is his second episode in 6 months. _____

Temperature is 101°F, skin hot and flushed. _____

He reports frequent, hacking cough with moderate amount of thick greenish mucus. _____

Auscultation of the chest reveals scattered rhonchi throughout. _____

His mucous membranes are pale, and his lips are dry and cracked. _____

He says when he was sick last month, the doctor prescribed an antibiotic, which he discontinued after 6 days because he was feeling better. _____

You determine Robert has an airway clearance problem and a fluid volume deficit, and is not managing his therapeutic regimen effectively and thus requires teaching to promote adequate self-care and to prevent recurrence. _____

You establish the following outcomes:

- Expectorates secretions completely with breath sounds clear and respirations noiseless _____
- Demonstrates adequate fluid balance with moist mucous membranes and loose respiratory secretions _____
- Verbalizes understanding of cause of condition and rationale for therapeutic regimen _____

You decide to set up a regular schedule for respiratory activities and fluid replacement. _____

In addition, you formulate a teaching plan to cover the identified concerns for self-care and illness prevention. _____

You provide a tube of petroleum jelly for Robert to use on his lips. _____

Every 2 hours, you visit Robert to encourage him to deep-breathe, cough, change his position, and drink a glass of fluid of his choice. _____

You use this time to discuss avoidance of crowds and individuals with upper respiratory infections and continuing the treatment plan after discharge. _____

The following day, Robert's skin is no longer hot and flushed, temperature is 99°F, secretions are loose and readily expectorated, and breath sounds are clearing. _____

Robert's lips and oral mucous membranes are moist. He is able to explain in his own words how to care for himself and how to prevent pneumonia. _____

You decide that the current treatment plan is achieving the identified outcomes and to continue the plan as written. _____

BIBLIOGRAPHY

American Nurses' Association. (1980). *Nursing: A Social Policy Statement*. Kansas City, MO: Author.

American Nurses' Association. (1991). *Standards of Clinical Nursing Practice*. Kansas City, MO: Author.

American Nurses' Association. (1995). *Nursing's Social Policy Statement*. Washington, DC: Author.

American Nurses' Association. (2001). *Code of Ethics for Nurses*. Washington, DC: Author.

Erickson, H. C., Tomlin, E. M., & Swain, M. A. P. (1983). *Modeling and Role-Modeling*. Englewood Cliffs, NJ: Prentice-Hall.

Johnson, M., Maas, M., & Moorhead, S. (2000). *Nursing Outcomes Classification (NOC)*, ed 3. St. Louis: Mosby.

King, L. (1971). *Toward a Theory for Nursing: General Concepts of Human Behavior*. New York: Wiley.

Martin, K. S., & Scheet, N. J. (1992). *Omaha System: Applications for Community Health Nursing*. Philadelphia: W. B. Saunders.

McCloskey, J. C., & Bulecheck, G. M. (2000). *Nursing Intervention Classification (NIC)*, ed 3. St. Louis: Mosby.

Nightingale, F. (1859). *Notes on Nursing: What It Is and What It Is Not* (facsimile edition). Philadelphia: J. B. Lippincott, 1946.

North American Nursing Diagnosis Association (2001). *Nursing Diagnoses: Definitions & Classification*. Philadelphia: Author.

Peplau, H. E. (1952). *Interpersonal Relations in Nursing: A Conceptual Frame of Reference for Psychodynamic Nursing*. New York: Putnam.

Shore, L. S. (1988). *Nursing Diagnosis: What It Is and How to Do It, a Programmed Text*. Richmond, VA: Medical College of Virginia Hospitals.

Travelbee, J. (1971). *Interpersonal Aspects of Nursing*, ed 2. Philadelphia: F. A. Davis.

Yura, H., & Walsh, M. B. (1988). *The Nursing Process: Assessing, Planning, Implementing, Evaluating*, ed 5. Norwalk, CT: Appleton & Lange.

SUGGESTED READINGS

Classical Publications

American Nurses' Association. (1973). *Standards of Nursing Practice*. Kansas City, MO: Author.

American Nurses' Association. (1987). *The Scope of Nursing Practice*. Kansas City, MO: Author.

Aspinall, M. J., & Tanner, C. A. (1981). *Decision Making for Patient Care: Applying the Nursing Process*. New York: Appleton-Century-Crofts.

Bloch, D. (1974). Some crucial terms in nursing: What do they really mean? *Nursing Outlook*, *22*(11):669–694.

Carlson, J. H., Craft, C. A., & McGuire, A. D. (1982). *Nursing Diagnosis*. Philadelphia: W. B. Saunders.

Carnevali, D. L. (1983). *Nursing Care Planning: Diagnosis and Management*, ed 3. Philadelphia: J. B. Lippincott.

Orem, D. E. (1971). *Nursing: Concepts of Practice*. New York: McGraw-Hill.

Orlando, I. J. (1961). *The Dynamic Nurse-Patient Relationship: Function, Process, and Principles*. New York: Putnam.

Patterson, J. G., & Zderad, L. T. (1976). *Humanistic Nursing*. New York: Wiley.

U.S. Department of Health and Human Services. (1980). A classification scheme for client problems in community health nursing. DHHS Publication No. HRA 80-16.

Wiedenbach, E. (1964). *Clinical Nursing: A Helping Art*. New York: Springer.

Yura, H., & Walsh, M. B. (Eds.). (1967). *The Nursing Process*. Washington, DC: Catholic University of America Press.

Current Publications

Alfaro-Lefevre, R. (2002). *Applying Nursing Process: A Step-by-Step Guide*, ed 5. Philadelphia: Lippincott.

Carnevali, D. L., & Thomas, M. D. (1993). *Diagnostic Reasoning and Treatment Decision Making in Nursing*. Philadelphia: J. B. Lippincott.

Carpenito, L. J. (2002). *Nursing Diagnosis: Application to Clinical Practice*, ed 9. Philadelphia: Lippincott.

Cox, H., et al. (2002). *Clinical Applications of Nursing Diagnosis: Adult, Child, Women's Psychiatric, Gerontic, and Home Health Considerations*, ed 4. Philadelphia: F. A. Davis.

Craft-Rosenberg, M. J., & Denehy, J. A. (Eds.). (2002). *Nursing Interventions for Infants and Children.* Philadelphia: W. B. Saunders.

Gordon, M. (1994). *Nursing Diagnosis: Process and Application,* ed 3. St. Louis: Mosby.

Hannah, K. J., Reimer, M., Mills, W. C., & Letourneau, S. (Eds.). (1987). *Clinical Judgment and Decision Making: The Future with Nursing Diagnosis.* New York: Wiley.

Iowa Intervention Project. (1997). Nursing interventions classification (NIC): An overview. In M. J. Rantz & P. LeMone (Eds.). *Classification of Nursing Diagnoses: Proceedings of the Twelfth Conference, North American Nursing Diagnosis Association.* Glendale, CA: Cinahl Information Systems, pp 32–41.

Leuner, J. D., Manton, A. M., Kelliher, D. B., Sullivan, S. P., & Doherty, M. (1990). *Mastering the Nursing Process: A Case Study Approach.* Philadelphia: F. A. Davis.

Maas, M. L. (1997). Nursing-sensitive outcomes classification (NOC): Completing the essential comprehensive languages of nursing. In M. J. Rantz & P. LeMone (Eds.). *Classification of Nursing Diagnoses: Proceedings of the Twelfth Conference, North American Nursing Diagnosis Association.* Glendale, CA: Cinahl Information Systems, pp 40–47.

Maas, M., Buckwalter, K. C., & Hardy, M. (1991). *Nursing Diagnosis and Interventions for the Elderly.* Menlo Park, CA: Addison-Wesley.

Martin, K. S. (1997). The Omaha System. In M. J. Rantz & P. LeMone (Eds.). *Classification of Nursing Diagnoses: Proceedings of the Twelfth Conference, North American Nursing Diagnosis Association.* Glendale, CA: Cinahl Information Systems, pp 16–21.

Martin, K. S., & Scheet, N. J. (1992). *Omaha System: A Pocket Guide for Community Health Nursing.* Philadelphia: W. B. Saunders.

Chapter 2

The Assessment Step: Developing the Client Database

■ **ANA STANDARD 1:** Assessment: The nurse collects client health data.

The Client Database

The ASSESSMENT step of the nursing process is an organized dynamic process involving three basic activities:

> **ASSESSMENT**: the first step of the nursing process, during which data are collected.

13

- Systematically gathering data
- Sorting and organizing the data collected
- Documenting the data in a retrievable format

Using a number of techniques, you focus on eliciting a profile of the client that allows you to identify client problems or needs and corresponding nursing diagnoses, plan care, implement interventions, and evaluate outcomes. This profile is called the CLIENT DATABASE, and it serves as the fundamental pool of knowledge about the client from which all other steps of the nursing process proceed.

CLIENT DATABASE: the compilation of data collected about a client; it consists of the nursing history, physical examination, and results of diagnostic studies.

The client database supplies a sense of the client's overall health status, providing a picture of the client's physical, psychological, sociocultural, spiritual, cognitive, and developmental levels; economic status; functional abilities; and lifestyle. It is a combination of data gathered from the history-taking interview (a method of obtaining SUBJECTIVE information by talking with the client and/or significant other[s] and listening to their responses); the physical examination findings (a "hands-on" means of obtaining OBJECTIVE information); and data gathered from the results of laboratory/diagnostic studies. To be more specific, subjective data are what the client/significant others perceive, and objective data are what you observe.

SUBJECTIVE DATA: what the client reports, believes, or feels.

OBJECTIVE DATA: what can be observed, for example, vital signs, behaviors, diagnostic studies.

Because consistency is important, the same data collection model should be used for both the client interview (history) and the physical examination, whether that model is a nursing framework, a systems approach, a head-to-toe review, or a combination defined by your own agency. Frequently, to enhance efficiency and effectiveness, these two activities are combined into one interactive process in which physical data are gathered while interview questions are asked.

FRAMEWORK FOR DATA COLLECTION

Several nursing models may be used to guide your data collection. Two of the commonly used models are shown in Table 2–1: Doenges and Moorhouse's Diagnostic Divisions, and Gordon's Functional Health Patterns.

MEDICAL DIAGNOSIS: illness/conditions for which treatment is directed by a licensed physician; medical diagnoses focus on correction/prevention of the pathology of specific organs/body systems.

The use of a nursing model as a framework for data collection rather than a body systems approach (assessing the heart, moving on to the lungs) or the commonly known head-to-toe approach has the advantage of identifying and validating nursing diagnoses as opposed to MEDICAL DIAGNOSES. An assessment model such as the Assessment Tool shown in Appendix C limits repetitious collection of medical data and focuses data collection on the nurse's phenomena of concern—the human responses to health and illness. Such responses include self-care limitations; impaired functioning in areas such as sleep, rest, nutrition, and elimination; pain; deficiencies in decision making; problematic relationships; or a desire simply to improve one's well-being (ANA, 1995).

THE INTERVIEW PROCESS

Information in the client database is obtained primarily from the client (who is the most important source) and then from family members/significant others (secondary sources), as appropriate, through conversation and by observation during a structured

TABLE 2–1. Comparison of Nursing Models for Data Collection

Diagnostic Divisions (Doenges and Moorhouse, 2002)	Functional Health Patterns (Gordon, 1995)
Activity/Rest: Ability to engage in necessary/desired activities of life (work and leisure) and to obtain adequate sleep/rest.	**Health Perception/Health Management:** Client's perception of general health status and well-being. Adherence to preventive health practices.
Circulation: Ability to transport oxygen and nutrients necessary to meet cellular needs.	**Nutritional-Metabolic:** Patterns of food and fluid intake, fluid and electrolyte balance, general ability to heal.
Ego Integrity: Ability to develop and use skills and behaviors to integrate and manage life experiences.	**Elimination:** Patterns of excretory function (bowel, bladder, and skin), and client's perception.
Elimination: Ability to excrete waste products.	**Activity/Exercise:** Pattern of exercise, activity, leisure, recreation, and ADL; factors that interfere with desired or expected individual pattern.
Food/Fluid: Ability to maintain intake of and use nutrients and liquids to meet physiological needs.	**Cognitive-Perceptual:** Adequacy of sensory modes, such as vision, hearing, taste, touch, smell, pain perception, cognitive functional abilities.
Hygiene: Ability to perform basic activities of daily living (ADL).	**Sleep/Rest:** Patterns of sleep and rest-relaxation periods during 24-hour day, as well as quality and quantity.
Neurosensory: Ability to perceive, integrate, and respond to internal and external cues.	**Self-Perception/Self-Concept:** Individual's attitudes about self, perception of abilities, body image, identity, general sense of worth and emotional patterns.
Pain/Discomfort: Ability to control internal/external environment to maintain comfort.	**Role/Relationship:** Client's perception of major roles and responsibilities in current life situation.
Respiration: Ability to provide and use oxygen to meet physiologic needs.	**Sexuality/Reproductive:** Client's perceived satisfaction or dissatisfaction with sexuality. Reproductive stage and pattern.
Safety: Ability to provide safe, growth-promoting environment.	**Coping/Stress Tolerance:** General coping pattern, stress tolerance, support systems, and perceived ability to control and manage situations.
Sexuality: (Component of Ego Integrity and Social Interaction) Ability to meet requirements/characteristics of male/female role.	**Value-Belief:** Values, goals, or beliefs that guide choices or decisions.
Social Interaction: Ability to establish and maintain relationships.	
Teaching/Learning: Ability to incorporate and use information to achieve healthy lifestyle/optimal wellness.	

interview. The nursing interview may take place over several contact sessions, but each contact should yield information, verify information already gathered, and/or clarify data. A well-conducted interview can be the first step in establishing a beneficial nurse-client relationship and the rapport needed for good communication.

However, the interview is not merely the routine completion of the items on a standardized form by whomever is available. Rather, it is a tool of communication that permits an interactive exchange of information, a process that produces a higher level of understanding than that which either person could achieve alone. The nursing interview thus has a specific purpose: the collection of a set of specific data (information) from the client and/or significant others through both conversation (subjective data) and observation (objective data). Box 2–1 provides some examples to clarify the distinction between these two forms of data.

Clearly, the interview involves more than simply exchanging and processing data. Nonverbal communication is as important as the client's choice of words in providing the data. The ability to collect data that are meaningful to the client's health concerns depends heavily on your own knowledge base; the choice and sequence of questions; and the ability to give meaning to the client's responses, integrate the data gathered, and prioritize the resulting information. Your knowledge, understanding, and insight into the nature and behavior of the client are essential elements as well.

Now take a few moments to read through Box 2–2, which identifies 10 key elements of a successful interview. As you begin to understand and apply these client-interviewing techniques, you will see that they provide an opportunity for the client to use descriptive terms and to explain more fully the meaning of an answer. You will want to keep these tips in mind as you complete the practice activities in this chapter.

The interview question is the major tool you will use to obtain information. How you phrase the question is a skill that is important in obtaining the desired results and

---

BOX 2–1

Subjective Data Compared with Objective Data

Subjective data are what the client/significant other(s) say reflecting their own thoughts, feelings, and perceptions:

"My hip hurts."	"I can't walk that far."
"I'm worried about surgery."	"I don't know what to do to lower
"She didn't sleep well."	my cholesterol level."
"I can't give my husband a shot."	"His usual weight is 160 pounds."
"I haven't had a bowel movement for 3 days."	"I don't think I'll ever get better."

Objective data are observable and measurable and include information gathered during the physical assessment and diagnostic studies:

Restless/agitated	Cardiac murmur
Temperature 99.2°F	Putrid odor
Old surgical scar	Bloody vomitus
Flabby muscle tone	Facial grimacing
Hb 12.4	Glucose 107

BOX 2–2

Elements of a Successful Interview

A successful interview has 10 key elements: (1) a clear sense of the underlying purpose for conducting the interview, (2) preliminary or background research before the interview begins, (3) a formal request of the interviewee to conduct the interview, (4) sound interviewing strategy, (5) effective use of icebreakers, (6) smoothly addressing the business of the interview, (7) good rapport between nurse and client, (8) sensitivity to the client's needs during the interview process, (9) adequate time for recovery following discussion of sensitive areas, and (10) closure.

1. **Underlying purpose:** The information gathered during the interview will be used in formulating the plan of care. Knowing the underlying purpose provides guidance in asking and answering questions, especially when areas that appear to be unrelated to the current situation may need to be pursued.

2. **Preliminary research:** Investigate the client's and the family's current and previous situation. You can use resources such as records from the doctor's office, receiving department (e.g., emergency department) or prior admissions, as well as other health-team members. Make notes to identify key points because research often generates questions that should be written down so they are not lost. This preparation will assist you when formulating questions in the interview. The end result of the interview depends on what is put into it.

3. **Request to conduct the interview:** Formally requesting the interview is courteous and can clearly promote a positive interaction. Identify yourself to the client and explain precisely the purpose of collecting the data and how those data will be used. Together, set a time for the interview, giving consideration to the needs and severity of the client's condition and the availability of significant others. Allow yourself as much time as possible to prepare. Your approach and attitude are important in helping the client be comfortable and understand the importance of the interview. "Mr. Jones, I would like to ask you some questions about yourself and your health status, so that together we may plan your care," is a more positive approach than, "I need to know your history." The first approach not only sells the interview but stimulates the client's thinking. The result is a more productive interview.

4. **Interview strategy:** Cover the details of the interview in accordance with the definition of its purpose with the client. Preparation and planning give a sense of security and a plan to fall back on if things go slowly or unexpectedly wrong. This also allows a comfortable departure from the plan when conversation takes an unexplored path into productive channels. A new twist and a refreshing insight are the gold nuggets of interviewing, leading to information that otherwise might not have been remembered or shared.

(Continued)

Elements of a Successful Interview (Continued)

5. **Icebreakers:** Icebreakers are the words and phrases that can put the client at ease, set the stage, and promote a relaxed situation. They are the first bond of human communication and trust in this new relationship. How the icebreakers are used during the first few minutes may determine how and if the interview proceeds because the participants make important decisions concerning the future of this relationship. The client and/or significant others are making judgments about you (that you are sincere, trustworthy, sensitive, professionally competent, or not).

   Some examples of icebreakers that might be used are the acknowledgement of what you know and see: "You've been admitted for surgery." A simple comment about the weather may also put the client at ease. Offering something to drink, if allowed, and asking the client how he or she prefers to be addressed also serve to promote an atmosphere of relaxation. When you sit down and appear relaxed and interested, this goal is more readily achieved.

6. **Business:** Get to the business at hand. Ask your prepared questions, using terminology the client understands. Listen for answers and clues that will lead to other questions that you may not have anticipated. The relaxed informality that you have achieved needs to continue through this phase. Do not expect insights immediately; they usually come with time, increased comfort level, and trust.

7. **Rapport:** Call the participants by name, and monitor reactions to questions. Be careful not to bore or intimidate them with embarrassing questions. It is important to know when to shift gears, speed up, or slow down, or when to ask more challenging questions. Do not hurry the interview, and maintain eye contact as appropriate based on cultural belief systems.

8. **Sensitivity:** It may be necessary to ask questions about issues that involve sensitive areas for the client. For example, questions about sexuality, lifestyle, or behaviors that put the person at risk for sexually transmitted diseases (STDs, including human immunodeficiency virus/acquired immunodeficiency syndrome [HIV/AIDS]) may be perceived as threatening. The nurse needs to proceed gently toward these sensitive areas. Be alert to verbal/nonverbal cues that may indicate that the area of discussion is particularly sensitive for the individual. Ceasing exploration at this point demonstrates respect for the individual's rights/privacy and can enhance the trust between participants. At a future point in the interview, the client's level of comfort may allow you to revisit the topic and gather necessary data.

9. **Recovery:** Recover the rapport. If the sensitive areas have been approached slowly, the recovery period should be fairly easy to accomplish. Warmth and caring evidenced by a smile and a touch of the hand are helpful.

10. **Closure:** Conclude the interview by summarizing the highlights of the interview and leave the door open for further communication by asking the client if he or she has anything else to add or any questions to ask of you.

getting the information necessary to make accurate nursing diagnoses. Nine effective data collection questioning techniques are:

- **Open-ended questions** allow the client maximum freedom to respond in his or her own way, impose no limitations on how the question may be answered, and can produce considerable information. For example, "How do you feel about your new medications?" or "Explain the injection technique to me."
- **Hypothetical questions** pose a situation and ask the client how it might be handled. You can learn whether the client has accurate information and can think about how a similar situation might be handled. For example, "What would you do if you felt dizzy?" These questions may be very useful in determining the extent to which the client has learned previously presented material.
- **Reflecting or "mirroring"** responses are useful techniques in getting at underlying meanings that might not be verbalized clearly. The client might say, "Some days I'd like to throw this needle out the window." A mirror response would be, "You feel angry about having to use the needle?" Now the client is encouraged to verbalize what he or she is actually angry about. This response is nonevaluative and nonthreatening.
- **Focusing** shows the client that you are attending to what is being said and consists of eye contact (within cultural limits), body posture, and verbal responses, that is, "Tell me more about that."
- **Giving broad openings** encourages the client to take the initiative about what is to be talked about: "Where would you like to begin?"
- **Offering general leads** encourages the client to continue: " . . . and then?"
- **Exploring** pursues a topic in more detail: "Would you describe it more fully?"
- **Verbalizing the implied** gives voice to what has been suggested; for instance, the client says, "It's no use taking this medicine anymore." You respond, "You're concerned that it isn't making a difference for you?"
- **Encouraging evaluation** helps the client to consider the quality of his or her own experience, such as: "How does that seem to you?"

However, be aware that even with a properly phrased question, there will be times when the answer you are seeking will not be given. It is important to remember, too, that the client has the right to refuse to answer any question at all, no matter how reasonably phrased. Some questioning strategies to be avoided because they are generally ineffective in eliciting information from clients include:

- **Closed-ended questions** (such as "Why?") allow little or no freedom in choosing a response, such as, "Do you take your medicine?" (client responds "No") or "How long have you been taking insulin?" (client responds "3 years"). Typically there are only one or two possible answers to the question. The interviewer remains in close control over the interview because of the rigid structure. Although the closed-ended question may be useful in an emergency situation (when it is necessary to gather information in a short time), it is important to provide an opportunity for asking the client to explain the answers to these questions in greater detail.
- **Leading questions** typically suggest the desired response, such as, "The infec-

tion seems to be getting better, don't you agree?" and thereby reduce the range of responses because the interviewee most commonly agrees with leading statements. Highly emotional questions, tone of voice, or inflection ("Where did you learn *that* injection technique?") may be heard as challenging, provoking the interviewee to "attack" or become defensive, thereby blocking communication.

- **Probing** is a persistent questioning, a demand for more information than is given willingly. "Now tell me about. . . ." This creates an uneasy feeling in the client and may be interpreted as an invasion of privacy, resulting in a defensive response or withholding of information.
- **Agreeing/disagreeing** implies that the client is "right" or "wrong" rather than promoting the client's idea as separate from your own. This can block exploration of an issue. "I agree, that would be the thing to do," or "You didn't mean to do that, did you?"

At this point, take a moment to complete Practice Activity 2–1.

The Nursing Interview: Questioning and Listening

The client's MEDICAL DIAGNOSIS can provide a starting point for the nursing interview. Your knowledge about the anatomy and physiology of the disease/condition helps in choosing and prioritizing questions. Remember, though, that when using a nursing model assessment tool, the results of the focused interview will point to the human responses to health and illness and to the development of nursing (rather than medical) diagnoses. Let us visit our first client, Robert. Although you will ask Robert about the signs and symptoms associated with his pneumonia, your nursing focus is:

- How does his shortness of breath affect his ability to care for himself? (Hygiene)
- Have the coughing episodes resulted in chest-wall pain or loss of sleep? (Pain/Discomfort, Activity/Rest)
- Has his appetite been affected by his frequent expectoration of purulent mucus? (Food/Fluid)
- How does he protect himself and others from transmission of infection? (Safety, Teaching/Learning)

In addition, you need to keep an open mind and pay attention to clues that may identify other human responses of concern requiring investigation.

THE CLIENT HISTORY

The history is more than simply recording information. You must review the data, organize and determine the relevance of each item (value the data), and document the facts. The quality of a history improves with your knowledge and experience with the history-taking process. Although such assessments are often lengthy and time-consuming in the beginning, more time is eventually saved by avoiding the necessity to retrace steps, correct misinformation, and undo actions. With practice, as you become skilled, the time required for this activity will decrease.

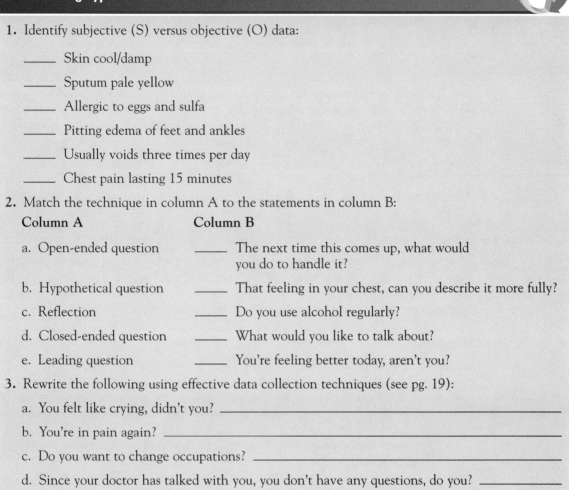

PRACTICE ACTIVITY 2–1
Determining Types of Data

1. Identify subjective (S) versus objective (O) data:

_____ Skin cool/damp

_____ Sputum pale yellow

_____ Allergic to eggs and sulfa

_____ Pitting edema of feet and ankles

_____ Usually voids three times per day

_____ Chest pain lasting 15 minutes

2. Match the technique in column A to the statements in column B:

Column A   **Column B**

a. Open-ended question   _____ The next time this comes up, what would you do to handle it?

b. Hypothetical question   _____ That feeling in your chest, can you describe it more fully?

c. Reflection   _____ Do you use alcohol regularly?

d. Closed-ended question   _____ What would you like to talk about?

e. Leading question   _____ You're feeling better today, aren't you?

3. Rewrite the following using effective data collection techniques (see pg. 19):

a. You felt like crying, didn't you? _____

b. You're in pain again? _____

c. Do you want to change occupations? _____

d. Since your doctor has talked with you, you don't have any questions, do you? _____

e. Did you eat lunch? _____

GUIDELINES FOR HISTORY-TAKING

Listen Carefully

Be a good listener: You need to listen attentively to what the individual is saying. Listen for whole thoughts and ideas, not merely isolated facts. Facts may not be as important as the ideas that bind them together. For example, Robert tells you, "Sure, my doctor ordered some pills for me [antibiotics for pneumonia], last month." But Robert's tone of voice, facial expression, and body language communicate the idea that he may not be following his treatment regimen. Robert's nonverbal communication requires validation by asking either reflecting or open-ended questions as described previously. For example, "You seem to have a lack of enthusiasm as you tell me about your medication. What is that about?"

ACTIVE LISTENING:
reflecting back what
the other person
has said to validate
your understanding of
the meaning. A
restatement of the
other person's total
communication,
including the words
and the feelings.

Active Listening

Use skills of active listening, silence, and acceptance to provide ample time for the person to respond: Give your full attention to the interview and do not interrupt. Save your own comments until the speaker is completely finished. Finally, ask related questions to stimulate the individual's memory if blocks occur. Once again, "facts" may not be as important as the client's perception of reality. As you gain more experience in professional practice, you will begin to understand how important the client's perception is. This is especially true in your assessment, understanding, management, and treatment of your client's reported perception of pain.

Objectivity

Be as objective as possible: Identify only the client's and/or significant others' contributions to the history, and do not try to interpret the data at this point. Record subjective data from the client/significant others just as they were stated during the interview. Failure to do so may cause confusion and lead to inaccurate diagnoses. However, lengthy responses may need to be paraphrased.

Your initial responsibility is to observe, collect, and record data without drawing conclusions or making judgments/assumptions. Your self-awareness is a crucial factor in the interaction because perceptions, judgments, and assumptions can easily color the assessment findings unless they are recognized. We all have a responsibility to understand how our biases affect the conclusions we draw from the data and not be influenced by them. It may be useful to review the beliefs cited in Chapter 1 (p 6) and the Code of Ethics for Nurses contained in Appendix E.

Manageable Detail

Keep the amount of detail manageable: The data collected about the client and/or significant others contain a vast amount of information, some of which may be repetitious. However, some of it will be valuable for eliciting information that was not recalled or volunteered previously.

Enough material needs to be noted in the history so that a complete picture is presented, and yet not so much that the information will not be read or used.

"Necessary" information includes all data (positive and negative) that are relevant to the situation. For example, let us return to your client Robert. He was admitted with the diagnosis of pneumonia. During the history, he reports, "I've been coughing a lot lately." Necessary information in this case would be to clarify what Robert means by "coughing a lot lately." You need to know the frequency and time of coughing and factors that bring about or terminate an episode of coughing. Along with knowing there was a cough, you would want the necessary information about whether or not the cough was productive. So you would want to know the descriptive characteristics of the mucus. What color was it? How much mucus does he expectorate? As you can see, the "necessary" information is that which clarifies and makes the communication of Robert's subjective data to other healthcare providers both useful and meaningful.

Sequence Information

Order is imperative: Develop and use a form that makes it easy to find information, identify problems, and choose nursing diagnoses. In addition, present the current health problems in chronological order and include relevant events from the past. It is also useful to express topics in a uniform manner. For example, expressing the age at which events/illnesses/surgery occurred instead of just the year events occurred: "age 70/born 1932"; or "hysterectomy, age 35/1968."

Document Clearly

Unless you have computerized data collection, you must write legibly: This required skill improves the communication and comprehension of your findings, decreasing the chance of misunderstanding, saving time for you and other healthcare professionals who rely on your records.

Record Data in a Timely Way

Record the data during the interview, or write the history as soon as possible after gathering the information: This helps ensure greater accuracy of the data. The longer you wait to record, the more likely it is the data and specific details will fade and be more difficult to recall. A word of advice: Data not recorded are data lost.

Physical Examination: The Hands-On Phase

You perform the physical examination to gather objective information and also as a screening device. For the data collected during the physical examination to be meaningful, you need to know the normal physical and emotional characteristics of human beings sufficiently well to be able to recognize deviations.

FOCUS AND PREPARATION

To gain as much information as possible from the assessment procedure, approach the client with a positive, sincere attitude. Such an attitude conveys competence, interest, kindness, thoroughness, orderliness, and confidence. It may be frightening for the client if you give the impression that you do not know what you are doing, or if you are awkward in performing assessment tasks. Give the client a clear explanation of the procedures you will be using. Then, proceed with the examination according to the format you have previously chosen to gather and record the data: a nursing model (as suggested earlier), a systems approach (cardiovascular, respiratory, gastrointestinal, and so on), a head-to-toe review (head, neck, chest, and so on), or a combination of these. The same format should be used each time you perform a physical examination, to lessen the possibility of omissions and to increase your confidence and efficiency in completing the task.

However, the client's state of health/severity of condition may require you to place priority on specific portions of your assessment. This priority in data collection is based in part on the measurement criteria developed by the ANA. "The priority of data collection is determined by the client's immediate condition or needs" (ANA, 1991). For example, when examining a client with severe chest pain, you would probably choose to evaluate the pain and the cardiovascular system before addressing other areas. Likewise, the duration and length of any physical examination depend on circumstances such as the condition of the client and the urgency of the situation.

During the examination, emotional support and care should be offered as indicated. Your professional judgment needs to be used in selecting the steps and sequencing the assessment to provide emotional support as needed. The client with resolving chest pain may want to talk about his or her embarrassment of being perceived as "weak" during the episode of chest pain. Interrupting your examination to support and listen to your client is not only a correct intervention, but also demonstrates the sensitive blending of the art and science of nursing. It is also important to provide the client with as much feedback as possible. While completing the examination process, you will find this is an excellent opportunity to provide education on associated procedures, assessment findings, and health teaching in general. Perceptual and observational skills are especially important in determining what your client needs.

ASSESSMENT METHODS

Four common methods used during the physical examination are inspection, palpation, percussion, and auscultation. These techniques incorporate the senses of sight, hearing, touch, and smell:

1. *Inspection* is a systematic process of observation that is not limited to vision but also includes the senses of hearing and smell.

    Sight: Observing the skin for color, discolorations, lacerations; the lesion for drainage; the respiratory pattern for depth and symmetry; body language, movement, and posture; use of extremities; presence of physical limitations; the face for expressions.

    Hearing: Listening to the nature of a cough, the integrity of a joint, the tone of a voice, or content of interactions with others.

Smell: Detecting significant odors.

2. **Palpation** is the touching or pressing of the external surface of the body with the fingers.

Touch: Feeling a lump; noting temperature, degree of moistness, and texture of skin; or determining strength of uterine contraction.

Pressure: Determining the character of a pulse, evaluating edema, noting position of the fetus, or pinching (tenting) to observe skin turgor.

Probing deeper: Reveals muscle tone/tension or an abnormal pain response.

3. **Percussion** is the direct or indirect tapping of a specific body surface to ascertain information about underlying tissues or organs.

Using fingertips: Tap the chest and listen for the sound indicating the presence or absence of fluid, masses, or consolidation.

Using a percussion hammer: Tap the knee and observe the presence or absence of lower leg movement/reflexes.

4. **Auscultation** is listening for sounds within the body with the aid of a stethoscope and describing or interpreting them.

Hearing: Listening at the antecubital space for blood pressure, the chest for heart/lung sounds, the abdomen for bowel sounds or fetal heart tones.

FOLLOW-UP CONSIDERATIONS

After completion of the physical examination, your client may require assistance. The client may need to be helped down off the examination table for safety reasons or may require help with dressing. Consideration of these sometimes forgotten needs enhances the rapport and trust developed during the examination. Including these interventions personalizes the client-nurse interaction and makes the assessment process much more than just your hasty gathering of required data.

You may need to verify or clarify communication associated with the physical examination. By repeating aloud what you have observed, you give the client the opportunity to validate the accuracy of the information obtained, and misunderstandings can be avoided. For example, Observation: "I noticed that you flinched when I felt your abdomen"; Response: "Yes, your hand was cold and I'm ticklish."

Laboratory Tests and Diagnostic Procedures: Supporting Evidence

Laboratory and other diagnostic studies are a part of the information-gathering stage. They aid in the management, maintenance, and restoration of health. Some tests are used to diagnose disease, whereas others are useful in following the course of a disease or adjusting therapy. Your knowledge about the purpose, procedure, and results of various scans, x-rays, performance tests (e.g., treadmill electrocardiogram, pulmonary function), and numerous laboratory studies is necessary for the success of the study and to promote timely nursing intervention and a positive client outcome through proper preparation and education of the client about the prescribed studies.

In reviewing and interpreting laboratory tests, it is important to remember that the origin of the test material does not always correlate to an organ or body system. For example, a urine test might be done to detect the presence of bilirubin and urobilinogen, which could indicate liver disease, biliary obstruction, or hemolytic disease. In some cases, the relationship of the test to the pathology is clear, whereas in others, such as obtaining renal function studies in the presence of cardiac failure, it is not. This is a result of the interrelationships between the various organs and systems of the body. In a few cases, the results of a test are nonspecific because they indicate only that there is a disorder or abnormality and do not indicate the location of the cause of the problem. For example, an elevated erythrocyte sedimentation rate (ESR) suggests the presence but not the location of an inflammatory process.

In evaluating laboratory tests, it is advisable to consider which drugs are being administered to the client, as well as over-the-counter (OTC) medications and herbal supplements, because these may have the potential to blur or falsify results, creating a misleading diagnostic picture.

FOR EXAMPLE:

- Heparin and aspirin products prolong blood clotting times.
- Oral iron preparations cause a false-positive result when the stool is tested for occult blood.
- Phenazopyridine (Pyridium) is a urinary tract analgesic that can color the urine red.
- Use of promethazine (Phenergan), an antiemetic, can cause a false-negative result in a pregnancy test.
- Ingestion of poppy seeds can provide a false-positive result for heroin; use of vitamin E can affect clotting times.

In some cases, it is necessary to note at what time medication was administered. Serum levels can be drawn to determine the varied concentrations of administered medications. Terms such as *peak* and *trough levels* are used to determine both the possible toxic effects and the therapeutic ranges of the medication.

There are also several mechanisms that may alter the laboratory results through the introduction of interfering materials.

FOR EXAMPLE:

- Foods that give a yellow color to blood serum (e.g., carrots, yams) alter a bilirubin test.
- Food may contribute to the presence of substances in body fluids/excretions, such as hemoglobin and myoglobin in meat, which may lead to a misdiagnosis of occult blood in the stool.
- Intramuscular injections can elevate creatine phosphokinase (CPK) levels used to diagnose acute myocardial infarction.

Organizing Information Elements

CLUSTERING THE COLLECTED DATA

Data gathered in the interview, in the physical examination, and from other records/sources are organized and recorded in a concise systematic way and clustered into similar categories. Various formats have been used to accomplish this, including a review of body systems. The body systems approach has been used by both medicine and nursing for many years but is actually more useful for the physician in making a medical diagnosis than for a nurse in identifying nursing diagnoses. Currently, nursing is developing and fine-tuning its own tools for recording and clustering data (e.g., Doenges & Moorhouse, 2002; Gordon, 2002; Guzzetta, et al., 1989). Organizing data using a nursing framework (Box 2–3) assists you in focusing your attention and in choosing specific nursing diagnosis labels to describe the data accurately. However, it is important to be aware of the advantages of each type of framework and to follow the approach recommended by your school or agency. Remember, consistency is the key. Before you meet Donald and complete Practice Activity 2–2, it is suggested that you read about Michelle in Box 2–4 and return to Table 2–1 to review the definitions of the 13 diagnostic divisions and the 11 functional health patterns.

REVIEWING AND VALIDATING FINDINGS

VALIDATION is an ongoing process that occurs during the data collection phase and on its completion, when the data are reviewed and compared. You review the data to be sure that what has been recorded is factual and to identify errors of omission or inconsistencies that require additional investigation. Validation is particularly important when the data are conflicting, when the source of the data may not be reliable, or when serious harm to the client could result from any inaccuracies. Ask questions of the client or others to verify your impressions; for example, "Tell me more about that." "What I heard you say is. . . ." Validating the information gathered can prevent the possibility that wrong inferences can be made or conclusions drawn that can lead to inaccurate nursing diagnoses, incorrect outcomes, and/or inappropriate nursing actions. This can be done by sharing your assumptions with the individuals involved and having them verify the accuracy of those conclusions. (Remember that data given in confidence should not be shared with other individuals unless the information is necessary for their evaluation of the client or for providing care. For example, information received in confidence regarding a client's sexual contacts should not be discussed with a parent or spouse without the client's consent but would be provided to public health officials in the presence of a reportable sexually transmitted disease.)

Data that are grossly abnormal are rechecked, and objective and subjective data are compared for congruencies and/or inconsistencies. For example, the client reports upper right abdominal pain, although musculature appears relaxed and the client does not flinch on abdominal palpation. Additional investigation reveals that the pain is episodic and usually follows meal times. Temporary factors that may affect the data are also identified and noted. For example, you note the client's right hand is cool in

BOX 2–3

Assessment Data for Robert with Application to Excerpt from Doenges and Moorhouse Diagnostic Divisions Assessment Tool

Respiration

Reports (Subjective)

Dyspnea, related to: Climbing stairs/walking more than 2 blocks, close places/crowds

    Cough/sputum: Thick, green, approximately 1/4 tsp, 6 to 10 times/day, especially with activity

History of:

    Bronchitis: Diagnosed 1994

    Asthma: No   **Tuberculosis:** No

    Emphysema: Diagnosed 1994

    Recurrent pneumonia: Yes; last admission approximately 6 months ago

    Exposure to noxious fumes: Not aware of past exposures (was a diesel trucker)

Smoker: Cigarettes (pack/day): 1×45 years, $^{1}/_{2} \times 8$ years (since 1994)

    Number of pack/years: 49

Use of respiratory aids: Inhaler and PO meds

Oxygen: No/"Doctor suggested I use oxygen at night, but I don't think I'm that bad."

Exhibits (Objective)

Respiratory: Rate: 28 at rest **Depth:** Shallow

    Symmetry: Increased AP diameter

Use of accessory muscles: Yes

Nasal flaring: None observed

Fremitus: Increased tactile   **Egophone:** Resonance increased

    Percussion: Hyperresonate

Breath sounds: Diminished, bronchovesicular, basilar inspiratory crackles bilateral, scattered rhonchi—limited clearing with cough

Cyanosis: Oral mucous membranes pale

Clubbing of fingers: Slight

Sputum characteristics: Green, tenacious, scant amount during assessment

Mentation/restlessness: Alert; responds to all questions; no restlessness

Other: Verbal responses slow; breathless—phrases four to five words long

Results chest x-ray: Bilateral lower lobe infiltrates

On reviewing the collected data for this client with pneumonia and noting cues (signs and symptoms) in the Respiration section of the database, you are referred to the Respiration section of the Diagnostic Divisions. Four possible labels are suggested: Airway Clearance, ineffective; Aspiration, risk for; Breathing Pattern, ineffective; and Gas Exchange, impaired.

BOX 2–4

Organizing Assessment Data for Michelle Using a Nursing Framework

You obtained the following information for the client database during your assessment of Michelle (following her admission to the orthopedic unit, having had an external fixation device applied for multiple compound fractures of the right lower leg). The data have been clustered in two nursing frameworks by means of the identifying numbers for each data element.

Assessment Data

1. 14-year-old female
2. High-school student
3. Practicing Buddhist
4. Single
5. Living with parents, one older brother, one younger sister
6. Temperature 100°F
7. Sharp severe pain, right lower leg, "toes to knees," rated "9" on 0 to 10 scale, and right-sided headache rated "4"
8. Hospitalized for tonsillectomy 4 years ago—1998/age 11
9. Alert and oriented, brief loss of consciousness at time of injury
10. Respirations 26, lungs clear, splinting with deep inspiration
11. Weight 98 pounds
12. Indwelling catheter in place, urine clear, amber
13. Independent in self-care
14. Usually sleeps 8 hours each night
15. Right lower leg—wound packed with sterile dressing; multiple puncture sites (external fixator in place)
16. Menarche at age 13
17. Manages stress by talking with friends, exercise (distance runner and mountain biking), meditation
18. States has no allergies
19. Concerned that injury will leave scars and affect participation in track activities
20. P 110, BP 100/78 (left arm/supine)

How you organize these data depends on the format you choose for recording. On occasion, data may be recorded in more than one section because the divisions/patterns are based on human responses instead of specific body systems. The above data could be recorded in two different nursing formats, thus:

(Continued)

Organizing Assessment Data for Michelle Using a Nursing Framework (Continued)

Doenges and Moorhouse: Diagnostic Divisions

Activity/Rest: 2, 9, 14, 17
Circulation: 20
Ego Integrity: 3, 4, 17, 19
Elimination: 12
Food/Fluid: 11
Hygiene: 13
Neurosensory: 9

Pain/Discomfort: 7
Respiration: 10
Safety: 6, 15, 18
Sexuality: 1, 4, 16
Social Interaction: 4, 5
Teaching/Learning: 2, 8

Gordon's: Functional Health Patterns

Health Perception/
   Health Management: 7, 8
Nutritional/Metabolic: 6, 10, 11,
   15, 18, 20
Coping/Stress Tolerance: 17
Value/Belief: 3
Cognitive/Perceptual: 9

Self-perception/
   Self-concept: 19
Role/Relationship: 1, 2, 4, 5
Sexuality/Reproductive: 4, 16
Elimination:12
Activity/Exercise: 10, 13, 17
Sleep/Rest: 14

comparison with the left hand. On questioning, you discover that the patient had been holding a glass of ice water in the right hand.

Finally, the client may remember something, or may feel more comfortable in sharing information with you, and as previously mentioned, although the data collected by any healthcare professional are confidential, it may be appropriate or necessary to share the information. For example, you may have a greater opportunity to observe interactions between family members during the assessment process that could have an impact on the diagnostic process and/or the plan of care. Some of these findings may need to be brought to the attention of other healthcare professionals, such as the physician, dietitian, or physical therapist. Sharing these additional data aids in collaborative planning of care.

Summary

The ASSESSMENT step of the nursing process emphasizes and should provide a holistic view of the client. The generalized assessment done during the overall gathering of data creates a profile of the client. A focused assessment may be done to obtain more information about a specific issue that needs expansion or clarification. Both types of assessment are important and complement each other. A successfully completed assessment provides data on the client's state of wellness, response to health problems, and risk factors.

PRACTICE ACTIVITY 2–2
Organizing Data: Diagnostic Divisions and Functional Health Patterns

Donald has been admitted to the psychiatric hospital acute substance abuse unit for treatment of depression and withdrawal from alcohol.

Organize the data below according to diagnostic divisions and functional health patterns. Place the number of the listed data next to the category where you believe it fits (see Table 2–1).

1. 46-year-old male
2. Divorced, not currently involved in a relationship
3. Loan banker, laid off 7 months ago
4. Unsteady gait
5. Clothes rumpled, has not shaved for 2 days, dry skin
6. Eats 1 or 2 meals a day—donuts, sandwiches, meat and potatoes, no vegetables or fruits; coffee 4+ cups/day
7. Stools have been loose, 3 to 4/day
8. BP 136/82 (right arm/sitting), radial pulse 92
9. Alert and oriented
10. Catholic, not practicing
11. Sleeps usually 3 to 4 hours a night, awakens around 5 AM
12. "I've been drinking a lot lately." (bourbon 1 fifth/day)
13. Worries about financial situation, unable to make child support payments
14. Congested nonproductive cough
15. Reports constant throbbing pain, left knee—old sports injury
16. Genogram

GENOGRAM: graphic representation of a family (may include several generations) reflecting medical data and relationships/roles.

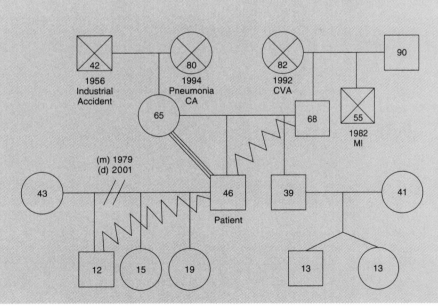

(Continued)

PRACTICE ACTIVITY 2–2 (Continued)
Organizing Data: Diagnostic Divisions and Functional Health Patterns

Diagnostic Divisions	Functional Health Patterns
Activity/Rest:	Health Perception/Health Management:
Circulation:	Nutritional/Metabolic:
Ego Integrity:	Elimination:
Elimination:	Activity/Exercise:
Food/Fluid:	Cognitive/Perceptual:
Hygiene:	Sleep/Rest:
Neurosensory:	Self-Perception/Self-Concept:
Pain/Discomfort:	Role/Relationship:
Respiration:	Sexuality/Reproductive:
Safety:	Coping/Stress Tolerance:
Sexuality:	Value/Belief:
Social Interaction:	
Teaching/Learning:	

To assist you in your assessment assignments and future applications of this first step of the nursing process, an extensive review of the current literature is provided. The Suggested Readings at the end of this chapter provide assessment references for adult health, the pediatric or geriatric client, telephone assessment, home health, and long-term care. Also included is a separate bibliography on genograms. A genogram is displayed in Practice Activity 2–2.

Now, before we briefly describe the next chapter, let us return to the first ANA Standard of Clinical Nursing Practice and review the measurement criteria necessary to achieve and ensure compliance with the standard. The knowledge and skills required to meet the criteria listed in Box 2–5 have been described in this chapter.

BOX 2–5

Measurement Criteria for ANA Standard I

Assessment: The nurse collects client health data.

1. Data collection involves client, significant others, and healthcare providers when appropriate.
2. The priority of data collection activities is determined by the client's immediate condition or needs.
3. Pertinent data are collected using appropriate assessment techniques and instruments.
4. Relevant data are documented in a retrievable form.
5. The data collection process is systematic and ongoing.

1. Rewrite the following questions so that they are open-ended:

   a. You're feeling better after the respiratory treatment, aren't you? _____

   _____

   b. Have you taken your medicine today? _____

   _____

   c. Do you understand these directions? _____

   _____

2. Using the technique of reflection, write a question to clarify these client statements:

   a. Do you think I should tell my doctor about my concern? _____

   _____

   b. What do you want to talk about today? _____

   _____

   c. I don't think I can go on without my husband. _____

   _____

   d. Do you think it is important to get married? _____

   _____

3. When might a closed-ended question be helpful? _____

   _____

4. Describe the three components of the client database:

   a. _____ b. _____ c. _____

5. The four activities involved in the physical assessment are:

   a. _____ b. _____ c. _____ d. _____

6. The client database is important to the provision of client care because _____

   _____

7. For assessment purposes, the difference between subjective data and objective data is _____

   _____

8. Underline the subjective data and circle the objective data in the following vignette. _____

   _____

VIGNETTE: Sally comes to the obstetric department for evaluation of her stage of labor. Back pains began about 3 hours ago (8 PM) while she was on her job as a respiratory therapist. Contractions are 5 minutes apart, lasting 30 seconds for the past 45 minutes. BP 146/84 (left arm/lying), P 110, respirations 24. Weight 155 pounds (up 4 pounds this week). Cervix dilated 4 cm, membranes intact. Fetal head engaged, heart tones slightly muffled in right lower quadrant, rate 132. Nauseated since a dinner of fried chicken 4 hours ago. Appears anxious and seems irritated that her physician is not here. Voided 1 hour ago, has not had a bowel movement for 2 days. Stopped smoking 8 months ago. Lungs clear. No allergies. Married, husband plans to attend the birth. Two children are in the care of their grandmother tonight. Appears well groomed with a well-fitting maternity uniform and low-heeled shoes. Requests to leave contacts in to observe the birth. Last physical examination 1 week ago. Gestation 37 weeks, with due date 3 weeks off—3/11/02.

9. An important benefit of doing "research" or reviewing available information before an interview is _____

_____

10. An interview should be "requested" because _____

_____

11. Check those information resources that can be useful in helping the nurse to prepare for the interview:

_____ Family/significant other _____ Physician notes

_____ Old medical records _____ Textbooks/reference journals

_____ Diagnostic studies _____ Other nurses/healthcare providers

12. Sensitivity of the nurse is important during the interview process to _____

_____

13. List three abilities of the nurse that are necessary in order to collect a relevant client database.

a. _____ b. _____ c. _____

14. In the following vignette, cluster and record the assessment data (following the numbers) into the appropriate diagnostic divisions listed below. Refer to Table 2–1 as needed for the type of data included in the specific divisions to assist you in clustering the data.

VIGNETTE: Robert, a 72-year-old (1) African-American male admitted to the medical unit at 1:00 PM for (2) bilateral lower lobe pneumonia. (3) has had liquids only by mouth for several days. (4) Last BM—2 days ago, brown/formed stool, (5) voided at 1:20 PM—clear, dark amber. He reports (6) "my chest hurts," as he splints chest while coughing. (7) Small amount thick, green sputum expectorated with cough. (8) Appears anxious, fidgeting with sheets, face tense, watching nurse intently. (9) Tympanic temperature (TMT) 101°F, (10) BP 178/102 (left arm/lying), P 100/regular, (11) Respirations 28/shallow. (12) Skin warm, moist; color pale. (13) Has difficulty hearing questions, left hearing aid (R ear) at home. (14) Reports, "This is the second episode in a month." (15) Doctor did prescribe antibiotic (drug unknown) a month ago; client did not complete treatment. (16) States he lives alone (widower) and is (17) responsible for meeting his own needs. In reviewing diagnostic studies, you note that the (18) chest x-ray reveals infiltrates in both lower lobes, and a (19) Gram stain of the sputum reveals Gram-negative bacteria.

DIAGNOSTIC DIVISIONS

Activity/Rest: _____   Hygiene: _____   Safety: _____

Circulation: _____   Neurosensory: _____   Sexuality: _____

Ego Integrity: _____   Pain/Discomfort: _____

Social Interaction: _____   Elimination: _____

Respiration: _____   Teaching/Learning: _____

Food/Fluid: _____

The next chapter presents the second step of the nursing process—DIAGNOSIS/NEED IDENTIFICATION. In this upcoming chapter, the diagnostic reasoning process is used to analyze/synthesize the information obtained from the client database and to identify the client healthcare needs or nursing diagnoses that form the basis for the development of the plan of care.

BIBLIOGRAPHY

American Nurses' Association. (1991). *Standards of Clinical Nursing Practice.* St. Louis: Author.

American Nurses' Association. (1995). *Nursing's Social Policy Statement.* Washington, DC: Author.

Doenges, M. E., Moorhouse, M. F., & Geissler-Murr, A. C. (2002). *Nurse's Pocket Guide: Diagnoses, Interventions, and Rationales,* ed 8. Philadelphia: F. A. Davis.

Doenges, M. E., Moorhouse, M. F., & Geissler-Murr, A. C. (2002). *Nursing Care Plans: Guidelines for Individualizing Patient Care,* ed 6. Philadelphia: F. A. Davis.

Fitzpatrick, J. J. (1991). In R. M. Carroll-Johnson (Ed.). *Classification of Nursing Diagnosis: Proceedings of the Ninth Conference.* Philadelphia: J. B. Lippincott.

Gordon, M. (1994). *Nursing Diagnosis: Process and Application,* ed 3. St. Louis: Mosby.

Gordon, T. (2000). *Parent Effectiveness Training.* New York: Three Rivers Press.

Guzzetta, C. E., Bunton, S. D., Prinkey, L. A., Sherer, A. P., & Seifert, P. C. (1989). *Clinical Assessment Tools for Use with Nursing Diagnoses.* St. Louis: Mosby.

SUGGESTED READINGS

Allen, J.E. (1997). *Long Term Care Facility Resident Assessment Instrument User's Manual: For Use with Version 2.0 of HCFA: Minimum Data Set Resident Assessment Protocols and Utilization Guidelines, October 1995, Plus HCFA's 249 Questions and Answers, August 1996.* New York: Springer.

Barkauskas, V. H., Staltenberg-Allen, K., & Baumann, L. (1998). *Health & Physical Assessment,* ed 2. St. Louis: Mosby.

Barry, P. D. (1989). *Psychosocial Nursing Assessment and Intervention: Care of the Physically Ill Person,* ed 2. Philadelphia: Lippincott.

Bates, B. (1995). *A Visual Guide to Physical Examination,* ed 3. Philadelphia: Lippincott.

Billings, P. C. (1996). *Instant Nursing Assessment: Pediatric.* Albany: Delmar.

Bowers, A. C., & Thompson, J. M. (1992). *Clinical Manual of Health,* ed 4. St. Louis: Mosby-Year Book.

Cole, S. A., & Bird, J. (2000). *The Medical Interview: The Three-Function Approach,* ed 2. St. Louis: Mosby.

Coulehan, J. L., & Block, M. R. (2001). *The Medical Interview: Mastering Skills for Clinical Practice,* ed 4. Philadelphia: F. A. Davis.

Eliopoulos, C. (1990). *Health Assessment of the Older Adult,* ed 2. Redwood City, CA: Addison-Wesley Nursing.

Engel, K. (2002). *Pocket Guide to Pediatric Assessment,* ed 3. St. Louis: Mosby.

Expert 10-Minute Physical Examinations. (1997). St. Louis: Mosby.

Fuller, J., & Schaller-Ayers, J. (2000). *Health Assessment: A Nursing Approach,* ed 3. Philadelphia: Lippincott.

Giger, J. N., & Davidhizar, R. E. (Eds.). (1995). *Transcultural Nursing: Assessment and Intervention,* ed 2. St. Louis: Mosby.

Guzzetta, C. E., Bunton, S. D., Prinkey, L. A., & Sherer, A. (1989). *Clinical Assessment Tools for Use with Nursing Diagnoses.* St. Louis: Mosby.

Hogstel, M. O., & Keen-Payne, R. (2001). *Practical Guide to Health Assessment: Through the Lifespan,* ed 3. Philadelphia: F. A. Davis.

Jackson, J. E., & Neighbors, M. (1990). *Home Care Client Assessment Handbook.* Rockville, MD: Aspen.

Jaffe, M. S., & Skidmore-Roth, L. (1997). *Home Health Nursing: Assessment and Care Planning,* ed 3. St. Louis: Mosby.

Leasia, M. S., & Monahan, F. D. (1997). *A Practical Guide to Health Assessment.* Philadelphia: W. B. Saunders.

Mezey, M. D., Hauckhorst, L. H., & Stokes, S. A. (1993). *Health Assessment of the Older Individual,* ed 2. New York: Springer.

Murray, R. B., & Zenter, J. P. (1997). *Nursing Assessment and Health Promotion Strategies Through the Life Span,* ed 6. Norwalk, CT: Appleton & Lange.

Pesut, D. F., & Herman, J. (1999). *Clinical Reasoning: The Art and Science of Critical and Creative Thinking.* Albany, NY: Delmar.

Seidel, H. M., Ball, J. W., Dains, J. E., & Benedict, G. W. (1999). *Mosby's Guide to Physical Examination,* ed 4. St. Louis: Mosby.

Simonsen, S. M. (2001). *Telephone Health Assessment: Guidelines for Practice,* ed 2. St. Louis: Mosby.

Thompson, J. M., & Wilson, S. F. (2000). *Health Assessment for Nursing Practice,* ed 2. St. Louis: Mosby.

Weber, J. (1997). *Nurses' Handbook of Health Assessment,* ed 3. Philadelphia: Lippincott.

Genogram References

Beauchesne, M., Kelley, B., & Gauthier, M. A. (1997). News, notes & tips. The genogram: A health assessment tool. *Nurse Educator, 2*(3):9, 16.

Beck, R. (1987). The genogram as process. *American Journal of Family Therapy,* 15:343–351.

Engelman, S. R. (1988). Use of the family genogram technique with spinal cord injured patients. *Clin Rehab,* 2: 7–15.

Friedman, H., Rohrbaugh, M., & Krakauer, S. (1988). The time-line genogram: Highlighting temporal aspects of family relationships. *Fam Process, 27*(3):293–303.

Herth, K. A. (1989). The root of it all: Genograms as a nursing assessment tool. *Journal of Gerontological Nursing,* 15:32–37.

Hurley, P. M. (1982). Family assessment: Systems theory and the genogram. *Children's Health Care,* 10:76–82.

Like, R. C., Rogers, J., & McGoldrick, M. (1988). Reading and interpreting genograms: A systematic approach. *J Fam Pract,* (4):407–412.

Marinelli, R. D. (1995). The genogram in health education. *Journal of Health Education, 26*(4):243–244.

Puskar, K., & Nerone, M. (1996). Genogram: A useful tool for nurse practitioners. *Journal of Psychiatric and Mental Health Nursing, 3*(1):55–60.

Richards, W. R., Burgess, D. E., Petersen, F. R., & McCarthy, D. L. (1993). Genograms: A psychosocial assessment tool for hospice. *Hospice Journal: Physical, Psychosocial, and Pastoral Care of the Dying, 9*(1):1–12.

Rogers, J. C., & Rohrbaugh, M. (1991). The SAGE-PAGE trial: Do family genograms make a difference? *J Am Board Fam Pract, 4*(5):319–326.

Rogers, J. C., Rohrbaugh, M., & McGoldrick, M. (1992). Can experts predict health risk from family genograms? *Fam Med, 24*(3):209–215.

Shore, W. B., Wilkie, H. A., & Croughan-Minihane, M. (1994). Family of origin genograms: Evaluation of a teaching program for medical students. *Fam Med, 26*(4):238–243.

Visscher, E. M., & Clore, E. R. (1992). The genogram: A strategy for assessment. *Journal of Pediatric Health Care,* 6(6):361–367.

Waters, I., Watson, W., & Wetzel, W. (1994). Genograms: Practical tools for family physicians. *Can Fam Physician,* 40:282–287.

Chapter 3

The Diagnosis or Need Identification Step: Analyzing the Data

---

■ **ANA STANDARD 2:** Diagnosis: The nurse analyzes the assessment data in determining diagnoses.

The second step of the nursing process is often referred to as **ANALYSIS**, as well as **NEED (OR PROBLEM) IDENTIFICATION** or **NURSING DIAGNOSIS**. Although all these terms may be used interchangeably, the purpose of this step of the nursing process is to draw conclusions regarding a client's specific needs or human responses of concern so that effective care can be planned and delivered. We have chosen to label this step of the nursing process **DIAGNOSIS** or **NEED IDENTIFICATION**. To be more specific, this is a process of data analysis using diagnostic reasoning (a form of clinical judgment) in which judgments, decisions, and conclusions are made about the meaning of the data collected to determine whether or not nursing intervention is indicated.

ANALYSIS: the process of examining and categorizing information to reach a conclusion about a client's needs.

NEED IDENTIFICATION: the second step of the nursing process, in which the data collected are analyzed and, through the process of diagnostic reasoning, specific client diagnostic statements are created.

DIAGNOSIS: Forming a clinical judgment identifying a disease/condition or human response through scientific evaluation of signs/symptoms, history, and diagnostic studies.

NURSING DIAGNOSES: Noun: a label approved by NANDA identifying specific client needs. The means of describing health problems amenable to treatment by nurses; may be physical, sociological, or psychological. **Verb:** the process of identifying specific client needs; used by some as the title of the second step of the nursing process.

The **DIAGNOSIS** of client needs has been determined by nurses on an informal basis since the beginning of the profession. The term came into formal use in the nursing literature during the 1950s (Fry, 1953), although its meaning continued to be seen in the context of medical diagnosis. A group of interested nursing leaders met and held a national conference in 1973 (Gebbie & Lavin, 1975). Their purpose was to identify the client needs that fall within the scope of nursing, label them, and develop a classification system that could be used by nurses throughout the world. This group called these labels **NURSING DIAGNOSES.** Regional, national, and international workshops and conferences continue to be held since the first conference. NANDA International Inc. (formerly North American Nursing Diagnosis Association) meets every 2 years to review its work on the development and classification of nursing diagnoses, as well as the work of other nursing groups worldwide, representing various clinical specialties and healthcare settings.

American Nurses' Association (ANA) standards of practice were first developed in 1973, and with the acceptance of the ANA Social Policy Statement in 1980, which defined nursing as the "diagnosis and treatment of human responses to actual or potential health problems," and the 1995 update description as the "diagnosis and treatment of human responses to health and illness" (ANA, 1995), the movement for broad use of a common language was enhanced. The system developed by NANDA provides a standard terminology that is accepted by ANA and various specialty groups and is being used across the United States and in many countries around the world. NANDA has established a liaison with the International Council of Nursing to support and contribute to the global effort to standardize the language of health care with the goal that NANDA labels will be included in the International Classification of Diseases (ICD-11). In the meantime, NANDA nursing diagnoses are included in the United States version of International Classification of Diseases–Clinical Modifications (ICD-10CM) and the NANDA, Nursing Interventions Classification (NIC), and Nursing Outcomes Classification (NOC) classifications have been coded into Systematized Nomenclature of Medicine (SNOMED). (Inclusion in an international coded terminology is essential if nursing's contribution to health care is to be recognized. Indexing of the entire medical record supports disease management activities, research, and analysis of outcomes for quality improvement for all healthcare disciplines. Coding also supports telehealth, the use of telecommunications technology to provide medical information and healthcare services over distance, and facilitates access to healthcare data across care settings and different computer systems.)

Today, the use of the nursing process and nursing diagnoses is rapidly becoming an integral part of an effective system of nursing practice. It is a system that can be used within existing conceptual frameworks, because it is a generic approach adaptable to all academic and clinical settings. In addition, as mentioned in the first chapter, organizing schemata of nursing problems other than NANDA are used within the profession. Additional schemata, such as the Omaha System, the Patient Care Data Set, the Home Health Care Classification, and the Perioperative Nursing Data Set (see individual bibliographies for each of these four additional schema), have been approved for use. In this edition, we introduce you to the Omaha System by presenting associated Omaha System problems with the NANDA diagnoses in the case studies.

Defining Nursing Diagnosis

The term *nursing diagnosis* has been used as both a verb and a noun. This may result in confusion. Nursing diagnosis is used as a noun in reference to the work of NANDA. For the purposes of this text, *nursing diagnosis* refers to the NANDA list of nursing diagnosis labels (Table 3–1) that form the stem of the **CLIENT DIAGNOSTIC STATEMENT.**

Although nurses work within the nursing, medical, and psychosocial domains, nursing's phenomena of concern are patterns of human response, not disease processes. Therefore, nursing diagnoses do not parallel medical/psychiatric diagnoses but do involve independent nursing activities, as well as collaborative roles and actions.

The nursing diagnosis is a conclusion drawn from the data collected about a client that serves as a means of describing a health need amenable to treatment by nurses. A uniform or standardized way of identifying, focusing on, and labeling specific phenomena allows the nurse to deal effectively with individual client responses.

Although there are different definitions of the term *nursing diagnosis*, NANDA has accepted the following:

> Nursing diagnosis is a clinical judgment about individual, family, or community responses to actual and potential health problems/life processes. Nursing diagnoses provide the basis for selection of nursing interventions to achieve outcomes for which the nurse is accountable.

The nursing diagnosis is as correct as the current data allow because it is supported by these data. It says what the client's situation is at the present time and reflects changes in the client's condition as they occur. Each decision the nurse makes is time dependent and, with additional information gathered later, decisions may change. Unlike medical diagnoses, nursing diagnoses change as the client progresses through various stages of illness/maladaptation, to resolution of the need for nursing intervention or to the conclusion of the condition. For example, for a client undergoing cardiac surgery, initial needs may be acute Pain; decreased Cardiac Output; ineffective Airway Clearance; and risk for Infection. As the client progresses, needs may shift to risk for Activity Intolerance; deficient Knowledge (Learning Need) (specify); and ineffective Role Performance.

The Use of Nursing Diagnoses

Although not yet comprehensive, the current NANDA list of diagnostic labels defines/refines professional nursing activity. The list of labels is now at a point where nurses need to use the proposed diagnoses on a daily basis, becoming familiar with the parameters of each individual diagnosis and identifying its strengths and weaknesses, thus promoting research and further development.

A frequently asked question is "Why should we use a nursing diagnosis … what is its value to the nursing profession?" The use of a nursing diagnosis can provide many benefits. The accurate choice of a nursing diagnosis to label a client need:

- **Gives Nurses a Common Language:** Promotes improved communication among nurses, other healthcare providers, and alternate care settings.

   FOR EXAMPLE: Using the nursing diagnosis "ineffective Airway Clearance"

CLIENT DIAGNOSTIC STATEMENT: the outcome of the diagnostic reasoning process; a three-part statement identifying the client's need, the cause of the need (or human response of concern), and the associated signs/symptoms. Distinguishing between Medical and Nursing Diagnoses....

- **Medical Diagnoses** are illnesses/conditions, such as diabetes, heart failure, hepatitis, cancer, and pneumonia, that reflect alteration of the structure or function of organs/systems and are verified by medical diagnostic studies. The medical diagnosis usually does not change

- **Nursing Diagnoses** address human responses to actual and potential health problems/life processes, such as Activity Intolerance (specify level); Health Maintenance, ineffective; Airway Clearance, ineffective; Self Care deficit (specify). The nursing diagnoses change as the client's situation or perspective changes/resolves.

TABLE 3–1. **Nursing Diagnoses (accepted for use and research [2001])**

Activity Intolerance [specify level]

Activity Intolerance, risk for

Adjustment, impaired

Airway Clearance, ineffective

Allergy, latex

Allergy, latex, risk for

Anxiety [specify level]

Anxiety, death

Aspiration, risk for

Attachment, risk for impaired parent/infant/child

Autonomic Dysreflexia

Autonomic Dysreflexia, risk for

Body Image, disturbed

Body Temperature, risk for imbalanced

Bowel Incontinence

Breastfeeding, effective

Breastfeeding, ineffective

Breastfeeding, interrupted

Breathing Pattern, ineffective

Cardiac Output, decreased

Caregiver Role Strain

Caregiver Role Strain, risk for

Communication, impaired verbal

Conflict, decisional (specify)

Confusion, acute

Confusion, chronic

Constipation

Constipation, perceived

Constipation, risk for

Coping, community, ineffective

Coping, community, readiness for enhanced

Coping, defensive

Coping, ineffective

Coping, family: compromised

Coping, family: disabling

Coping, family: readiness for enhanced

Denial, ineffective

Dentition, impaired

Development, risk for delayed

Diarrhea

Disuse Syndrome, risk for

Diversional Activity, deficient

Energy Field, disturbed

Environmental Interpretation Syndrome, impaired

Failure to Thrive, adult

Falls, risk for

Family Processes, dysfunctional: alcoholism

Family Processes, interrupted

Fatigue

Fear

[Fluid Volume, deficient (hyper/hypotonic)]

Fluid Volume, deficient [isotonic]

Fluid Volume, excess

Fluid Volume, risk for deficient

Fluid Volume, risk for imbalanced

Gas Exchange, impaired

Grieving, anticipatory

Grieving, dysfunctional

Growth, risk for disproportionate

Growth & Development, delayed

Health Maintenance, ineffective

Health-Seeking Behaviors [specify]

Home Maintenance, impaired

Hopelessness

Hyperthermia

Hypothermia

Infant Behavior, disorganized

Infant Behavior, readiness for enhanced, organized

Infant Behavior, risk for disorganized

Infant Feeding Pattern, ineffective

Infection, risk for

Injury, risk for

Injury, risk for perioperative positioning

Intracranial Adaptive Capacity, decreased

Knowledge, deficient [Learning Need] [specify]

TABLE 3–1. Nursing Diagnoses (accepted for use and research [2001]) (Continued)

Loneliness, risk for

Memory, impaired
Mobility, impaired bed
Mobility, impaired physical
Mobility, impaired wheelchair
Nausea
Noncompliance [Adherence, ineffective] [specify]
Nutrition: imbalanced, less than body requirements
Nutrition: imbalanced, more than body requirements
Nutrition: imbalanced, risk for more than body requirements

Oral Mucous Membrane, impaired

Pain, acute
Pain, chronic
Parental Role Conflict
Parenting, impaired
Parenting, risk for impaired
Peripheral Neurovascular Dysfunction, risk for
Personal Identity, disturbed
Poisoning, risk for
Post-Trauma Syndrome
Post-Trauma Syndrome, risk for
Powerlessness
Powerlessness, risk for
Protection, ineffective

Rape-Trauma Syndrome
Rape-Trauma Syndrome: compound reaction
Rape-Trauma Syndrome: silent reaction
Relocation Stress Syndrome
Role Performance, ineffective

Self Care Deficit, bathing/hygiene
Self Care Deficit, dressing/grooming
Self Care Deficit, feeding
Self Care Deficit, toileting

Self Esteem, chronic low
Self Esteem, risk for situational low
Self Esteem, situational low
Self Mutilation
Self Mutilation, risk for
Sensory Perception, disturbed (specify: visual, auditory, kinesthetic, gustatory, tactile, olfactory)
Sexual Dysfunction
Sexuality Patterns, ineffective
Skin Integrity, impaired
Skin Integrity, risk for impaired
Sleep Deprivation
Sleep Pattern, disturbed
Social Interaction, impaired
Social Isolation
Sorrow, chronic
Spiritual Distress
Spiritual Distress, risk for
Spiritual Well-being, readiness for enhanced
Suffocation, risk for
Suicide, risk for
Surgical Recovery, delayed
Swallowing, impaired

Therapeutic Regimen: community, ineffective management
Therapeutic Regimen: family, ineffective management
Therapeutic Regimen, effective management
Therapeutic Regimen, ineffective management
Thermoregulation, ineffective
Thought Processes, impaired
Tissue Integrity, impaired
Tissue Perfusion, ineffective (specify type: cerebral, cardiopulmonary, renal, gastrointestinal, peripheral)
Transfer Ability, impaired
Trauma, risk for

Unilateral Neglect
Urinary Elimination, impaired

(Continued)

TABLE 3–1. **Nursing Diagnoses (accepted for use and research [2001])** (Continued)	
Urinary Incontinence, functional	Ventilation, impaired spontaneous
Urinary Incontinence, reflex	Ventilatory Weaning Response, dysfunctional
Urinary Incontinence, stress	Violence, [actual/]risk for, directed at others
Urinary Incontinence, total	Violence, [actual/]risk for, self-directed
Urinary Incontinence, risk for urge	
Urinary Incontinence, urge	Walking, impaired
Urinary Retention [acute/chronic]	Wandering [specify sporadic or continual]

Information that appears in brackets has been added by the authors to clarify and facilitate the use of nursing diagnoses.

SIGN: objective or observable evidence or manifestation of a health need.

SYMPTOM: subjectively perceptible change in the body or its functions that indicates disease or the kind or phases of disease.

REMEMBER ...nursing diagnoses may represent a physical, sociological, or psychological finding. **Physical Nursing Diagnoses** include those that pertain to circulation (e.g., ineffective peripheral Tissue Perfusion), ventilation (e.g., ineffective Airway Clearance), elimination (e.g., Constipation), and so on.

instead of saying "difficulty breathing" conveys a distinct image. When the former is heard, a clear picture begins to develop in your mind, as your thoughts focus on the musculature of the upper airway, mucus production, and cough effort. With the second label, you do not have a clear idea as to what is happening with this client, and you question whether the client is experiencing an airway maintenance problem, movement of the chest, or perfusion to the lungs.

This improved communication may result in improved quality and continuity of the care provided to the client.

- **Promotes Identification of Appropriate Goals:** Aids in the choice of correct nursing interventions to alleviate the identified need and provides guidance for evaluation. Whereas nursing actions were once based on variables such as SIGNS and SYMPTOMS, test results, or a medical diagnosis, nursing diagnosis is a uniform way of identifying, focusing on, and dealing with specific client responses to health and illness (i.e., the phenomena of concern for nurses).

  FOR EXAMPLE: "Risk for Infection" compared with "presence of urinary catheter." The risk or potential threat of an infection brings to mind specific goals/outcomes and interventions to protect the client, but what is your concern, if any, with the urinary catheter?

- **Provides Acuity Information:** Ranks the amount of work that involves nursing care and can serve as a basis for client classification systems. This method of ranking can be used to determine individual staffing needs. It can also serve as documentation to provide justification for third-party reimbursement.

  FOR EXAMPLE: Nursing diagnoses can be given different, weighted values according to the degree of nursing involvement required; that is, "impaired Gas Exchange" may require a considerable amount of skilled nursing time to promote adequate ventilation, to provide oxygen and respiratory treatments, and to monitor laboratory studies. "Acute Urinary Retention" may require a much shorter period to insert a catheter into the bladder and periodically measure the urine output.

In addition, some third-party payors (such as Medicare and other insurance companies) include nursing diagnoses when considering extended length of stay or delayed discharge.

- **Can Create a Standard for Nursing Practice:** Provides a foundation for quality assurance programs, a means of evaluating nursing practice, and a mechanism of costing-out delivery of nursing care.

  FOR EXAMPLE: Did the nursing interventions address and resolve the need? Did the client experience the desired result (e.g., alleviation of pain)? Were the goals met, or is there documentation of the reasons why they were not met? Were the expected outcomes changed to meet changing client needs?

- **Provides a Quality Improvement Base:** Clinicians, administrators, educators, and researchers can document, validate, or alter the process of care delivery, which then improves the profession.

  FOR EXAMPLE: The use of universally understood labels enhances retrieval of specific data for review to determine accuracy, to validate and/or change nursing actions related to specific nursing diagnoses, and to evaluate an individual nurse's performance.

Psychosocial Nursing Diagnoses include those that pertain to the mind (e.g., disturbed Thought Processes), emotion (e.g., Anxiety [specify level]), or lifestyle/relationships (e.g., ineffective Sexuality Patterns, or Social Isolation).

Identifying Client Needs

During the ASSESSMENT step, the collection, clustering, and validation of client data flow directly into the DIAGNOSIS or NEED IDENTIFICATION step of the nursing process, where you sense needs or problems and choose nursing diagnoses.

DIAGNOSTIC REASONING: ANALYZING THE CLIENT DATABASE

Identifying client needs and then selecting a nursing diagnosis label involves the use of experience, expertise, and intuition on your part. There are six steps involved in need identification that constitute the activities of diagnostic reasoning. The result is the creation of a client diagnostic statement that identifies the client need, suggests its potential cause or etiology, and notes its signs and symptoms. This is known as the PES format, reflecting Problem, Etiology, and Signs/symptoms (Gordon, 1976).

PES: format for combining a nursing diagnosis label, client-specific cause, and signs/symptoms to create an individualized diagnostic statement.
CUE: a signal that indicates a possible need/direction for care.

Step 1: Problem-Sensing

Data are reviewed and analyzed to identify CUES (signs and symptoms) suggesting client needs that can be described by nursing diagnosis labels. If the data have been recorded in a nursing format (e.g., Diagnostic Divisions or Functional Health Patterns), the nurse is automatically guided to specific groups of nursing diagnoses when certain cues from the data are identified (Box 3–1). This helps to focus attention on appropriate diagnoses. Reviewing the NANDA definitions of specific diagnoses (see Appendix A) can be of further assistance in deciding between two or more similar diagnostic labels; for instance, there are five different diagnoses for urinary incontinence (see step 4).

  FOR EXAMPLE: When the Diagnostic Divisions format is used, body temperature is recorded in the Safety section. When the client's temperature rises, the nurse reviews the diagnostic labels under Safety to find a possible fit, such as Hyperthermia or risk for Infection. At the same time, cues are noted in other

BOX 3–1

Nursing Diagnoses Organized According to Diagnostic Divisions

After data have been collected and areas of concern/need identified, consult the Diagnostic Divisions framework to review the list of nursing diagnoses that fall within the individual categories. This will assist with the choice of specific diagnostic labels to accurately describe data from the client database. Then, with the addition of etiology (when known) and signs and symptoms, the client diagnostic statement emerges.

Diagnostic Division: Activity/Rest

Ability to engage in necessary/desired activities of life (work and leisure) and to obtain adequate sleep/rest

Diagnoses

Activity Intolerance [specify level]
Activity Intolerance, risk for
Disuse Syndrome, risk for
Diversional Activity, deficient
Fatigue
Mobility, impaired bed
Mobility, impaired wheelchair
Sleep Deprivation
Sleep Pattern, disturbed
Transfer Ability, impaired
Walking, impaired

Diagnostic Division: Circulation

Ability to transport oxygen and nutrients necessary to meet cellular needs

Diagnoses

Autonomic Dysreflexia
Autonomic Dysreflexia, risk for
Cardiac Output, decreased
Intracranial Adaptive Capacity, decreased
Tissue Perfusion, ineffective (specify type: cerebral, cardiopulmonary, renal, gastrointestinal, peripheral)

Diagnostic Division: Ego Integrity

Ability to develop and use skills and behaviors to integrate and manage life experiences

Nursing Diagnoses Organized According to Diagnostic Divisions

Diagnoses

Adjustment, impaired
Anxiety [specify level]
Anxiety, death
Body Image, disturbed
Conflict, decisional (specify)
Coping, defensive
Coping, ineffective
Denial, ineffective
Energy Field, disturbed
Fear
Grieving, anticipatory
Grieving, dysfunctional
Hopelessness
Personal Identity, disturbed
Post-Trauma Syndrome
Post-Trauma Syndrome, risk for
Powerlessness
Powerlessness, risk for
Rape-Trauma Syndrome
Rape-Trauma Syndrome: compound reaction
Rape-Trauma Syndrome: silent reaction
Relocation Stress Syndrome
Relocation Stress Syndrome, risk for
Self-Esteem, chronic low
Self-Esteem, risk for situational low
Self-Esteem, situational low
Sorrow, chronic
Spiritual Distress
Spiritual Distress, risk for
Spiritual Well-being, readiness for enhanced

Diagnostic Division: Elimination

Ability to excrete waste products

(Continued)

Nursing Diagnoses Organized According to Diagnostic Divisions (Continued)

Diagnoses

  Bowel Incontinence
  Constipation
  Constipation, perceived
  Constipation, risk for
  Diarrhea
  Urinary Elimination, impaired
  Urinary Incontinence, functional
  Urinary Incontinence, reflex
  Urinary Incontinence, risk for urge
  Urinary Incontinence, stress
  Urinary Incontinence, total
  Urinary Incontinence, urge
  Urinary Retention [acute/chronic]

Diagnostic Division: Food/Fluid

Ability to maintain intake of and use nutrients and liquids to meet physiological needs

Diagnoses

  Breastfeeding, effective
  Breastfeeding, ineffective
  Breastfeeding, interrupted
  Dentition, impaired
  Failure to Thrive, adult
  Fluid Volume, deficient [hyper/hypotonic]
  Fluid Volume, deficient [isotonic]
  Fluid Volume, excess
  Fluid Volume, risk for deficient
  Fluid Volume, risk for imbalanced
  Infant Feeding Pattern, ineffective
  Nausea
  Nutrition: imbalanced, less than body requirements
  Nutrition: imbalanced, more than body requirements
  Nutrition: imbalanced, risk for more than body requirements
  Oral Mucous Membrane, impaired
  Swallowing, impaired

Diagnostic Division: Hygiene

Ability to perform basic activities of daily living

Nursing Diagnoses Organized According to Diagnostic Divisions

Diagnoses

> Self-Care Deficit, bathing/hygiene
> Self-Care Deficit, dressing/grooming
> Self-Care Deficit, feeding
> Self-Care Deficit, toileting

Diagnostic Division: Neurosensory

Ability to perceive, integrate, and respond to internal and external cues

Diagnoses

> Confusion, acute
> Confusion, chronic
> Infant Behavior, disorganized
> Infant Behavior, readiness for enhanced, organized
> Infant Behavior, risk for disorganized
> Memory, impaired
> Peripheral Neurovascular Dysfunction, risk for
> Sensory Perception, disturbed (specify: visual, auditory, kinesthetic, gustatory, tactile, olfactory)
> Thought Processes, disturbed
> Unilateral Neglect

Diagnostic Division: Pain/Discomfort

Ability to control internal/external environment to maintain comfort

Diagnoses

> Pain, acute
> Pain, chronic

Diagnostic Division: Respiration

Ability to provide and use oxygen to meet physiological needs

Diagnoses

> Airway Clearance, ineffective
> Aspiration, risk for
> Breathing Pattern, ineffective
> Gas Exchange, impaired
> Ventilation, impaired spontaneous
> Ventilatory Weaning Response, dysfunctional

(Continued)

Nursing Diagnoses Organized According to Diagnostic Divisions (Continued)

Diagnostic Division: Safety

Ability to provide safe, growth-promoting environment

Diagnoses

Allergy Response, latex
Allergy Response, risk for latex
Body Temperature, risk for imbalanced
Environmental Interpretation Syndrome, impaired
Falls, risk for
Home Maintenance, impaired
Health Maintenance, ineffective
Hyperthermia
Hypothermia
Infection, risk for
Injury, risk for
Injury, risk for perioperative positioning
Mobility, impaired physical
Poisoning, risk for
Protection, ineffective
Self-Mutilation
Self-Mutilation, risk for
Skin Integrity, impaired
Skin Integrity, risk for impaired
Suffocation, risk for
Surgical Recovery, delayed
Thermoregulation, ineffective
Tissue Integrity, impaired
Trauma, risk for
Violence, [actual/]risk for, directed at others
Violence, [actual/]risk for, self-directed
Wandering [specify sporadic or continual]

Diagnostic Division: Sexuality

(Component of Ego Integrity and Social Interaction) Ability to meet requirements/characteristics of male/female role

Diagnoses

Sexual Dysfunction
Sexuality Patterns, ineffective

Nursing Diagnoses Organized According to Diagnostic Divisions

Diagnostic Division: Social Interaction

Ability to establish and maintain relationships

Diagnoses

Attachment, risk for impaired parent/infant/child
Caregiver Role Strain
Caregiver Role Strain, risk for
Communication, impaired verbal
Coping, community, ineffective
Coping, community, readiness for enhanced
Coping, family: compromised
Coping, family: disabling
Coping, readiness for enhanced
Family Processes, dysfunctional: alcoholism
Family Processes, interrupted
Loneliness, risk for
Parental Role Conflict
Parenting, impaired
Parenting, risk for impaired
Role Performance, ineffective
Social Interaction, impaired
Social Isolation

Diagnostic Division: Teaching/Learning

Ability to incorporate and use information to achieve healthy lifestyle/optimal wellness

Diagnoses

Development, risk for delayed
Growth, risk for disporportionate
Growth and Development, delayed
Health-Seeking Behaviors [specify]
Knowledge, deficient [Learning Need] [specify]
Noncompliance [Adherence, ineffective] [specify]
Therapeutic Regimen: community, ineffective management
Therapeutic Regimen: family, ineffective management
Therapeutic Regimen, effective management
Therapeutic Regimen, ineffective management

sections of the database that may be combined with fever or may be totally unrelated. In fact, cues may have relevance in more than one section, as you can see in Box 3–2.

BOX 3–2

Walking Through the Use of Diagnostic Divisions

During the Assessment phase, the following data were obtained from Robert:

Activity/Rest

Reports (Subjective)

Occupation: Retired truck driver
Usual Activities/Hobbies: Used to like to hunt and fish
Leisure Time Activities: Mostly watches baseball on TV, takes short walks—one to two blocks
Feelings of Boredom/Dissatisfaction: "Wish I could do more; just getting too old"
Limitations Imposed by Condition: "I get short of breath; stay at home mostly"
Sleep: Hours: 5 **Naps:** After lunch **Aids:** None
Insomnia: Only if short of breath (1 or 2 ×/wk) or needs to void (1 ×/night)
Rested on Awakening: Not always; "feel weak most of the time"
Other: "Sometimes, it feels like there isn't enough air"

Exhibits (Objective)

Observed Response to Activity: Cardiovascular: BP 178/102, P 100 after walking half-length of corridor from floor scale
Respiratory: 32, rapid, leaning forward ("to catch breath")
Mental Status (i.e., withdrawn/lethargic): Alert, responding to all questions
Neuromuscular Assessment: Muscle mass/tone: Decreased/bilaterally equal/diminished Posture: Leans forward to breathe
Tremors: No **ROM:** Movement in all extremities **Strength:** Moderate
Deformity: No

Having previously noted respiratory cues of dyspnea with activity when you reviewed the respiratory data in Box 2–3, you return to the Activity/Rest section of the Diagnostic Divisions, where the effects/limitations of this condition on both activity and sleep would also be considered. You are referred to the following nursing diagnoses: Activity Intolerance [specify level]; Activity Intolerance, risk for; Mobility, impaired bed; Disuse Syndrome, risk for; Diversional Activity, deficient; Fatigue; Sleep Deprivation; Sleep Pattern, disturbed; Walking, impaired; Mobility, impaired wheelchair; and Transfer Ability, impaired, as possible choices to describe or label Robert's needs.

Step 2: Rule-Out Process

Alternative explanations are considered for the identified cues to determine which nursing diagnosis label may be the most appropriate. This step is crucial in establishing an adequate list of diagnostic statements. As you compare and contrast the relationships among and between data, etiologic factors are identified within or between categories based on an understanding of the biologic, physical, and behavioral sciences.

> **FOR EXAMPLE:** Although Hyperthermia or risk for Infection was suggested during the first step of diagnostic reasoning, another consideration might be deficient Fluid Volume. In another example, cues of increased tension, restlessness, elevated pulse rate, and reported apprehension may initially be thought to indicate Anxiety (specify level). However, a similar diagnosis of Fear should be considered, as well as the possibility that these cues may be physiologically based, requiring medical treatment and nursing interventions related to education and monitoring.

If you encounter difficulty in choosing a nursing diagnosis label, asking yourself the following questions may provide additional guidance:

1. What are my concerns about this client?
2. Can I/am I doing something about it?
3. Can the overall risk be reduced by nursing intervention?

For example, in the teen client with bulimia, electrolyte imbalance may occur. Questions to ask might be:

- What is a major concern about electrolyte imbalance?

The client may develop a cardiac dysrhythmia or even arrest.

- Can I do something about it?

Monitor signs of imbalance, encourage foods/fluids rich in necessary electrolytes, administer supplements, and educate client regarding nutritional needs.

- Can the overall risk be reduced by nursing interventions?

Yes, the risk of cardiac dysrhythmias can be reduced if electrolyte balance is maintained/restored.

Conclusion: The Nursing Diagnosis would be risk for decreased Cardiac Output; and the client diagnostic statement would be risk for decreased Cardiac Output, risk factor of decreased potassium intake/excessive loss.

Step 3: Synthesizing the Data

A view of the data as a whole (including information collected by other members of the healthcare team) can provide a comprehensive picture of the client in relation to past, present, and future health status. This is called **SYNTHESIZING** the data. The suggested nursing diagnosis label is combined with the identified related factor(s) and cues to create a hypothesis.

> **FOR EXAMPLE:** Sally had a period of bleeding during delivery of the placenta following the unexpected delivery of twins. Blood loss was estimated to be approximately 600 ml. In addition, she experienced several episodes of vomiting

SYNTHESIZING: reviewing all data as a whole to obtain a comprehensive picture of the client.

before delivery and reduced oral intake because of nausea. The nursing diagnosis label: deficient Fluid Volume (isotonic); related factors of hemorrhage, vomiting, poor oral intake; cues of dark urine, dry mouth/lips, low blood pressure.

Step 4: Evaluating or Confirming the Hypothesis

ETIOLOGY: identified causes and/or contributing factors responsible for the presence of a specific client need.

RELATED FACTOR: the conditions/ circumstances that contribute to the development/ maintenance of a nursing diagnosis; forms the "related to" component of the client diagnostic statement.

RISK FACTOR: environmental factors and physiological, psychological, genetic, or chemical elements that increase the vulnerability of an individual, family, or community to an unhealthy event.

Test the hypothesis for appropriate fit; that is, review the NANDA nursing diagnosis and definition. Then, compare the assessed possible ETIOLOGY with NANDA's RELATED FACTORS or RISK FACTORS. Next, compare the assessed client cues with NANDA's Defining Characteristics, which are used to support and provide an increased level of confidence in your selected nursing diagnosis. Appendix A provides a complete listing of NANDA nursing diagnostic labels, definitions, defining characteristics, and related factors. This listing will be helpful as you work through the Practice Activities and Work Pages contained in each chapter. Take a moment to review Box 3–3. The information contained within the box provides a beginning effort in assessing the appropriateness of a specific nursing diagnosis label.

Lunney (1989, 1990) addressed the self-monitoring task of accuracy determination, defining the characteristics of accuracy and providing an ordinal scale for measurement. The scale ranges from a high assigned accuracy point value describing a diagnosis that is consistent with all the cues, to the lowest point value, which describes a diagnosis indicated by more than one cue but recommended for rejection based on the presence of at least two disconfirming cues (see Appendix F).

BOX 3–3

Elements of NANDA Nursing Diagnostic Labels

Appendix A supplies a complete listing of NANDA nursing diagnosis labels, which will be helpful to you as you work through the exercises in this chapter and throughout the book. It is important to become familiar with this list, so that you can find information quickly in the clinical setting. Take a moment to identify the key elements of the diagnostic label, "Deficient Fluid Volume" as excerpted below.

Deficient Fluid Volume [isotonic]
Definition: Decreased intravascular, interstitial, and/or intracellular fluid. This refers to dehydration—water loss alone without change in sodium.
Related Factors: Active fluid volume loss, failure of regulatory mechanisms.
Defining Characteristics: Decreased urine output; increased urine concentration; weakness; sudden weight loss (except in third-spacing); decreased venous filling; increased body temperature; change in mental state; elevated hematocrit; decreased skin/tongue turgor; dry skin/mucous membranes; thirst; increased pulse rate; decreased blood pressure; decreased pulse volume/pressure.

Additionally, Appendix G, Lunney's Integrated Model for Self-Monitoring of Accuracy of the Diagnostic Process, is an excellent self-evaluation of your progress in diagnostic efforts. (Also, a separate section in the Suggested Readings is dedicated to the topic of accuracy of nursing diagnoses.) The completed evaluation provides feedback regarding your diagnostic abilities. Reflection and self-monitoring are tools to assist you in developing your critical thinking skills. The attention you give to measuring the accuracy of your suggested nursing diagnosis is time well spent. Comparing the subjective and objective data gathered from the client with the defining characteristics of the possible nursing diagnoses that are listed not only helps ensure the accuracy of your statement, but also stresses the importance of objectivity in this diagnostic process.

Now return to Box 3–2. In reviewing Robert's database, you sense that he may have a problem with activity. After reviewing the NANDA nursing diagnosis labels and definitions relevant to the Activity/Rest Diagnostic Division, you choose risk for Activity Intolerance. Next, to confirm your hypothesis, compare the cues from the database with the related factors and defining characteristics noted in Appendix A. Practice Activity 3–1 presents an Interactive Care Plan Worksheet for the client problem of Activity Intolerance, on which you can document the identified cues.

Step 5: List the Client's Needs

Based on the data obtained from steps 3 and 4, the accurate nursing diagnosis label is combined with the assessed etiology and signs/symptoms, if present, to finalize the client diagnostic statement.

> **FOR EXAMPLE,** Sally is diagnosed with deficient Fluid Volume (isotonic) related to hemorrhage, vomiting, reduced intake as evidenced by dark urine, dry mucous membranes, hypotension, and hemoconcentration. This individualized diagnosis reflects the PES format for a three-part diagnostic statement, as described in Box 3–4. A diagnostic statement is needed for each need or problem you identify. Take a moment here to complete Practice Activity 3–2.

Step 6: Re-evaluate the Problem List

Be sure all areas of concern are noted. Once all nursing diagnoses are identified, list them according to priority and classify them according to status: an actual need; a risk need; or a resolved need.

- **Actual Diagnoses:** describe human responses to health conditions/life processes that currently exist in an individual, family, or community. They are supported by defining characteristics (manifestations/signs and symptoms) that cluster in patterns of related cues or inferences (NANDA, 2001). They are expressed by the use of a three-part PES statement.

  > **FOR EXAMPLE:** A client is admitted for a medical workup because of difficulties with bladder function related to her diagnosis of multiple sclerosis. An actual diagnosis might be Urinary Retention.

Record the cues from Box 3–2 that are relevant to the problem of Activity Intolerance, identified for Robert, in the appropriate spaces on this worksheet.

INTERACTIVE CARE PLAN WORKSHEET

Student Name:

ACTIVITY INTOLERANCE

Client's Medical Diagnosis:

DEFINITION: Insufficient physiological or psychological energy to endure or complete required or desired daily activities.

DEFINING CHARACTERISTICS: Verbal report of fatigue or weakness; abnormal heart rate or blood pressure response to activity; exertional discomfort or dyspnea; ECG changes reflecting dysrhythmias or ischemia.

RELATED FACTORS: Bedrest and/or immobility; generalized weakness; sedentary lifestyle; imbalance between oxygen supply and/or demand.

STUDENT INSTRUCTIONS: In the space below, enter the subjective and objective data gathered during your client assessment.

ASSESSMENT

Subjective Data Entry

Objective Data Entry

TIME OUT! **Student Instructions:** To be sure your client diagnostic statement written below is accurate, you need to review the defining characteristics and related factors associated with the nursing diagnosis and see how your client data match. Do you have an accurate match or are additional data required, or does another nursing diagnosis need to be investigated?

DIAGNOSIS

CLIENT DIAGNOSTIC STATEMENT:

Activity Intolerance (specify) _____

_____

Related to _____

BOX 3–4

Components of the Client Diagnostic Statement: Problem (Need), Etiology, and Signs and Symptoms (PES)

P = Problem (Need) is the name or diagnostic label identified from the NANDA list. The key to accurate nursing diagnosis is need identification that focuses attention on a current risk or potential physical or behavioral response to health or illness that may interfere with the client's quality of life. It deals with concerns of the client/significant other(s) and the nurse that require nursing intervention and management.

E = Etiology is the suspected cause or reason for the response that has been identified from the assessment (client database). The nurse makes inferences based on knowledge and expertise, such as understanding of pathophysiology, and situational or developmental factors. The etiology is stated as "related to." *Note:* One problem or need may have several suspected causes, such as Self Esteem, chronic low, related to lack of positive feedback and dysfunctional family system.

S = Signs and Symptoms are the manifestations (or cues) identified in the assessment that substantiate the nursing diagnosis. They are stated as "evidenced by," followed by a list of subjective and objective data. It is important to note that risk diagnoses are not accompanied by signs and symptoms because the need has not yet actually occurred. In this instance, the "S" component of the diagnostic statement is omitted, and the "E" component would be replaced by an itemization of the identified risk factors that suggest that the diagnosis could occur (e.g., risk for Infection, risk factors of Malnutrition and Invasive Procedures).

- **Wellness Diagnoses:** provide another form of an actual diagnosis that has a wellness focus that is more of an opportunity than a need. In such cases, clients (i.e., individuals, family, or community) have an assessed opportunity to improve an aspect of their health or well-being. (**Note:** See section on Wellness and Health Promotion in Suggested Readings.) The diagnostic statement would be written as readiness for enhanced ....

  FOR EXAMPLE: A client's need to improve his or her sense of harmony with others (i.e., family members) could be labeled readiness for enhanced Spiritual Well-being. Or, the family of a client with multiple sclerosis (MS) has been very supportive during periods of exacerbated symptoms; however, they want to learn to optimize the client's health status and enrich their lifestyle. A wellness diagnosis of readiness for enhanced Family Coping is appropriate.

- **Risk Diagnoses:** refer to human responses to health conditions/life processes that may develop in a vulnerable individual, family, or community. They are supported by risk factors that contribute to increased vulnerability (NANDA,

PRACTICE ACTIVITY 3–2
Identifying the PES Components of the Client Diagnostic Statement

Instructions (questions 1–5): Identify the "PES" components of each of these diagnostic statements:

1. Severe Anxiety, related to changes in health status of fetus/self and threat of death as evidenced by restlessness, tremors, focus on self/fetus.

   P = _____ E = _____ S = _____

2. Disturbed Thought Processes, related to pharmacological stimulation of the nervous system as evidenced by altered attention span, disorientation, and hallucinations.

   P = _____ E = _____ S = _____

3. Ineffective Coping, related to maturational crisis as evidenced by inability to meet role expectations and alcohol abuse.

   P = _____ E = _____ S = _____

4. Hyperthermia, related to increased metabolic rate and dehydration as evidenced by elevated temperature, flushed skin, tachycardia, and tachypnea.

   P = _____ E = _____ S = _____

5. Acute Pain, related to tissue distention and edema as evidenced by verbal reports, guarding behavior, and changes in vital signs.

   P = _____ E = _____ S = _____

6. Explain the difference between actual and risk diagnoses: _____

   _____

7. Give an example of an actual and a risk need for a client with second-degree burns of the hand.

   _____

2001). They represent a need that you believe could develop, but because it has not yet occurred, there are no signs or symptoms—only "risk factors"—so it would be written as a two-part statement.

FOR EXAMPLE: The client's MS has been in remission; however, she has had difficulty in the past with physical mobility. This past problem must be considered when planning this client's care to minimize the possibility of recurrence. A potential problem would then be identified as risk for impaired Physical Mobility.

- **Resolved Diagnoses:** are those that no longer require intervention. Because the need no longer exists, no diagnostic statement is needed.

> **BOX 3–5**
>
> *Potential Errors in Choosing a Nursing Diagnosis*
>
> - **Overlooking Cues** resulting in a missed diagnosis can lead to worsening of the problem.
>
>   FOR EXAMPLE: A client reports discomfort at the insertion site of an intravenous (IV) catheter. You notice that the area is slightly reddened but fail to consider the risk for infection. As a result, the client develops sepsis or a blood infection, requiring emergency intervention and longer hospital stay.
>
> - **Making a Diagnosis with an Insufficient Database** can lead in the wrong direction, wasting valuable time and resources.
>
>   FOR EXAMPLE: The client displays signs of anxiety. Without additional assessment, you administer a tranquilizer on the belief that the signs and symptoms are psychologically based. Later, when checking the client, you find signs of cyanosis, suggesting inadequate oxygenation. Thus, the anxiety probably was at least in part physiologically based and needed other nursing interventions.
>
> - **Stereotyping** leads to treatment of all clients in the same way and negates individualization.
>
>   FOR EXAMPLE: In a medical-surgical setting, the assumption is often made that a client with a psychiatric diagnosis is apt to become violent.

FOR EXAMPLE: Your client once suffered a decubitus ulcer (impaired Skin Integrity); however, she has learned techniques to prevent recurrence of this problem, and her skin is in good condition. Therefore, as long as she is able to participate in or direct her own care, this is of no significant concern to you at this time.

Finally, validate the diagnostic conclusions/impressions with the client and/or a colleague. This helps reduce the possibility of **DIAGNOSTIC ERRORS** and/or omissions as discussed in Box 3–5. Inclusion of the client/significant others promotes understanding and participation in the planning of individualized care.

DIAGNOSTIC ERROR: a mistaken assumption leading to a wrong conclusion.

As you can see, the process of need identification is more complex than simply attaching a label to your client. In reviewing the definition of nursing, it can be seen that "the human responses to health and illness" are complex, and the process of accurately diagnosing these human responses attests to the complexity of nursing.

OTHER CONSIDERATIONS FOR NEED IDENTIFICATION

The medical/psychiatric diagnosis can provide a starting point for identifying associated client needs (problem-sensing). Review Box 3–6 for several medical/psychiatric diagnoses with examples of associated nursing diagnoses. Although the presence of a

BOX 3-6

Applicable Nursing Diagnoses Associated with Selected Medical/Psychiatric Disorders

Certain nursing diagnoses may be linked to specific health problems (e.g., medical disorders). This linkage is often presented as choices in a diagnostic database, in various types of clinical pocket manuals, or on preprinted or computerized care planning forms. The purposes are to assist the clinician in rapidly identifying other applicable nursing diagnoses, based on the changing needs of the client, and to develop a decisive plan of care.

Because the nursing process is cyclical and ongoing, other nursing diagnoses may become appropriate as the individual client situation changes. Therefore, you must continually assess, identify, and validate new needs and evaluate the effectiveness of subsequent care. Keep in mind that the client may have needs unrelated to the medical diagnosis.

AIDS (Acquired Immunodeficiency Syndrome)

Risk for Infection, progression to sepsis/opportunistic overgrowth: risk factors may include depressed immune system, inadequate primary defenses, use of antimicrobial agents, broken skin, malnutrition, and chronic disease processes.

Risk for Deficient Fluid Volume: risk factors may include excessive losses (copious diarrhea, profuse sweating, vomiting, hypermetabolic state, and fever) and impaired intake (nausea, anorexia, lethargy).

Fatigue, may be related to disease state, malnutrition, anemia, negative life events, stress/anxiety possibly evidenced by inability to maintain usual routines, decreased performance, lethargy/listlessness, and disinterest in surroundings.

Labor Stage I (Active Phase)

Acute Pain/[Discomfort], may be related to contraction-related hypoxia, dilation of tissues, and pressure on adjacent structures combined with stimulation of both parasympathetic and sympathetic nerve endings, possibly evidenced by verbal reports, guarding/distraction behaviors (restlessness), muscle tension, and narrowed focus.

Impaired Urinary Elimination, may be related to retention of fluid in the prenatal period, increased glomerular filtration rate, decreased adrenal stimulation, dehydration, pressure of the presenting part, and regional anesthesia, possibly evidenced by increased/decreased output, decreased circulating blood volume, spasms of glomeruli and albuminuria, and reduced sensation.

Risk for Ineffective Coping [Individual/Couple]: risk factors may include stressors accompanying labor, personal vulnerability, use of ineffective coping mechanisms, inadequate support systems, and pain.

Applicable Nursing Diagnoses Associated with Selected Medical/Psychiatric Disorders

Fractures

Acute Pain, may be related to movement of bone fragments, muscle spasms, tissue trauma/edema, traction/immobility device, stress, and anxiety, possibly evidenced by verbal reports, distraction behaviors, self-focusing/narrowed focus, facial mask of pain, guarding/protective behavior, alteration in muscle tone, and autonomic responses (changes in vital signs).

Deficient Knowledge [Learning Need] regarding healing process, therapy requirements, potential complications, and self-care needs, may be related to lack of information, possibly evidenced by statements of concern, questions, and misconceptions.

Impaired Physical Mobility, may be related to neuromuscular/skeletal impairment, pain/discomfort, restrictive therapies (bedrest, extremity immobilization), and psychological immobility, possibly evidenced by inability to purposefully move within the physical environment, imposed restrictions, reluctance to attempt movement, limited range of motion, and decreased muscle strength/control.

Depressive Disorders (Mood Disorders)

Major Depression/Dysthymia

Risk for Violence, directed at self/others: risk factors may include depressed mood and feelings of worthlessness and hopelessness.

Anxiety [moderate to severe]/Disturbed Thought Processes, may be related to psychological conflicts, unconscious conflict about essential values/goals of life, unmet needs, threat to self-concept, sleep deprivation, interpersonal transmission/contagion, possibly evidenced by reports of nervousness or fearfulness, feelings of inadequacy, agitation, angry/tearful outbursts, rambling/discoordinated speech, restlessness, hand rubbing or wringing, tremulousness, poor memory/concentration, decreased ability to grasp ideas, inability to follow/impaired ability to make decisions, numerous/repetitious physical complaints without organic cause, ideas of reference, hallucinations/delusions.

Disturbed Sleep Pattern, may be related to biochemical alterations (decreased serotonin levels), unresolved fears and anxieties, and inactivity, possibly evidenced by difficulty in falling/remaining asleep, early morning awakening/awakening later than desired (hypersomnia), reports of not feeling well rested, and physical signs (e.g., dark circles under eyes, excessive yawning).

* A risk diagnosis is not evidenced by signs and symptoms because the problem has not occurred, and nursing interventions are directed at prevention.

Extracted from Doenges, M. E., Moorhouse, M. F., & Geissler-Murr, A. C. (2002). *Nurse's Pocket Guide, Nursing Diagnoses with Interventions*, ed 8 . Philadelphia: F. A. Davis.

medical/psychiatric diagnosis can suggest several nursing diagnoses, these nursing diagnoses must be supported by cues in the client database.

> **FOR EXAMPLE:** In the experience of a myocardial infarction, the client often suffers pain, anxiety, and activity intolerance and requires teaching activities. In addition, the client may be at risk for decreased Cardiac Output, ineffective Tissue Perfusion, and excess Fluid Volume. These needs do not necessarily occur in each client with this condition. One client may actually be pain-free, whereas another could demonstrate a sleep disturbance or report spiritual distress. Therefore, a medical diagnosis can provide an initial point for problem-sensing, but the validity of a nursing diagnosis depends on the presence of individually appropriate supporting data.

The client's or family member's understanding of normal body function, individual expectations (including cultural), or mistaken perceptions may result in the belief that a need exists, even in the absence of diagnostically appropriate supporting data. Even though the need seems to exist only in the mind of the client/significant other, it needs to be addressed and resolved in order to promote optimal wellness and allow the client to focus on the supported needs.

> **FOR EXAMPLE:**
> 1. The parent of a child with cancer may believe that the child is incapable of self-care activities even though the child's level of function and development would indicate otherwise. This then is not a client problem with self-care but rather the parent's problem—possibly, compromised Family Coping.
> 2. A female client may believe that sexual desire normally disappears after menopause/hysterectomy, and the fact that it does not indicates to her that something is wrong. Although sexual dysfunction may have occurred, the assessment reveals inadequate information and misconceptions. Therefore, the nursing diagnosis is deficient Knowledge of normal sexual functioning.
> 3. An elderly, confused client with a diagnosis of Alzheimer's disease is found wandering in the day room. She has soiled herself and is smearing feces on the walls and couch. The problem would not be one of bowel elimination but of disturbed Thought Processes. Interventions would be addressed to behavioral management, rather than only to a bowel control program.

As noted in the previous examples, it is important to "reduce" the need to its basic component in order to focus interventions on the "roots" of the human response. It is also important to take the related factors and the defining characteristics to the lowest "denominator" possible so the client and nurse are better able to formulate individually specific goals/outcomes and can identify more clearly the appropriate interventions/actions to be taken to correct or alleviate the need.

> **FOR EXAMPLE:** Impaired Social Interaction related to neurological impairment and the resulting sequelae (i.e., cognitive, behavioral, and emotional changes) is better stated, "related to skill deficit about ways to enhance mutuality, commu-

nication barriers, limited physical mobility as evidenced by family report of change in pattern of interacting, dysfunctional interactions with peers and family, observed discomfort in social situations." This simplifies care and increases the likelihood of a timely and satisfactory resolution.

Neurological impairment is a broad umbrella that reflects general pathophysiology and lacks the specificity that is necessary to guide nursing actions/interventions. By identifying specific responses, you focus attention directly on issues that can be corrected or altered by nursing interventions.

For beginners, it is advisable to use the NANDA list in Appendix A when choosing a diagnostic label. Because the list is still evolving, "holes" may exist. With practice and experience, you may very well identify a need that is treatable with nursing interventions but for which there is no appropriate NANDA label. In this situation, the diagnosis should be stated clearly using the PES format and then reviewed with other nursing colleagues to verify that the meaning and intent are accurately communicated. Finally, the work should be documented and submitted to NANDA for consideration.

Nursing knowledge is both objective and subjective, and it is the combination of intuition and analysis that guides nursing's methodology. Experienced nurses may use **INTUITION** to arrive at a conclusion as an integral part of critical thinking. This skill is difficult to teach, and it may not develop in all nurses; however, it needs to be respected, valued, and encouraged. Intuition is grounded in both knowledge and experience and is involved in nursing judgments.

INTUITION: a sense of something that is not clearly evidenced by known facts.

Paying attention to the feelings or sense of something for which there are no visible data can add an important dimension to the diagnostic reasoning process. Intuition, responsibly applied by checking, rechecking, and validating these impressions (to avoid errors in judgment), can lead to insights not available in any other way.

Finally, identification of a client's needs may be assisted by entering the client database into a computer. On-line diagnostic software programs are available that contain lists of frequently used nursing diagnoses correlated to specific medical diagnoses. Other programs may suggest possible nursing diagnoses based on cues that the program identifies in the client database. Such programs are support tools and do not eliminate your need to use the diagnostic reasoning process to identify and formulate appropriate client diagnostic statements *independently* of computer recommendations.

Writing a Client Diagnostic Statement: Using PES Format

As NANDA's list of nursing diagnosis labels has increased, issues of **WELLNESS** are being addressed. The focus of a nursing diagnosis is no longer limited solely to "problems" but may also include the client's needs and strength areas for potential enhancement. For this reason, although we use the PES format, we have chosen to identify the outcome of the diagnostic reasoning process as the *Client Diagnostic Statement* instead of the commonly used term *Client Problem*.

WELLNESS: a state of optimal health, physical and psychosocial.

According to the PES format as previously outlined, the problem (need), etiology, and signs and symptoms (or risk factors) are combined into a "neutral" statement that avoids value-laden or judgmental language. The use of ambiguous or judgmental terms such as "too often," "uncooperative," or "manipulative" can lead to misunderstanding on the part of the reader. Clients may become defensive, or readers may be influenced to make an inaccurate or biased decision, resulting in a negative treatment outcome.

The *need* and *etiology* sections of the diagnostic statement are joined by the phrase "related to." Phrases such as "due to" or "caused by" indicate a specific/limited causal link that should therefore be avoided. "Related to" suggests a connection between the nursing diagnosis and the identified factors, leaving open the possibility that there may be other contributing factors not yet recognized.

When writing a diagnostic statement, remember to include qualifiers or quantifiers as appropriate. NANDA has provided for some flexibility of the nursing language by creating a multi-axial taxonomy. An *axis* is defined as a dimension of the human response that is considered in the diagnostic process. The first axis is the diagnostic concept. The other six axes (time, unit of care, age, health status, descriptor, and topology) can be used to modify the diagnostic concept (see Appendix B). Some modifiers are already included in the label.

FOR EXAMPLE: *Ineffective family Coping.* Coping (diagnostic concept) is the principal element or human response of concern. It has been modified by a descriptor (ineffective) and a unit of care (family). Or, in *adult Failure to Thrive*, "adult" reflects an age modifier.

If the term "specify" is noted with a diagnostic label, it is important that the correct information for the individual client be provided to make the communication clear.

FOR EXAMPLE: In *ineffective Tissue Perfusion (specify)*, the modifier to be specified is from the topology axis (e.g., cerebral, renal). However, in the diagnostic label *deficient Knowledge (specify)*, the modifier is actually the area or topic for which the client has deficient knowledge, such as *regarding care of the newborn*. In the case of *Decisional Conflict (specify)*, the modifier is the subject of the conflict or life crisis. The client diagnostic statement might read "Decisional Conflict regarding divorce related to perceived threat to value system as evidenced by vacillation between alternative choices, increased muscle tension, and reports of distress."

PROTOCOL: written guidelines of steps to be taken for providing client care in a particular situation/condition.

COLLABORATIVE PROBLEM: a need identified by another discipline that contains a nursing component requiring nursing intervention and/or monitoring and therefore is an element of the interdisciplinary plan of care.

By definition, nursing diagnoses identify client needs that can be positively affected, or possibly prevented, by nursing actions. Some diagnoses permit greater independent function, whereas others are more collaborative. This may be visualized as a continuum without a fixed midpoint differentiating independent from dependent actions (Fig. 3–1). Furthermore, the extent of independent function is influenced by the individual nurse's experience, level of expertise, and work setting and the presence of established **PROTOCOLS**, or standards of care. For this reason, the authors recommend that nurses identify the nursing component and appropriate interventions for any client need, instead of labeling independent versus **COLLABORATIVE PROBLEMS** or potential complications.

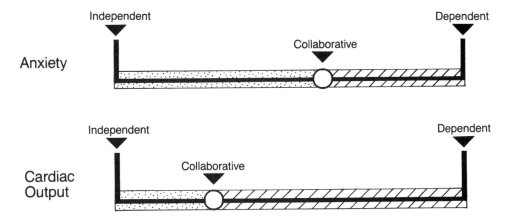

FIGURE 3–1. Representative comparison of the degree of independent nursing function in two nursing diagnoses. Nursing diagnoses have a varying degree of independent function, and nursing actions can be identified for any client situation. As shown in this diagram, the nursing diagnosis Anxiety has a high degree of independent nursing action, whereas Cardiac Output has a lower degree.

FOR EXAMPLE:

- During and following Sally's bleeding episode, the nursing component would be deficient Fluid Volume [isotonic] and the nurse not only would monitor the problem, but would take action to control/prevent further blood loss (e.g., fundal massage), increase fluid intake (oral, IV, or both), and provide assurance to the client.
- A low serum potassium level may result in dysrhythmias that can be addressed in risk for decreased Cardiac Output requiring electrocardiographic (ECG) interpretation, possible limiting of activities, provision of potassium-containing foods/fluids as appropriate, and possibly other interventions based on protocols.
- Michelle has a subclavian intravenous catheter. You might be concerned with risk for Infection with implications for sterile dressing changes, observation of the site, and monitoring of vital signs.

Debate concerning the amount of independent function associated with nursing diagnoses and the interpretation of the definition of nursing diagnoses has been ongoing. These debates attest to the perceived and actual importance that nursing diagnoses have had and continue to have in the structuring of both the education and the practice of nursing. A bifocal model of nursing diagnosis and collaborative problems has existed for many years (Carpenito, 2002; Wallace et al., 1989). Also, a trifocal model of nursing diagnosis (Kelly et al., 1995) that reinforces the wellness diagnoses has been proposed (Fig. 3–2).

In creating a diagnostic statement, it is important to be aware of common errors that can result in an incorrect nursing diagnosis. An incorrect nursing diagnosis or misstatement of needs can lead to incorrect goals/outcomes and inappropriate nursing interventions. This can result in inappropriate/inadequate treatment of the client

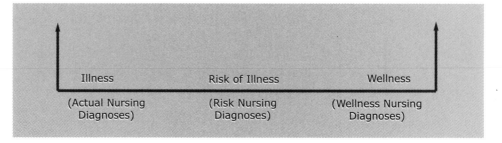

FIGURE 3–2. Trifocal model for client assessment. Adapted from Kelly, Frisch, & Avant, 1995.

that may not resolve the need and that may occasionally place the nurse at risk for legal liability.

- **Using the Medical Diagnosis:** Self Care deficit related to stroke.
  Correct: Self Care deficit related to neuromuscular impairment.
- **Relating the Problem to an Unchangeable Situation:** Risk for Injury related to blindness.
  Correct: Risk for Injury, risk factors of unfamiliarity with surroundings.
- **Confusing the Etiology or Signs/Symptoms for the Need:** Postoperative lung congestion related to bedrest.
  Correct: Ineffective Airway Clearance related to general weakness and immobility.
- **Use of a Procedure Instead of the "Human Response":** Catheterization related to urinary retention.
  Correct: Urinary Retention related to perineal swelling.
- **Lack of Specificity:** Constipation related to nutritional intake.
  Correct: Constipation related to inadequate dietary bulk and fluid intake.
- **Combining Two Nursing Diagnoses:** Anxiety and Fear related to separation from parents.
  Correct: Fear related to separation from parents, or Moderate Anxiety related to change in environment and unmet needs.
- **Relating One Nursing Diagnosis to Another:** Ineffective Coping related to anxiety.
  Correct: Severe Anxiety related to change in role functioning and socioeconomic status.
- **Use of Judgmental/Value-Laden Language:** Chronic Pain related to secondary/monetary gain.
  Correct: Chronic Pain related to recurrent muscle spasms and psychosocial disability.
  Note: The patient's report is valid, but the issue of secondary gain may require additional assessment to reveal other appropriate nursing diagnoses and interventions.
- **Making Assumptions:** Risk for impaired Parenting, risk factors of inexperience (new mother).

Correct: Deficient Knowledge regarding child care issues related to lack of previous experience, unfamiliarity with resources.

Note: The label "Deficient Knowledge" can have negative connotations for the client and may result in defensive responses. The authors support the use of a substitute label "Learning Need."

- **Writing a Legally Inadvisable Statement:** Impaired Skin Integrity related to not being turned every 2 hours.

  Correct: Impaired Skin Integrity related to prolonged pressure and altered circulation.

  Note: If a client complication occurs as a result of poor care/failure to meet standards of care, an incident report would be completed to document what happened.

With this in mind, review In a Nutshell before proceeding to Practice Activity 3–3.

In a Nutshell ...

How to Write a Client Diagnostic Statement

1. Using physical assessment and history-taking interview techniques, collect both subjective and objective data from the client, significant other, family members, other healthcare professionals, and/or client records as appropriate. A nursing framework is recommended, such as Diagnostic Divisions (Doenges and Moorhouse) or Functional Health Patterns (Gordon).

2. Organize the collected data using a nursing framework (see item 1, above), a body systems approach (cardiovascular, gastrointestinal, and so on), a head-to-toe review (head, neck, thorax, and so on), or a combination of these. Your institution may use its own clustering model. If you have used a nursing framework, however, you will discover that information in the client database is already conveniently structured for ease in identifying applicable nursing diagnoses.

3. Using diagnostic reasoning skills, review and analyze the database to identify cues (signs and symptoms) suggesting needs that can be described by nursing diagnostic labels. Check the NANDA definitions of specific diagnoses for further assistance in distinguishing between two or more potentially applicable labels (see Appendix A).

4. Consider alternative rationales for the identified cues by comparing and contrasting the relationships among and between data, and isolating etiologic factors. This will allow you to determine which nursing diagnostic labels may be most appropriate, while ruling out those that are not.

5. Test your selection of nursing diagnostic label(s) and associated etiology(ies) for appropriate "fit" by:

    - Confirming the NANDA nursing diagnosis and definition for your choice of diagnostic label [P]

    - Comparing your proposed etiology with the NANDA "Related Factors" or "Risk Factors" associated with that particular diagnosis [E]

(Continued)

In a Nutshell ... (Continued)

- Comparing your identified signs and symptoms (cues) with the NANDA "Defining Characteristics" for the selected diagnosis [S]
6. Re-evaluate your list of selected diagnoses to be sure that all client needs are accounted for. Then, order your list according to a needs priority model (the Maslow or Kalish model is usually used) with validation from the client, and classify each diagnosis as actual (signs and symptoms supporting it are already present), risk for (risk factors are present, but the problem has not yet occurred), potential for enhanced (there is a desire to move to a higher state), or resolved (need no longer requires nursing action).
7. Write the client diagnostic statement for each diagnosis on your list. A three-part statement using the PES format is indicated for actual or wellness diagnoses, and an adaptation of the PES format is used to create the two-part statement for risk diagnoses. Resolved diagnoses do not require diagnostic statements.

Three-Part Client Diagnostic Statement

To write the client diagnostic statement for actual/wellness diagnoses, combine (1) the confirmed nursing diagnosis label [P], (2) related factors [E], and (3) defining characteristics [S]. These elements are linked together by the phrases "related to" and "as evidenced by":

NEED (PROBLEM): [nursing diagnostic label]
ETIOLOGY: Related to [etiologic factors]
SIGNS AND SYMPTOMS: As evidenced by [defining characteristics]

Two-Part Client Diagnostic Statement

To write the diagnostic statement for risk diagnoses, combine (1) the confirmed risk nursing diagnosis label [P] and (2) the associated risk factors [E]. These elements are linked together by the phrase "risk factors of."

NEED (PROBLEM): [risk nursing diagnosis label]
ETIOLOGY: Risk factors of [associated risk factors]

Finally, although the PES format is a commonly recognized way of structuring the client diagnostic statement, other formats may be appropriate when a different standardized language is used. For example, the Omaha System identifies four levels of a diagnostic statement: Level 1—Domain, Level 2—Problem Classification, Level 3—Modifier, and Level 4—Signs/Symptoms (Box 3–7).

Summary

Although identification of an accurate nursing diagnosis requires time to analyze the gathered data and to validate the diagnosis, this process is critical and essential because it is the pivotal part of the nursing process. The time you take to formulate an accurate client diagnostic statement and to plan the required care results in increased nursing efficiency, better use of time for all nursing staff, and the delivery of appropriate client care, with the end result of better client outcomes.

PRACTICE ACTIVITY 3-3
Identifying Correct and Incorrect Client Diagnostic Statements

Label each client diagnostic statement as correct or incorrect. Identify why a statement is incorrect

_____ 1. Ineffective Airway Clearance, related to increased pulmonary secretions and bronchospasm, evidenced by wheezing, tachypnea, and ineffective cough. _____

_____ 2. Impaired Thought Processes, related to delusional thinking or reality base, evidenced by persecutory thoughts of "I am victim," and interference with ability to think clearly and logically. _____

_____ 3. Impaired Gas Exchange, related to bronchitis, evidenced by rhonchi, dyspnea, and cyanosis. _____

_____ 4. Deficient Knowledge regarding diabetic care, related to inaccurate follow-through of instructions, evidenced by information misinterpretation and lack of recall. _____

_____ 5. Acute Pain, related to tissue distention and edema, evidenced by reports of severe colicky pain in right flank, elevated pulse and respirations, and restlessness. _____

Some nurses still organize care directly around medical diagnoses, spending most of their time following medical orders. Medical diagnoses have a narrower focus than nursing diagnoses because they are based on pathology. A nursing diagnosis takes into account the psychological, social, spiritual, and physiological responses of the client and family. NANDA diagnostic labels listed in Appendix A are used in formulating diagnostic statements that are structured in a three-part Problem (Need), Etiology, and Signs/Symptoms (PES) format. Two-part statements may be used for risk diagnoses.

At times, something that appears easy to do in theory may seem difficult to achieve in practice. Nurses often have visionary ideas for the delivery of quality care to all clients. All too frequently, turning those ideas into actions can seem to be an exercise in futility. However, as you work with and become more familiar with nursing diagnoses, the client goals, related outcomes, and nursing interventions for attaining these goals and outcomes become more readily apparent. As you can see, an accurate and complete nursing diagnosis serves as the basis for the activities of the Planning step of the nursing process, discussed in Chapter 4.

Before continuing, let us return to the second ANA Standard of Clinical Nursing Practice and review the measurement criteria necessary to achieve and ensure compliance with the standard as discussed in this chapter (Box 3–8).

BOX 3–7

Omaha System Example

In Box 3–2, Robert is assessed using the Activity/Rest Diagnostic Division, revealing a range of possible NANDA nursing diagnosis labels:

Activity Intolerance
Disuse Syndrome, risk for
Diversional Activity, deficient
Fatigue
Mobility, impaired bed
Sleep Deprivation
Sleep Pattern, disturbed
Walking, impaired

These lead to a client diagnostic statement of: Activity Intolerance related to imbalance between oxygen supply/demand as evidenced by dyspnea and tachycardia with exertion, weakness, and limitation of desired activities. If we apply the Omaha System to the assessment data for Robert's level of physical activity, his problem would be documented as:

Level 1—Domain IV, Health-Related Behaviors
Level 2—Problem Classification, No. 37. Physical Activity
Level 3—Modifier, Individual Impairment
Level 4—Signs/Symptoms, No. 3. Inappropriate Type/Physical Condition

You are encouraged to read the articles and texts included in the Omaha System section of the Suggested Readings at the end of this chapter.

BOX 3–8

Measurement Criteria for ANA Standard II

ANA Standard II: Diagnosis: The nurse analyzes the assessment data in determining diagnoses.

1. Diagnoses are derived from the assessment data.
2. Diagnoses are validated with the client, family, and healthcare providers, when possible and appropriate.
3. Diagnoses are documented in a manner that facilitates the determination of expected outcomes and plan of care.

1. What is the definition of Need Identification? _____
   _____

2. What two factors influenced the development and acceptance of *nursing diagnosis* as the language
   of nursing? _____
   _____

3. List three reasons for using nursing diagnosis.

   a. _____

   b. _____

   c. _____

4. List the six steps of diagnostic reasoning.

   a. _____

   b. _____

   c. _____

   d. _____

   e. _____

   f. _____

5. Name the components of the Client Diagnostic Statement.

   a. _____

   b. _____

   c. _____

6. If a risk diagnosis is identified, how is the Client Diagnostic Statement altered?
   _____
   _____

7. What is the difference between a medical and a nursing diagnosis?
   _____
   _____

8. Which of these client diagnostic statements are stated correctly? Indicate by placing a C before
   correct or an I before incorrect statements. Then, differentiate actual (A) from risk (R) needs by
   placing an A or R by each statement.

   _____ a. Deficient Knowledge regarding drug therapy, related to misinterpretation and unfamiliarity with resources as evidenced by request for information and statement of misconception.

_____ b. Risk for Infection, risk factors of altered lung expansion, decreased ciliary action, decreased hemoglobin, and invasive procedures.

_____ c. Impaired Urinary Elimination, related to indwelling catheter evidenced by inability to void.

_____ d. Anxiety (moderate), related to change in health status, role functioning, and socioeconomic status evidenced by apprehension, insomnia, and feelings of inadequacy.

9. Underline the cues in the following client database that indicate that a need may exist, and write a Client Diagnostic Statement based on your findings.

VIGNETTE: Sally is 2 days post delivery. She reports that her bowels have not moved but says she has been drinking plenty of fluids, including fruit juices, and has been eating a balanced diet.

ELIMINATION (EXCERPT FROM THE CLIENT DATABASE)

Subjective

Usual bowel patterns: every morning
Laxative use: rare/MOM PM
Character of stool: brown, formed
Last BM: 4 days ago
History of bleeding: No
Hemorrhoids: last 5 weeks
Constipation: currently
Diarrhea: No
Usual voiding pattern: 3–4 ×/day
Character of urine: Yellow
Incontinence: No
Urgency: No
Pain/burning/difficulty voiding: No
History of kidney/bladder disease: several bladder infections, last one 6 years ago
Associated concerns: pain with stool, nausea, "I just can't go no matter what I do."

Objective

Abdomen tender: Yes
Soft/firm: somewhat firm
Palpable mass: No
Size/girth: enlarged/postpartal
Bowel sounds: present all four quadrants, hypoactive every 1 to 2 minutes
Hemorrhoids: Visual examination not done
Now, write the Client Diagnostic Statement. Refer to the listing of Nursing Diagnoses in Appendix A to compare diagnostic labels addressing bowel elimination.

_____

_____

_____

_____

BIBLIOGRAPHY

American Nurses' Association. (1980). *Nursing: A Social Policy Statement*. Kansas City, MO: Author.

American Nurses' Association. (1995). *Nursing's Social Policy Statement*. Washington, DC: Author.

Carpenito, L. J. (2002). *Nursing Diagnosis: Application to Clinical Practice*, ed 9. Philadelphia: J. B. Lippincott.

Fry, V. S. (1953). The creative approach to nursing. *Am J Nurs*, 53:301–302.

Gebbie, K. M., & Lavin, M. A. (1975). *Classification of Nursing Diagnoses: Proceedings from the First National Conference*. St. Louis: Mosby.

Gordon, M. (1976). Nursing diagnosis and the diagnostic process. *American Journal of Nursing*, 76 (8):1298–1300.

Kelly, J., Frisch, N., & Avant, K. (1995). A trifocal model of nursing diagnosis: Wellness reinforced. *Nursing Diagnosis*, 6(3):123–128.

Lunney, M. (1989). Self-monitoring of accuracy using an integrated model of diagnostic process. *J Adv Med Surg Nurs*, 1(3):43–52.

Lunney, M. (1990). Accuracy of nursing diagnosis: Concept development. *Nursing Diagnosis*, 1(1):12–17.

North American Nursing Diagnosis Association. (2001). *Nursing Diagnoses: Definition & Classification*. Philadelphia: Author.

Wallace, D., & Ivey, J. (1989). The bifocal clinical nursing model: Descriptions and applications to patients receiving thrombolytic or anticoagulant therapy. *Journal of Cardiovascular Nursing*, 4(1): 33–45.

SUGGESTED READINGS

Nursing Language, Classification, Theory, and Taxonomy

Advant, K. C. (1990). The art and science in nursing diagnosis development. *Nursing Diagnosis*, 1(1):51–56.

Dobryzn, J. (1995). Components of written nursing diagnostic statements. *Nursing Diagnosis*, 6(1):29–38.

Kerr, M. (1991). Validation of taxonomy. In R. M. Carroll-Johnson (Ed.). *Classification of Nursing Diagnoses: Proceedings of the Ninth Conference North American Nursing Diagnosis Association*. Philadelphia: J. B. Lippincott.

Kerr, M., et al. (1992). Development of definitions for taxonomy II. *Nursing Diagnosis*, 3(2):65–71.

Kerr, M., et al. (1993). Taxonomic validation: An overview. *Nursing Diagnosis*, 4(1):6–14.

Loomis, M. E., & Conco, D. (1991). Patients' perception of health, chronic illness, and nursing diagnosis. *Nursing Diagnosis*, 2(4):162–170.

Miers, L. J. (1991). NANDA's definition of nursing diagnosis: A plea for conceptual clarity. *Nursing Diagnosis*, 2(1):9–18.

Mills, W. C. (1991). Nursing diagnosis: The importance of a definition. *Nursing Diagnosis*, 2(1):3–8.

Shoemaker, J. (1984). Essential features of a nursing diagnosis. In M. Kim, G. K. McFarland, & A. M. McLane (Eds.). *Classification of Nursing Diagnoses: Proceedings of the Fifth Conference, North American Nursing Diagnosis Association*. St. Louis: Mosby.

Spackman, K. (2000). SNOMED RT and SNOMED CT: The promise of an international clinical terminology. *MD Computing*, 17(6):29.

Warren, J. J., & Hoskins, L. M. (1990). The development of NANDA's nursing diagnosis taxonomy. *Nursing Diagnosis*, 1(4):162–168.

Whitley, G. G., & Gulanick, M. (1995). Barriers to use of nursing diagnosis in clinical settings. *Nursing Diagnosis*, (5):25–32.

Texts

Carpenito, L. J. (2002). *Nursing Diagnosis: Application to Clinical Practice*, ed 9. Philadelphia: J. B. Lippincott.

Cox, H., et al. (2002). *Clinical Applications of Nursing Diagnosis: Adult, Child, Women's, Psychiatric, Gerontic, and Home Health Considerations*, ed 4. Philadelphia: F. A. Davis.

Doenges, M. E., Moorhouse, M. F., & Geissler, A. C. (2002). *Nursing Care Plans: Guidelines for Individualizing Patient Care*, ed 6. Philadelphia: F. A. Davis.

Leuner, J. D., Manton, A. K., Kelliher, D., Sullivan, S. D., & Doherty, M. (1990). *Mastering the Nursing Process: A Case Study Approach*. Philadelphia: F. A. Davis.

Maas, M., Buckwalter, K. C., & Hardy, M. (1991). *Nursing Diagnosis and Interventions for the Elderly*. Menlo Park, CA: Addison-Wesley.

Validation of Nursing Diagnoses

Brukwitzki, G., Holmgen, C., & Maibusch, R. M. (1996). Validation of the defining characteristics of the nursing diagnosis Ineffective Airway Clearance. *Nursing Diagnosis, 7*:63–69.

Chiang, L., Ku, N., & Lo, C. K. (1994). Clinical validation of the etiologies and defining characteristics of Altered Nutrition: Less than body requirements in patients with cancer. In R. M. Carroll-Johnson & M. Paquette (Eds.). *Classification of Nursing Diagnoses: Proceedings of the Tenth Conference, North American Nursing Diagnosis Association*. Philadelphia: J. B. Lippincott.

Chung, L. (1997). The clinical validation of defining characteristics and related factors of fatigue in hemodialysis patients. In M. J. Rantz & P. Lemone (Eds.). *Classification of Nursing Diagnoses: Proceedings of the Twelfth Conference, North American Nursing Diagnosis Association*. Glendale, CA: Cinahl.

Dougherty, C. (1997). Reconceptualization of the nursing diagnosis decreased cardiac output. *Nursing Diagnosis: The Journal of Nursing Language and Classification, 8*:29–36.

Ennen, K. A., Komorita, N. I., & Pogue, N. (1997). Validation of defining characteristics of the nursing diagnosis: Fluid volume excess. In M. J. Rantz & P. Lemone (Eds.). *Classification of Nursing Diagnoses: Proceedings of the Twelfth Conference, North American Nursing Diagnosis Association*. Glendale, CA: Cinahl.

Fowler, S. B. (1997). Impaired verbal communication: During short-term oral intubation. *Nursing Diagnosis: The Journal of Nursing Language and Classification, 8*:93–98.

Hensley, L. D. (1994). Spiritual distress: A validation study. In R. M. Carroll-Johnson & M. Paquette (Eds.). *Classification of Nursing Diagnoses: Proceedings of the Tenth Conference, North American Nursing Diagnosis Association*. Philadelphia: J. B. Lippincott.

Kerr, M., et al. (1993). Development of definitions for taxonomy II. *Nursing Diagnosis, 3*(2):65–71.

Kraft, L. A., Maas, M., & Hardy, M. A. (1994). Diagnostic content validity of impaired physical mobility in the older adult. In R. M. Carroll-Johnson & M. Paquette (Eds.). *Classification of Nursing Diagnoses: Proceedings of the Tenth Conference, North American Nursing Diagnosis Association*. Philadelphia: J. B. Lippincott.

Lemone, P. (1993). Validation of the defining characteristics of altered sexuality. *Nursing Diagnosis, 4*(2): 56–62.

Lemone, P., & Weber, J. (1995). Validating gender specific defining characteristics. *Nursing Diagnosis, 6*(2):64–72.

Lemone, P., & James, D. (1997). Nursing assessment of altered sexuality: A review of salient factors and objective measures. *Nursing Diagnosis: The Journal of Nursing Language and Classification, 8*:120–128.

Levin, R. F., Krainovich, B. C., Bahrenburg, E., & Mitchell, C. A. (1988). Diagnostic content validity of nursing diagnosis. *Image J Nurs Schol, 21*(1):40–44.

Morton, N. (1997). Validation of the nursing diagnosis decreased cardiac output in a population without cardiac disease. In M. J. Rantz & P. Lemone (Eds.). *Classification of Nursing Diagnoses: Proceedings of the Twelfth Conference, North American Nursing Diagnosis Association*. Glendale, CA: Cinahl.

Sidani, S., & Woodtli, M. A. (1994). Testing and validating an instrument to assess the defining characteristics of stress and urge incontinence. In R. M. Carroll-Johnson & M. Paquette (Eds.). *Classification of Nursing Diagnoses: Proceedings of the Tenth Conference, North American Nursing Diagnosis Association*. Philadelphia: J. B. Lippincott.

Simon, J., Baumann, M. A., & Nolan, L. (1995). Differential diagnostic validation: Acute and chronic pain. *Nursing Diagnosis, 6*(2):73–79.

Smith, J. E., et al. (1997). Risk for suicide and risk for violence: A case study approach for separating the current violence diagnoses. *Nursing Diagnosis: The Journal of Nursing Language and Classification, 8*:67–77.

Tiesinga, L. J., Dassen, T. W. N., & Halfens, R. J. G. (1997). Validation of the nursing diagnosis fatigue among patients with chronic heart failure. In M. J. Rantz & P. Lemone (Eds.). *Classification of Nursing Diagnoses: Proceedings of the Twelfth Conference, North American Nursing Diagnosis Association*. Glendale, CA: Cinahl.

Wall, B., Howard, J., & Perry-Phillips, J. (1995). Validation of two nursing diagnoses: Increased intracranial pressure and high risk for increased intracranial pressure. In M. J. Rantz & P. Lemone (Eds.). *Classification of Nursing Diagnoses: Proceedings of the Eleventh Conference, North American Nursing Diagnosis Association*. Glendale, CA: Cinahl.

Whitley, G. G. (1992). Concept analysis of anxiety. *Nursing Diagnosis, 3*(3):107–116.

Whitley, G. G. (1992). Concept analysis of fear. *Nursing Diagnosis, 3*(4):155–161.

Specific Nursing Diagnoses

Bakker, R. H., Kastermans, M. C., & Dassen, T. W. N. (1997). Noncompliance and ineffective management of therapeutic regimen: Use in practice and theoretical implications. In M. J. Rantz & P. Lemone (Eds.). *Classification of Nursing Diagnoses: Proceedings of the Twelfth Conference, North American Nursing Diagnosis Association.* Glendale, CA: Cinahl.

Bakker, R. H., Kastermans, M.C., & Dassen, T. W. N. (1995). An analysis of the nursing diagnosis Ineffective Management of Therapeutic Regimen compared to Noncompliance and Orem's Self-Care Deficit theory. *Nursing Diagnosis, 6:*161–168.

Harness-DoGloria, D., & Pye, C. G. (1995). Risk for impaired skin integrity: Incorporation of the risk factors from AHCPR guidelines. In M. J. Rantz & P. Lemone (Eds.). *Classification of Nursing Diagnoses: Proceedings of the Eleventh Conference, North American Nursing Diagnosis Association.* Glendale, CA: Cinahl.

Heliker, D. (1992). Reevaluation of the nursing diagnosis: Spiritual distress. *Nurs Forum, 27*(4):15–20.

Mahon, S. M. (1994). Concept analysis of pain: Implications related to nursing diagnoses. *Nursing Diagnosis, 1*(5):15–25.

Minton, J. A., & Creason, N. S. (1991). Evaluation of admission nursing diagnoses. *Nursing Diagnosis, 2*(1):119–125.

Schmelz, J. O. (1997). Ineffective airway clearance: State of the science. In M. J. Rantz & P. Lemone (Eds.). *Classification of Nursing Diagnoses: Proceedings of the Twelfth Conference, North American Nursing Diagnosis Association.* Glendale, CA: Cinahl.

Smucker, C. (1995). A phenomenological description of the experience of spiritual distress. In M. J. Rantz & P. Lemone (Eds.). *Classification of Nursing Diagnoses: Proceedings of the Eleventh Conference, North American Nursing Diagnosis Association.* Glendale, CA: Cinahl.

Tiesinga, L. J., Dassen, T. W. N., & Halfens, R. J. G. (1995). Fatigue: A summary of definitions, dimensions, and indicators. *Nursing Diagnosis, 7:*51–62.

Whitley, G. G. (1997). A comparison of two methods of clinical validation of nursing diagnosis. In M. J. Rantz & P. Lemone (Eds.). *Classification of Nursing Diagnoses: Proceedings of the Twelfth Conference, North American Nursing Diagnosis Association.* Glendale, CA: Cinahl.

Whitley, G. G., & Tousman, S. A. (1996). A multivariate approach for the validation of anxiety and fear. *Nursing Diagnosis, 7:*116–124.

Woodtli, M. A., & Yocum, K. (1994). Urge incontinence: Identification and clinical validation of defining characteristics. In R. M. Carroll-Johnson and M. Paquette (Eds.). *Classification of Nursing Diagnoses: Proceedings of the Tenth Conference, North American Nursing Diagnosis Association.* Philadelphia: J. B. Lippincott.

Woodtli, A. (1995). Stress incontinence: Clinical identification and validation of defining characteristics. *Nursing Diagnosis, 6:*115–122.

Woolridge, J., et al. (1998). A validation study using the case-control method of the nursing diagnosis Risk for Aspiration. *Nursing Diagnosis: The Journal of Nursing Language and Classification, 9:*5–14.

Accuracy of Nursing Diagnoses

Lunney, M. (1992). Divergent productive thinking factors and accuracy of nursing diagnoses. *Res Nurs Health, 15*(3):303–311.

Lunney, M. (1994). Measurement of accuracy of nursing diagnosis. In R. M. Carroll-Johnson & M. Paquette (Eds.). *Classification of Nursing Diagnoses: Proceedings of the Tenth Conference, North American Nursing Diagnosis Association.* Philadelphia: J. B. Lippincott.

Lunney, M., & Paradiso, C. (1995). Accuracy of interpreting human responses. *Nursing Management, 26*(10):48H–48K.

Lunney, M., Karlik, B. A., Kiss, M., & Murphy, P. (1995). Accuracy of nursing diagnosis in clinical settings. In M. J. Rantz & P. Lemone (Eds.). *Classification of Nursing Diagnoses: Proceedings of the Eleventh Conference, North American Nursing Diagnosis Association.* Glendale, CA: Cinahl.

Lunney, M., Karlik, B. A., Kiss, M., & Murphy, P. (1997). Accuracy of nursing diagnosis of psychosocial responses. *Nursing Diagnosis: The Journal of Nursing Language and Classification*, 8:157–166.

Wellness (Health Promotion)

Allen, C. (1989). Incorporating a wellness perspective for nursing diagnosis in practice. In R. M. Carroll-Johnson (Ed.). *Classification of Nursing Diagnoses: Proceedings of the Eighth Conference, North American Nursing Diagnosis Association*. Philadelphia: J. B. Lippincott.

Appling, S. E. (1997). Wellness issues. Sleep: Linking research to improved outcomes. *MEDSURG Nursing*, 6(3):159–161.

Armentrout, G. (1993). A comparison of the medical model and the wellness model: The importance of knowing the difference. *Holistic Nursing Practice, 7*(4):57–62.

Carpenito, L. J. (2002). *Nursing Diagnosis: Application to Clinical Practice*, ed 9. Philadelphia: J. B. Lippincott.

Fleury, J. (1991). Empowering potential: A theory of wellness motivation. *Nursing Research, 40*:286–291.

Fleury, J. (1991). Wellness motivation in cardiac rehabilitation. *Heart & Lung: Journal of Critical Care, 20*(1):3–8.

Fleury, J. (1996). Wellness motivation theory: An exploration of theoretical relevance. *Nurs Res, 45*:277–283.

Kelly, J., Frisch, N., & Avant, K. (1995). A trifocal model of nursing diagnosis: Wellness reinforced. *Nursing Diagnosis, 6*(3):123–128.

Moch, S. (1989). Health within illness: Conceptual evolution and practice possibilities. *Advances in Nursing Science, 11*:230–231.

Murdaugh, C. L., & Vanderboom, C. (1997). Individual and community models for promoting wellness. *J Cardiovasc Nurs, 11*(3):1–14.

Pender, N. (1987). *Health Promotion in Nursing Practice*, ed 2. Norwalk, CT: Appleton-Century.

Popkess-Vawter, S. (1991). Wellness nursing diagnoses: To be or not to be? *Nursing Diagnosis, 2*(1):19–25.

Ryan, J. P. (1993). Wellness and health promotion of the elderly. *Nurs Outlook, 41*(3):143.

Stolte, K. M. (1994). Health-oriented nursing diagnoses: Development and use. In R. M. Carroll-Johnson & M. Paquette (Eds.). *Classification of Nursing Diagnoses: Proceedings of the Tenth Conference, North American Nursing Diagnosis Association*. Philadelphia: J. B. Lippincott.

Stolte, K. M. (1996). *Wellness Nursing Diagnosis for Health Promotion*. Philadelphia: Lippincott-Raven.

Omaha System

Elfrink, V. L., Martin, K. S., & Davis, L. S. (1997). The nightingale tracker: Information technology for community nursing education. In U. Gerdin, M. Tallberg, & P. Wainright (Eds.). *Nursing Informatics: The Impact of Nursing Knowledge on Health Care Informatics*. Amsterdam, The Netherlands: IOS Press, pp 364–368.

Elfrink, V. L., & Martin, K. S. (1996). Educating for community nursing practice: Point of care technology. *Healthcare Information Management, 10*(2):81–89.

Lang, N., et al. (1997). *Nursing Practice and Outcomes Measurement*. Oakbrook Terrace, IL: Joint Commission on Accreditation of Healthcare Organizations, pp 17–34.

Martin, K. S. (1989). The Omaha System and NANDA: A review of similarities and differences: In R. M. Carroll-Johnson (Ed.). *Classification of Nursing Diagnoses: Proceedings of the Eighth Conference, North American Nursing Diagnosis Association*. Philadelphia: J. B. Lippincott, pp 171–172.

Martin, K. S. (1997). The Omaha System. In M. J. Rantz & P. Lemone (Eds.). *Classification of Nursing Diagnoses: Proceedings of the Twelfth Conference, North American Nursing Diagnosis Association*. Glendale, CA: Cinahl, pp 16–21.

Martin, K. S., Leak, G. K., & Aden, C. A. (1992). The Omaha System: A research based model for decision making. *J Nurs Adm, 22*:44–52.

Martin, K. S., & Martin, D. L. (1997). How can the quality of nursing practice be measured? In J. C. McCloskey & H. K. Grace (Eds.). *Current Issues in Nursing*, ed 5. St. Louis: Mosby, pp 315–321.

Martin, K. S., & Norris, J. (1996). The Omaha System: A model for describing practice. *Holistic Nursing Practice, 11*(1):75–83.

Martin, K. S., & Scheet, N. J. (1992). The Omaha System: *Applications for Community Health Nursing*. Philadelphia: W. B. Saunders.

Martin, K. S., & Scheet, N. J. (1992). *The Omaha System: A Pocket Guide for Community Health Nursing.* Philadelphia: W. B. Saunders.

Martin, K. S., Scheet, N. J., & Stegman, M. R. (1993). Home health care clients: Characteristics, outcomes of care, and nursing interventions. *Am J Public Health* 83:1730–1734.

Merrill, A. S., Hiebert, V., Moran, M., & Weatherby, F. (1998). Curriculum restructuring using the practice-based Omaha System. *Nurse Educator, 23*(3):41–44.

Westra, B. (1995). Implementing nursing diagnoses in community settings. In M. J. Rantz & P. Lemone (Eds.). *Classification of Nursing Diagnoses: Proceedings of the Eleventh Conference, North American Nursing Diagnosis Association.* Glendale, CA: Cinahl, pp 47–51.

Home Health Care Classification

Saba, V. K. (1997). An innovative Home Health Care Classification (HHCC) System. In M. J. Rantz & P. Lemone (Eds.). *Classification of Nursing Diagnoses: Proceedings of the Twelfth Conference, North American Nursing Diagnosis Association.* Glendale, CA: Cinahl.

Saba, V. K. (1994). *Home Health Care Classification (HHCC) of Nursing Diagnoses and Interventions. (Revised).* Washington, DC: Author.

Saba, V. K. (1992). The classification of home health care nursing: Diagnoses and interventions. *Caring, 11*(3):5–57.

Saba, V. K. (1992). Home health care classification. *Caring, 11*(5):58–60.

Saba, V. K., & Zucherman, A. E. (1992). A new home health care classification method. *Caring, 11*(10):27–34.

Patient Care Data Set

Ozbolt, J. G. (1997). From minimum data to maximum impact: Using clinical data to strengthen patient care. *MD Computing, 14*:295–301. [**Note**: Adapted from *Advanced Practice Nursing Quarterly* (1996:1:62–69).]

Ozbolt, J. G., Russo, M., & Schultz, M. P. (1995). Validity and reliability of standard terms and codes for patient care data. In R. M. Gardner (Ed.). *Proceedings of the Nineteenth Annual Symposium on Computer Applications in Medical Care,* pp 37–41. Philadelphia: Hanley & Belfus

Ozbolt, J. G., Fruchtnicht, J. N., & Hayden, J. R. (1994). Toward data standards for clinical nursing information. *J Am Med Inform Assoc* 1:175–185.

Perioperative Nursing Care Data Set

Beyea, S. C. (2002). *Perioperative Nursing Data Set (PNDS),* ed. 2. Denver: AORN.

Beyea, S. C. (2001). Data fields for intraoperative records using the Perioperative Nursing Data Set. *AORN Journal, 73*(5):952, 954.

Dawes. B. S. (2001). Communicating nursing care and crossing language barriers. *AORN Journal, 73*(5):892, 894.

Chapter 4

The Planning Step: Creating the Plan of Care

■ **ANA STANDARD 3:** Outcome identification: The nurse identifies expected outcomes individualized to the client.

■ **ANA STANDARD 4:** Planning: The nurse develops a plan of care that prescribes interventions to attain expected outcomes.

PLANNING: third step of the nursing process, during which goals/outcomes are determined and interventions chosen.

Once the etiology, signs, and symptoms previously identified are incorporated into a client diagnostic statement, you can proceed to the PLANNING step of the nursing

PLAN OF CARE: written evidence of the second and third steps of the nursing process that identifies the client's needs, goals/outcomes of care, and interventions to treat the need and achieve the outcomes.

process. Now, attention is focused on the actions that are most appropriate to effectively address the client's needs. You begin to set priorities, establish goals, identify desired outcomes, and determine specific nursing interventions. These actions are documented as the **PLAN OF CARE**, which then serves to guide the activities of all healthcare workers who are involved in the client's care. It is a priority that the client and/or significant others be included in the process of planning, so that they may contribute to, participate in, and take responsibility for their own care and the achievement of the desired outcomes and goals.

Setting Priorities for Client Care

Generally, the starting point for planning care is ranking the client's needs, so that the nurse's attention and subsequent actions are properly focused. Although there are many ways of prioritizing client needs, a useful framework is one developed by Abraham Maslow (Fig. 4–1). In 1943, Maslow theorized that human behavior is motivated by a hierarchy arranged from basic to progressively higher-level needs (Maslow, 1970). According to Maslow, physiological needs are generally considered baseline survival needs because they must be met in order for life to continue. When these base-level needs (such as food, fluid, and oxygen) are not satisfied, it is difficult or impossible to focus on, or attempt to meet, higher-level needs (such as love, belonging, and self-esteem). Once base-level needs are satisfied, however, it becomes possible for higher-level needs to be addressed. Keep in mind that some clients with chronic problems may achieve higher-level needs even though baseline survival needs may be compromised. This is possible because as clients learn to function within physiological limitations, they may be able to refocus some energy on other needs.

Richard Kalish (1983) expanded and further subdivided the structure of Maslow's hierarchy, resulting in a more comprehensive description of the specific

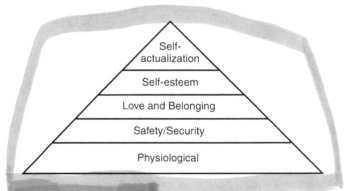

FIGURE 4–1. Maslow's hierarchy of needs. The pyramid of Maslow's hierarchy is a model that allows us to look at human behavior in a structured way to determine physiological and psychological needs. Physiological needs appear at the bottom or base of the pyramid. Maslow's theory tells us that these lower-level needs must be met before higher-level needs (such as self-esteem) can be addressed. This knowledge of the needs that must be met first can help the nurse determine the priorities of client care.

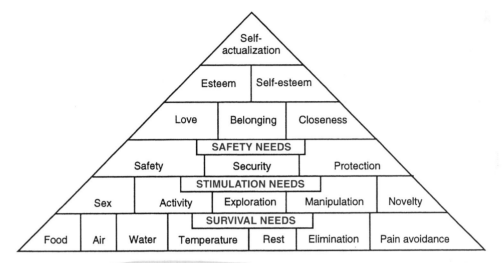

FIGURE 4–2. Kalish's expanded hierarchy. In an expansion of Maslow's model, Kalish restructured the first two levels of Maslow's pyramid (physiological and safety/security needs) into three levels and identified more-specific subcategories. The base level is labeled survival, the second level stimulation, and the third level safety. The refinement of these subcategories can further assist the nurse in identifying the priorities for planning client care.

need categories. This expanded hierarchy can help you, as a nurse, to identify and prioritize client needs more and to plan desired outcomes and the associated nursing interventions (Fig. 4–2). Failure to meet human needs at any level can dramatically interfere with a client's overall progress. Clearly, it is difficult to use active listening techniques (meeting a higher-level client need for self-esteem) to explain the importance of maintaining a patent airway to a client who is choking (a basic need of survival).

Once you have determined the priorities of care, the client's care needs can also be ranked according to a system (such as Maslow's hierarchy; see Appendix D) that can help you identify basic to higher-level actions/interventions. This is necessary because it is usually difficult to plan and provide care effectively when more than three to five nursing diagnoses exist at one time, depending on their complexity. By ranking the client's needs, you can proceed in a logical way to facilitate your client's recovery.

FOR EXAMPLE:

- Basic survival needs (i.e., air, water, and food) must be met before other needs can be considered. Sample diagnostic labels involving basic survival needs include ineffective Airway Clearance, and imbalanced Nutrition: less than body requirements.
- Safety needs are next in order of importance. Nursing diagnostic labels relating to safety needs include risk for self-directed Violence, risk for Injury, and ineffective Health Maintenance.

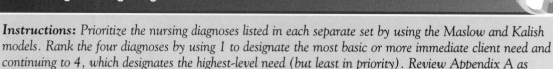

PRACTICE ACTIVITY 4–1
Prioritizing Nursing Diagnoses

Instructions: Prioritize the nursing diagnoses listed in each separate set by using the Maslow and Kalish models. Rank the four diagnoses by using 1 to designate the most basic or more immediate client need and continuing to 4, which designates the highest-level need (but least in priority). Review Appendix A as needed to compare definitions of these nursing diagnoses.

a. _____ Urinary Incontinence, stress

_____ Sexuality Patterns, ineffective

_____ Airway Clearance, ineffective

_____ Skin Integrity, risk for impaired

b. _____ Gas Exchange, impaired

_____ Knowledge, deficient

_____ Hypothermia

_____ Infection, risk for

c. _____ Pain, acute

_____ Self Esteem, chronic low

_____ Mobility, impaired physical

_____ Social Isolation

- Once these categories of client care needs are met, concerns regarding needs in the social, self-esteem, and self-actualization categories can be considered. Examples of nursing diagnostic labels related to these categories of needs include impaired Social Interaction (a need for relationships with others); Self-Esteem [specify] (the need to feel good about oneself); and readiness for enhanced Family Coping (a need for family and belonging).

Setting priorities for client care is a complex and dynamic challenge. What you may perceive today as the number one client care need or appropriate nursing intervention could change tomorrow or, for that matter, within minutes. Practice Activity 4–1 gives you some experience in prioritizing client concerns based on levels of need.

ESTABLISHING CLIENT GOALS

GOALS: broad guidelines indicating the overall direction for movement as a result of the interventions of the healthcare team; divided into long-term goals and short-term goals.

Once you have prioritized client needs, establish the **GOALS** for treatment/discharge. The client care goal(s) is a broad description of the general direction in which your client is expected to progress in response to treatment.

Goals may be either long term or short term. **LONG-TERM GOALS** indicate the overall direction or end result of care and may very well not be achieved before discharge from your care. Examples of long-term goals might be "Maintains control of blood glucose level" or "Uses resources/supports to prevent rehospitalization." **SHORT-**

TERM GOALS are more specific guides for care and must usually be met before discharge or transfer to a less acute level of care, supervision, or support. Short-term goals may be building blocks for attaining the long-term goals. Nursing care can then be planned more accurately when the focus is directed to the short-term goals. Depending on the client's anticipated length of stay/care, a short-term goal may be evaluated within a few hours or over the period of several therapeutic sessions. This period could be as long as several calendar weeks if the client is seen for counseling/therapy on a weekly, or even monthly, basis. Examples of short-term goals might be "Learns to use blood glucose monitoring system" or "Uses two support agencies within the community appropriately."

    If the short-term goal is to be met within the nursing shift or visit during which it is identified, it is not necessary to write the goal on the plan of care; it can be noted in the progress note. If the goal is not accomplished by the end of the shift/visit, it is added to the plan of care with a new timeframe, so that those involved in the patient's care can continue to work toward it.

LONG-TERM GOALS: those goals that may not be achieved before discharge from care but may require continued attention by client and/or others.

SHORT-TERM GOALS: those goals that usually must be met before discharge or movement to a less acute level of care.

IDENTIFYING DESIRED OUTCOMES

The next step in developing the plan of care is to determine specific OUTCOMES, which are defined as client responses that are achievable and desired by the client and that can be attained within a defined period, given the present situation and resources. Planned outcomes are the desired results of actions taken to achieve the broader goal; they are the measurable steps toward achieving the treatment/discharge criteria that were established earlier. Because they must be measurable, outcome statements need to:

- Be specific
- Be realistic
- Consider the client's circumstances and desires
- Indicate a definite timeframe
- Provide measurable evaluation criteria for determining success or failure

OUTCOMES: measurable steps to achieve the goals of treatment and to meet discharge criteria; the results of actions undertaken to achieve a broader goal.

    Desired outcomes are written by listing items/behaviors that can be observed and monitored to determine whether or not a positive/acceptable outcome has been achieved within the indicated timeframe (for example, "Verbalizes understanding of disease process and potential complications..."). A broad goal for a client with chronic obstructive pulmonary disease (COPD) might be "Ventilation/oxygenation adequate to allow a functional lifestyle"; the integral outcomes needed for this goal to be achieved could include:

- Maintains patent airway with breath sounds clear . . .
- Demonstrates techniques to improve airway clearance with use of pursed-lip breathing, liquefying secretions, and/or nebulizer therapy. . .
- Initiates necessary lifestyle changes and participates in treatment regimen. . .

    This itemized listing of outcomes then serves as the evaluation tool, which is discussed more fully in Chapter 6.

    Measurable action verbs are used to describe outcomes. Some examples of this type of verb include *discusses*, *states*, *identifies*, *administers*, *explains*, and *reports*. For

NURSING-SENSITIVE OUTCOMES: neutral concepts that reflect a client's status; they are influenced by nursing care and are measured as a continuum, rather than as discrete goals that are met/not met. They are useful in monitoring nursing practice, advancing standards of care, and documenting nursing's contributions to health care (Johnson & Maas, 2000).

instance, "Client will: Ambulate with use of cane." (Refer to Box 4–1 for additional examples.) Passive words are generally avoided. Specific time elements in outcome statements also provide measurable criteria, such as: "Client will: Ambulate with cane without assistance within 3 days." Some outcomes may be ongoing because they do not include a specific timeframe other than discharge from care. Examples of these ongoing outcomes are statements such as "Client will: Maintain a patent airway" or "Client will: Be free of skin breakdown." It is your job to monitor each of these situations and document regularly any client findings. However, the situation may not be resolved until the client's condition/status changes or discharge has occurred.

When outcomes are properly written, they provide direction for planning and validating the choice of appropriate nursing interventions.

FOR EXAMPLE:

- Client will: Identify individual nutritional needs within 2 visits.
- Client will: Formulate a dietary plan based on these needs within 3 days.

From these desired outcomes, you know that the client's level of dietary knowledge should be assessed and individual client needs identified; in addition, client teaching information should be presented to provide the client with the tools necessary to formulate a dietary plan.

Remember, though, that interventions can be wide ranging. The outcome state-

---

BOX 4–1

Action Verbs Useful in Writing Measurable Outcomes

Using active rather than passive verbs provides a clearer method for determining client progress. The following are examples of action verbs that can be measured or observed:

List, Record, Name, State
Describe, Explain, Identify
Demonstrate, Use, Schedule
Differentiate, Compare, Relate
Design, Prepare, Formulate, Calculate
Select, Choose, Compare
Increase/Decrease, Stand, Walk, Participate

> **FOR EXAMPLE:** The client will: *List* three things he understands about his diagnosis. The client will: *Walk* to the end of the hall and back three times today.

Below are a few samples of "passive" verbs. Notice that the "actions" described by the verbs are not measurable:
Understand, Feel, Learn, Know, Accept

> **FOR EXAMPLE:** The client will: *Understand* his treatment plan. How will the nurse measure achievement and *know* that the client understands?

ment "Client will: Verbalize acceptance of actual body image within 2 weeks" may call for interventions ranging from learning to recognize and express own feelings about body changes, to developing a program of diet and exercise to promote weight loss, to instruction in the use of makeup, hairstyles, and ways of dressing that maximize figure assets/minimize perceived faults.

All outcomes should tell the reader specifically what the client is working on or doing. If the outcome does not seem to logically relate to the goals for treatment/discharge, it should be questioned. Is the outcome, in fact, a valid component of the plan of care? With this in mind, there is a simple and straightforward method of determining whether or not an outcome is correctly written: Ask yourself if you could observe the client in the performance of the behavior indicated. If the answer is no, the desired, measurable outcome you have written should be modified. Below are several pairs of correctly and incorrectly written outcomes with notations to identify the desired elements. When you have finished looking them over, work through the exercises in Practice Activity 4–2.

1. **Incorrect**: "Understands insulin therapy within 48 hours."

   > *Rationale:* This client outcome states a clear time line, but can you measure a client's "understanding"? This outcome needs a measurable action verb.

PRACTICE ACTIVITY 4–2
Identifying Correctly Stated Outcomes

Instructions: *Identify which of the following outcome statements is written correctly, or if written incorrectly, state why it is incorrect. Modify those statements that are not correct.*

1. Client will: List individual risk factors and appropriate interventions. _____

   _____

2. Identify four adaptive/protective measures for individual situation by discharge.

   _____

3. Client will: Understand behaviors, lifestyle changes necessary to promote physical safety within

   72 hours. _____

   _____

4. Airway patent, aspiration prevented, ongoing. _____

   _____

5. Client will: Assume responsibility for own learning by participating in group discussions twice a

   day no later than 10/29/02. _____

   _____

    Correct: "Demonstrates correct insulin administration techniques within 48 hours."

    or

"Explains reasons for the steps of insulin administration within 48 hours."

      Rationale: These are well-written outcomes that are observable, measurable, and time limited.

2. **Incorrect:** "Requires no reminders from staff regarding dietary restrictions within 3 days."

      Rationale: This outcome tells what the staff will do, not what the client will do.

[handwritten margin note: Do not make 2 statements in one] *[handwritten: Incorrect]*

    ~~**Correct:**~~ "Lists individual dietary restrictions and makes appropriate choices from daily menu within 3 days."

      Rationale: This outcome is observable and easy to document.

3. **Incorrect:** "Receives fewer restrictions for defying staff instructions during the next 2 weeks."

      Rationale: What exactly is the definition of "fewer"? A specific number is clearer. What constitutes "defiance," and what is the client doing? According to this outcome, the client "receives" fewer restrictions, which places the client in an essentially passive role. Good measurable outcomes state what the client actively does.

    Correct: "Follows rules so that infractions decrease from the current rate of one per day to no more than two per week within 7 days."

      Rationale: Incidents of violation of unit rules are events that are observable, well documented, and easy to track. This outcome is also time limited.

As mentioned in Chapter 1, a classification of outcomes associated with both nursing diagnoses and nursing interventions has been researched and developed. The Nursing Outcomes Classification (NOC) was developed by a research team at the University of Iowa's College of Nursing. The current edited work, including the 260 nursing outcomes, is entitled *Iowa Outcomes Project: Nursing Outcomes Classification (NOC)*. A sample of NOC labels includes Abuse Cessation, Bone Healing, Cardiac Pump Effectiveness, Child Adaptation to Hospitalization, Dignified Dying, Hope, Leisure Participation, Oral Health, Quality of Life, Social Support, and Will to Live.

The Outcomes Classification is designed to describe the client state following the implementation of nursing interventions. Whereas the nursing diagnosis Activity Intolerance is defined by NANDA as "Insufficient physiological or psychological energy to endure or complete required or desired daily activities," the nursing outcome of "Endurance: Extent that energy enables a person's activity" describes the state (or status) the client would achieve after the implementation of selected nursing interventions (Box 4–2).

Each outcome then has an associated list of indicators that are measured by a variety of specific Likert scales (see Appendix K). Thus, the outcome is a variable state, with indicators used to measure the client response to the care provided. For example, Robert, with questioned disturbed Sleep Pattern as possibly diagnosed in the last chapter, can have an outcome state of "Sleep," and indicators of "sleep quality" and "hours of sleep," which, measured on a 1–5 scale, reveal the degree of compromise.

BOX 4-2

Pairing NANDA with NOC Outcomes

In the last chapter, your client Robert had the possible nursing diagnosis of either Activity Intolerance or Disturbed Sleep Pattern. Possible nursing outcomes identified in NOC associated with these diagnoses include:

Nursing Diagnosis:	Activity Intolerance
Outcomes:	Endurance
	Mobility level
	Pain: Disruptive effect
Nursing Diagnosis:	Disturbed Sleep Pattern
Outcomes:	Comfort level
	Rest
	Sleep

Source: Johnson, M., & Maas, M. (Eds.). (2000). *Iowa Outcomes Project: Nursing Outcomes Classification (NOC)*. St. Louis: Mosby.

Now that we have introduced you to NOC, let's go back and revisit your client Robert and review how another language of nursing, the Omaha System, assists in goal development. See Box 4–3 for the application of the Omaha System to Robert's NANDA Activity Intolerance nursing diagnosis and the Omaha System Problem: No. 37, Physical Activity.

Selecting Appropriate Nursing Interventions

NURSING INTERVENTIONS are prescriptions for behaviors, treatments, activities, or actions that assist the client in achieving the expected outcomes. Nursing interventions, like nursing diagnoses, are key elements of the knowledge of nursing; in fact, the scientific body of knowledge of nursing interventions, like that of nursing diagnoses, continues to grow as research supports the connection between actions and outcomes (McCloskey & Bulechek, 2000). In Chapter 3, we discussed the need to select the right nursing diagnosis. Selecting the appropriate nursing intervention so that your client can achieve the desired outcomes is as important as accuracy in diagnosing. It also is another method of individualizing your client's care. The Nursing Interventions Classification (NIC) contains a list of 486 intervention labels such as Infant Care, Organ Procurement, Blood Products Administration, and Code Management.

Naturally your expectation is that the interventions you select will benefit the client and/or family/significant other in a predictable way. You need to base your nursing interventions on the client's nursing diagnosis; the established goals and desired

NURSING INTERVENTIONS: any direct care treatment that a nurse performs on behalf of a client, including nurse- and physician-initiated treatments (resulting from nursing and medical diagnoses), and provision of essential daily functions for the client who cannot do them (Bulechek & McCloskey, 2000).

BOX 4–3

Application of the Omaha System: Goal Development—Part I

NANDA Nursing Diagnosis: Activity Intolerance
Omaha System Problem: No. 37, Physical Activity
The Omaha System has a Problem Rating Scale for Outcomes. This scale rates three conceptual components: knowledge, behavior, and status. Each scale has a Likert-scale ranging from 1–5. As with NOC, each concept has an associated scale. For example, Robert's knowledge of his level of physical activity can range from the following:

1—No knowledge
2—Minimal knowledge
3—Basic knowledge
4—Adequate knowledge
5—Superior knowledge

When Robert is questioned about his current medical condition and its effect on cardiac activity, we may find that Robert's knowledge of his physical activity is rated at 1, no knowledge.
Robert's behavior is also rated using the following:

1—Not appropriate
2—Rarely appropriate
3—Inconsistently appropriate
4—Usually appropriate
5—Consistently appropriate

Robert's behavior toward physical activity is assessed at 3, inconsistently appropriate. The assessed data indicate that Robert does try to complete some activities, but data do not confirm that he participates in a routine exercise program.
Robert's status is rated as follows:

1—Extreme signs/symptoms
2—Severe signs/symptoms
3—Moderate signs/symptoms
4—Minimal signs/symptoms
5—No signs/symptoms

Further assessment data would be required to assess his level of independence. For this example, however, we could assign a rating of 3, moderate signs/symptoms, based on the decrease in physical activity due to current medical condition and past health history of limited physical activity and no routine exercise program.

outcomes; the ability of the nurse to successfully implement the intervention; the ability and willingness of the client to undergo the intervention; and the appropriateness of the intervention. Interventions need to be age/situation appropriate and must promote identified client strengths, when possible.

FOR EXAMPLE:

- Discussion of fears may help to reduce the adult client's level of anxiety, whereas an infant may respond more positively to holding and cuddling.
- Although a walk down the hall to take a shower or bath may be desired by many new mothers, cultural beliefs may dictate that the new mother remain on bedrest for 7 days, or refrain from a full shower for 2 to 4 weeks.
- Orange juice is a good choice for fluid replacement unless the client has open lesions on the oral mucosa, in which case mild fruit nectars would be preferred because acidic juices cause pain.
- Visualization to assist with stress or pain management may be the appropriate intervention for the client assessed as having creative abilities, but it may not be successful in clients who are concrete thinkers.

You are accountable for being current and accurate in identifying nursing interventions. Therefore, you must be familiar with the body of scientific knowledge (rationale) that supports these interventions (in addition to respecting your client's personal preferences and cultural/religious beliefs).

NURSING STANDARDS and agency policy must also be considered during the choice of specific interventions. For example, one nursing standard describes the minimum level for nursing care related to urinary catheterization. The standard also contains the policies and procedures required to meet that standard. The policy identifies the level of educational preparation that is required for the nurse to perform the procedure, and the procedural section lists the needed equipment and suggested method of performing the procedure. The interventions must be deliberate and purposeful; they must include information on independent nursing activities (such as frequency of monitoring activities/focused assessments, whether counseling and/or teaching will be provided, the need to suction an airway), as well as any collaborative activities necessary for the nurse to carry out orders from other healthcare providers (including consultation by and referral to other providers).

NURSING STANDARD: identified criterion against which nursing care is compared and evaluated; generally reflects the minimum level of nursing care.

To be communicated accurately, nursing interventions, like nursing diagnoses and client care goals and outcomes, must be developed in the correct format, and they must be specifically and clearly stated. The following items must be included when one is creating and documenting the intervention in the client's plan of care:

- The date when the intervention is written
- An action verb describing the activity to be performed
- Qualifiers of how, when (time/frequency), where, and amount
- Signature and/or initials of originating nurse

FOR EXAMPLE:

- 1/27 Assist as needed with self-care activities each AM. AG
- 6/12 Record respiratory and pulse rates before, during, and after activity. BB
- 3/13 Inspect wound during each dressing change. MR
- 10/12 Measure intake and output hourly. SP

Note: Depending on agency policy, when the original plan of care is written, a single date and signature are sufficient. As subsequent interventions are added, the entry should be individually dated and initialed or signed. Now, take a moment to complete Practice Activity 4–3 before proceeding to Box 4–4, which walks you through the first three steps of the nursing process. Client data are presented, and a client need is identified. Then a goal, outcomes, and appropriate interventions are chosen to address the need.

Having completed that activity, consider how you would identify appropriate interventions using the Omaha System. You recall that in Robert's case the Omaha System first presented a problem based on the assessed signs/symptoms. When the planning of care was begun for Robert, the Outcome Rating Scales were used to assess knowledge, behavior, and status. The next portion of the Omaha System, the Intervention Scheme, is used to complete the plan of care (Box 4–5).

The three standardized nursing languages—NANDA, NIC, and NOC—have been combined into the NNN Alliance for a comprehensive classification of nursing. Having chosen the NANDA diagnosis of Activity Intolerance and the NOC of Endurance for your client Robert, you next determine the appropriate nursing intervention (NIC) to address Robert's problem (Box 4–6).

PRACTICE ACTIVITY 4–3
Identifying Correctly Stated Interventions

Instructions: Identify which of the following interventions are correctly stated, and rewrite those that are not.

1. Walk length of hall 2 ×/day with assistance from two staff members. _____
   _____

2. Force fluids. _____
   _____

3. Provide pericare after each BM. _____
   _____

4. Encourage deep-breathing exercises and cough q2h. _____
   _____

5. Reduce environmental stimuli. _____
   _____

6. Provide written handout for side effects of medications before discharge. _____
   _____

BOX 4-4

Application of the Nursing Process Through the Planning Step

Step I: Assessment

On 6/11/02 at 5:30 PM, Michelle, a 14-year-old female (DOB 3/2/88), is admitted with compound multiple fractures of the right tibia and fibula and a mild concussion following a mountain bike accident.

Assessment Data

Pain/Discomfort:

Subjective
Location: R lower leg, as well as general muscle aches and right-sided headache.
Intensity (0–10): 9
Frequency: Since accident
Quality: Sharp stabbing and aching R leg (headache dull, throbs)
Duration: Constant
Radiation: Toes to knee
Precipitating factors: Movement
How relieved: Morphine sulfate in ED
Associated symptoms: Muscle spasms

Objective
Facial grimacing: Yes
Guarding affected area: Yes
Emotional response: Tearful
Narrowed focus: Yes

Step II: Need Identification

Based on this assessment (and additional data recorded in other sections of the Assessment Tool), using the diagnostic reasoning process and working with Appendix A, you choose the nursing diagnosis label "Acute Pain" and write the plan of care.

    6/11/02 6 PM
Client Diagnostic Statement: Acute Pain related to movement of bone fragments R lower leg, soft tissue injury/edema, and use of external fixator as evidenced by verbal reports, guarding, muscle tension, narrowed focus, and tachycardia.

Step III: Planning

Goal: Pain-free or controlled.

(Continued)

Application of the Nursing Process Through the
Planning Step (Continued)

Outcomes:
Client will:

- Verbalize relief of pain within 30 minutes of administration of medication.
- Use relaxation skills to reduce level of pain by 6/12, 9 AM.
- Identify methods that provide relief by 6/12, 4 PM.

Interventions:

- Maintain limb rest of R leg × 24 hours.
- Elevate lower leg with folded blanket.
- Apply ice to area 20 minutes on/20 minutes off, as tolerated × 48 hours.
- Place cradle over foot of bed.
- Document reports and characteristics of pain.
- Medicate with Demerol 75 mg and Phenergan 25 mg IM q4h, prn, or Vicodin 5 mg PO q4h, prn.
- Demonstrate/encourage use of progressive relaxation techniques, deep-breathing exercises, and visualization.
- Provide alternate comfort measures, position change, backrub. *BB*

(*Note:* Michelle has reported a dull headache associated with the concussion, but it is not a major concern for her at this time; some of the interventions noted previously will be effective in relieving this pain as well.)

The Client Plan of Care

Planning care can save valuable time when the goals of care, client outcomes, and nursing interventions to achieve them are clearly identified, and then recorded, for all to see. The documentation of the planning process is provided in the client's plan of care, which some nurses refer to as the "care plan." This plan of care is written to:

- *Provide continuity of care* from nurse to nurse, from one nursing shift to the next, or from one unit/care setting to another.
- *Enhance communication* as the written plan becomes a permanent part of the client record and supplies consistent information for each person who reads it.
- *Assist with determination of agency or unit staffing needs,* as well as setting of priorities for the work schedule and individual client assignments.
- *Document the nursing process* by providing reminders of what needs to be charted and when evaluations should be done.
- *Serve as a teaching tool* that supports the sharing of nurses' expertise and fosters professional growth as nurses learn what interventions are successful.
- *Coordinate provision of care among disciplines,* maximizing effort and use of resources to enhance quality of care and client outcomes.

BOX 4–5

Application of the Omaha System: Goal Development—Part II

NANDA Nursing Diagnosis: Activity Intolerance
  Omaha System Problem: No. 37, Physical Activity
  Knowledge Rating Scale = 1
  Behavior Rating Scale = 3
  Status Rating Scale = 3

The Omaha System also has an Intervention Scheme. The scheme has 62 specific targets or objects of nursing actions. For example, Behavioral Modification No. 2 may be selected to assist Robert in his lack of an exercise program.

The scheme has four categories of intervention application:

1. Health teaching, guidance, and counseling
2. Treatments and procedures
3. Case management
4. Surveillance

Based on the assessed data and the outcome ratings on Robert's physical activity, the selection of the category Health teaching, Guidance, and Counseling would be appropriate. The actual target for the nursing actions could be No. 2, Behavioral Modification, or No. 19, Exercises.

Authors' Note: This is just an example of one possible application of the Omaha System. The Omaha System is a comprehensive nursing language system, and different problems, ratings, intervention categories, and targets could apply to Robert's case and would attest to your critical thinking skills. Our purpose is merely to introduce you to the Omaha System.

The term *health care* is not synonymous with medicine or nursing, but includes many professional disciplines, each of which has its own definite characteristics and independent, but overlapping, functions. The fields of nursing and medicine are closely related. The relationship includes the exchange of data, the sharing of ideas/thinking, and the development of a plan of care that reflects all data pertinent to the individual client/family/significant others. The same type of relationship extends to all healthcare disciplines in which the provider has contact with the client.

The implication of this relationship is seen in what is contained in the plan of care; it is more than simply a description of the actions initiated by medical orders (collaborative actions). It also includes a combination of nursing orders (independent actions) and describes in writing the coordination of care given by all health-related disciplines. The nurse becomes the person responsible for seeing to it that all of the different activities are coordinated. This is essential to the delivery of holistic, cost-effective health care that promotes optimal client recovery in a timely manner.

Exercises in "care planning" are assigned to students to enhance their mastery of the nursing process and application of related knowledge from other scientific

---

BOX 4-6

Pairing NANDA with NIC Interventions

To continue the process of planning care for Robert, you have chosen the NANDA diagnosis of Activity Intolerance and the NOC outcome of Endurance with the following indicators as measured by the 1–5 scale of "extremely compromised" to "not compromised."

1. Performance of usual routine
2. Activity
3. Exhaustion not present
4. Blood oxygen level within normal limits (WNL)

After reviewing NIC, you might choose Activity Therapy (*Definition*: Prescription of and assistance with specific physical, cognitive, social, and spiritual activities to increase the range, frequency, or duration of an individual's activity) and the following nursing activities:

Assist with regular physical activities (e.g., ambulation, transfers, turning, and personal care), as needed.

Assist client to identify deficits in activity level.

Assist to focus on what client can do rather than on deficits.

Assist client to identify meaningful activities.

Assist to choose activities consistent with physical, psychological, and social capabilities.

Assist to identify and obtain resources required for the desired activity.

Refer to community centers or activity programs.

Assist to obtain transportation to activities, as appropriate.

JCAHO: Joint Commission on Accreditation of Healthcare Organizations; surveying body that certifies clinical and organizational performance of an institution according to established guidelines.

disciplines. The need to identify and prepare for every possible client need in a given situation results in the creation of a case study, instead of the more abbreviated and succinct plan of care that is usually found in the nursing unit Kardex or computer database in most hospitals, or in the case plans maintained in community-based and/or home health agencies. However, the length of time and degree of detail required to complete these "case studies" often causes nursing students to develop a negative attitude toward planning care. It is important to keep this activity in perspective because, as a professional nurse, you will need to plan care for your clients, sometimes on a daily basis for the inpatient and for weeks, months, or even years for community-based and/or home health clients. Mastery of the skills of planning care will allow you to complete this activity in a timely fashion as you gain experience.

The plan of care is primarily a communication tool that directs the client's care. However, newly formulated requirements of outside agencies (for example, JCAHO, CMS [Medicare and Medicaid], and private insurance companies) stipulate that the nurse must be responsible for the planning of client care and that the plan is to be documented in the client's record. The plan of care is now a permanent part of the client's record for these reasons and because it contains the outline for the care provided.

Discharge Planning

As you plan for the client's current needs, you must also consider future needs, especially eventual discharge from the healthcare facility/setting. Discharge planning begins when the client enters the healthcare setting. It is crucial to ensure continuity of care as appropriate, and to take into account the anticipated discharge destination (e.g., home, assisted living, or skilled nursing facility). You are responsible for planning continuity of care between nursing personnel, between services within the care setting, and between the care setting and the community. You may also be responsible for initiating/cooperating in referrals to other community services and providing needed direction for client/family members who are learning to facilitate recovery and promote wellness.

Documenting the Plan of Care

The plan of care may be recorded on a single page or in a multiple-page format, which may include one page for each diagnostic statement for a particular client. The page (or pages) may be kept in a folder (Kardex) at the nursing station, in the patient's chart, or at the bedside to communicate and provide direction on a daily basis.

CLINICAL PATHWAYS: are a type of abbreviated plan of care; they provide outcome-based guidelines for goal achievement within a designated length of stay (see Appendix H).

The format for documenting the plan of care is determined by agency policy. Student plans of care (case studies) are individually generated and are very detailed. As a practicing professional, you might use a computer with a plan of care database, standardized care plan forms, or CLINICAL PATHWAYS (e.g., Critical Pathway, Care Map, etc.). Whichever you use, the plan of care must reflect the basic nursing standards of care; personal client data, nonroutine care, and qualifiers such as time or amount are added, as appropriate.

MIND MAPPING: a care planning technique that uses a graphic representation to illustrate the interconnections between all components of client care.

> **FOR EXAMPLE:**
>
> Measure intake and output [insert frequency]
>
> Increase oral fluids [insert amount and frequency]
>
> Medicate with [insert name of medication, dose, and frequency] for [insert reason].
>
> Weigh with bedscale [insert time, frequency]

Some computerized systems for plans of care generate an updated plan at the beginning of each shift. The care provided during the new shift is then recorded directly on the on-line plan of care throughout that shift. This method serves two purposes: (1) It documents the planning and implementation steps of the nursing process, and (2) it continuously updates the plan of care and the client's record. Other formats require the nurse to document updates to the plan of care through a notation on the Kardex or in the progress or nursing notes.

As was previously noted, the plan of care enables visualization of the nursing process. As such, it is preserved as part of the client's permanent record. Therefore, all entries need to be dated and initialed or signed. Key words should be used instead of complete sentences, and only agency-approved abbreviations/symbols should be included (see Appendix I).

FOR EXAMPLE:

- 8/15 Routine urinary catheter care q (every) shift. RE
- 9/2 NPO (nothing by mouth) after 6 AM, 9/13. PR
- 3/7 Maintain subarachnoid bolt per protocol. MT

Regardless of the format used, the plan of care contains identifying client data (including medical diagnosis), client diagnostic statements, goals/outcomes, and interventions; it also provides space for the healthcare provider to record the status of the outcomes (i.e., achieved, revised, or deleted), as shown in Figure 4–3. After you have reviewed the figure, take a moment to complete Practice Activity 4–4.

Validating the Plan of Care

Before the plan of care is implemented, it should be reviewed to ensure that:

- It is based on accepted nursing practice, reflecting knowledge of scientific principles, nursing standards of care, and agency policies.
- It provides for the safety of the client by ensuring that the care provided will do no harm.
- The client diagnostic statements are supported by the client data.
- The goals and outcomes are measurable/observable and can be achieved.
- The interventions can benefit the client/family/significant others in a predictable way in achieving the identified outcomes, and they are arranged in a logical sequence.
- It demonstrates individualized client care by reflecting the concerns of the client and significant others, as well as their physical, psychosocial, and cultural needs and capabilities.

Professional Concerns Related to the Plan of Care

Professional concerns associated with the identification of client needs in the construction of the plan of care include the following:

- What is the nurse's responsibility once a nursing diagnosis is made if the client is discharged from care before all short-term outcomes are met or problems are resolved?
- Who is responsible for follow-through in providing and evaluating care once the client has been discharged?
- Who is responsible for monitoring client progress toward long-term outcomes?
- Should this information be shared with the client's admitting/primary physician or office nurse?

Client: Donald Age: 46 DOB: 2/4/56 Gender: M Admission 11/12/02 3:40 Dx: Acute Alcoholism/Depression

Date	Client Diagnostic Statement	Goal	Intervention	Outcomes	Status
11/12	Coping, ineffective, related to situational crisis of unemployment, personal vulnerability evidenced by reported inability to cope, use of alcohol, insomnia, and diminished problem-solving.	short term: Managing own situation effectively long term: Expresses sense of self-worth. Maintains sobriety.	1. Asseses level of anxiety and Donald's perception of situation 2. Note verbal/nonverbal behaviors of anxiety 3. Look in q 2 hr and PRN 4. Encourage verbalization, expression of feelings of denial depression/anger 5. Discuss normalcy of these feelings 6. Identify current coping mechanisms 7. Note effectiveness/ need for change 8. Discuss/refer to resources: social worker, alcohol counselor, support group, AA	Verbalizes awarenes of sources of anxiety (1000 11/14) Demonstrates congruency between feelings/behavior (1000 11/15) Demonstrates initial problem-solving skills (1000 11/15) Identifies options and resourses available for assistance (1000 11/16) R. Smith, RN	Achieved 11/14 1030 R.S. Achieved 11/15 1000 P.D. Achieved 11/15 1000 P.D.

FIGURE 4–3. Sample documentation of a plan of care.

- Is the nurse who has made a nursing diagnosis responsible for follow-through to its resolution?

On a national level, these questions are unresolved, and client outcomes may remain unmet. Ethically, it is up to the nursing community and the healthcare industry to formulate policies that promote optimal client recovery and health maintenance. As a healthcare professional, you need to consider these issues because they affect the care you provide and the way you develop the plan of care for your client. It is important to remember that the plan of care is not developed in a vacuum but rather with input from the client and possibly the significant other/family. Therefore these individuals should be included in determining how to deal with unresolved needs. (Further discussion regarding termination of care is provided in Chapter 6.)

PRACTICE ACTIVITY 4–4
Documenting the Plan of Care

Instructions: Record the plan of care information from Box 4–4 on pages 89–90 using the following documentation format.

Date	Client Diagnostic Statement	Goal	Interventions	Outcomes	Status

Putting It All Together

Practice Activity 4–5 presents the back page of the interactive plan-of-care worksheet described and used in Chapter 3. The information included on the worksheet and in the TIME OUT sections should give you another view of the steps of the nursing process described in this chapter. Return to Practice Activity 3–1 in Chapter 3 and see what portion of the information you can include based on the subjective and objective data of your client Robert, who, as you remember, was diagnosed with Activity Intolerance. What desired outcome would you identify for Robert? The TIME OUT sections will give you evaluation criteria to ensure that Robert's outcome statement is correctly written. Once again, the TIME OUT sections give you guidance in correctly writing your nursing interventions.

A Complementary Approach—Mind Mapping

Some educators (Mueller, Johnston & Bligh, 2001) have been concerned that their students spend so much time and energy focusing on filling the columns of traditional clinical care plans that a holistic view of the client never develops. These educators have addressed this concern by adding a new technique or learning tool, called "mind mapping," to the planning step. In this process, as the student analyzes the client's assessment data and identifies appropriate nursing diagnoses, a visual picture is formed, with the client at the center. The nurse no longer focuses on a single client need but considers how each need interacts with other identified needs. The left brain is useful in linear problem–based thinking; the visualization process promotes right-brain thinking and assists the student in recognizing relationships or interconnections between the data sets (signs and symptoms), the client's needs (nursing diagnoses), desired outcomes, and nursing actions, thus creating a "whole" picture of the client. The focus is always on the client rather than on a disease process. The client data, outcomes, nursing diagnoses, and interventions, along with evaluation data and collaborative treatments, are of equal importance (rather than being subsumed under one another, as occurs in another care-planning technique, called "concept mapping").

Mind mapping encourages students to maintain a holistic view of the client in that the client is encouraged to participate in the care-planning process by sharing his or her own expectations; students are expected to validate findings. This supports the client's independence and enhances adherence to the plan, thus maximizing desired outcomes. Proponents believe that by combining mind mapping with care planning, students develop enhanced thinking skills, that is, both critical, whole-brain thinking, and client-centered thinking, which is so necessary for effective client care (Fig. 4–4.) Regardless of the technique used (traditional clinical care plans or mind maps), an understanding of the nursing process remains essential if competent client care is to be provided.

Summary

Healthcare providers have a responsibility to plan care with the client and family, whether the desired outcome is an optimal state of wellness or a dignified death.

PRACTICE ACTIVITY 4–5

PLANNING

Desired Outcome and Client Criteria: The Client will:

TIME OUT! The desired outcome must meet criteria to be accurate. The outcome must be specific, realistic, and measurable, and include a time frame for completion. Does the action verb describe the client's behavior to be evaluated? Can the outcome be used in the evaluation step of the nursing process to measure the client's response to the nursing interventions listed below?

Interventions	Rationale for Selected Intervention and References

EVALUATION

TIME OUT! Do your interventions assist the client in achieving outcomes? Do your interventions address further monitoring of the client's response to your interventions and to the achievement of the desired outcome? Are qualifiers: **when, how, amount, time,** and **frequency** used? Is the focus of the action's verb on the nurse's actions and not on the client? Do your rationales provide sufficient reason and directions?

What was your client's response to the interventions?

Was the desired outcome achieved?   ☐ Yes ☐ No   If no, what revisions to either the desired outcome or interventions would you make?

DOCUMENTATION

Documentation Focus: Now that you have completed the evaluation, the next step is to document your care and the client's response. Use the areas below to enter your progress note information.

Reassessment Data:

Interventions Implemented:

Patient's Response:

INSTRUCTOR'S COMMENTS:

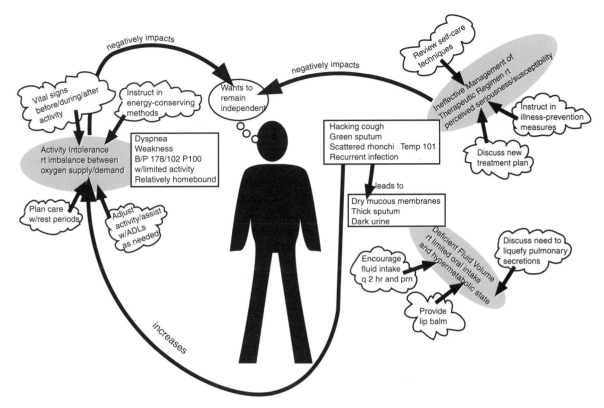

FIGURE 4–4. Initial mind map for Robert. Primary diagnosis: Recurrent bilateral lower lobe pneumonia.

Planning care by setting goals, determining outcomes, and choosing appropriate interventions is essential to the delivery of quality nursing care. These nursing activities make up the **PLANNING** step of the Nursing Process, and they are documented in the plan of care for a particular client. As a part of the client's permanent record, the plan of care not only provides a means for the nurse who is actively caring for the client to be aware of the needs (nursing diagnoses), goals, and actions to be taken; it also substantiates the plan of care for third-party payors, as well as for the accreditation process and legal review.

This chapter introduced you to how the work of the Iowa Outcomes and Interventions Projects as well as the Omaha System can be used to assist you in providing a research-based approach to designing a plan of care. Both systems provide the structure, terms, and definitions to assist you in planning client care in any healthcare environment. In Chapter 6, The Evaluation Step, you will see how helpful the standardized languages and accompanying rating and measurement scale are in evaluating the effectiveness of your plan of care.

Now, return to the third and fourth standards of the ANA Standard of Clinical Nursing Practice and review the measurement criteria necessary to achieve and ensure compliance with each standard. The knowledge and skill required to meet the criteria listed in Box 4–7 have been described in this chapter.

The next chapter provides information on the fourth step of the nursing process, **IMPLEMENTATION**. You will have an opportunity to see how the plan of care can be implemented. You will learn what mechanisms help to prioritize the nursing interventions that were selected during the **PLANNING** step. Finally, you will practice effective communication methods to help ensure the required continuity of care described in the client plan of care.

BOX 4–7

Measurement Criteria for ANA Standards III and IV

ANA Standard III: Outcome identification: The nurse identifies expected outcomes individualized to the client.

1. Outcomes are derived from the diagnoses.
2. Outcomes are mutually formulated with the client and healthcare providers, when possible and appropriate.
3. Outcomes are culturally appropriate and realistic in relation to the client's present and potential capabilities.
4. Outcomes are attainable in relation to resources available to the client.
5. Outcomes include a time estimate for attainment.
6. Outcomes provide direction for continuity of care.
7. Outcomes are documented as measurable goals.

ANA Standard IV: Planning: The nurse develops a plan of care that prescribes interventions to attain expected outcomes.

1. The plan is individualized to the client (e.g., age appropriate, culturally sensitive) and the client's condition or needs.
2. The plan is developed with the client, family, and other healthcare providers, as appropriate.
3. The plan reflects current nursing practice.
4. The plan provides for continuity of care.
5. Priorities for care are established.
6. The plan is documented.

1. List three reasons why the plan of care is important:

   a. _____

   b. _____

   c. _____

2. Briefly explain why setting priorities is necessary: _____

   _____

   _____

3. What is the difference between a goal and an outcome? _____

   _____

   _____

   _____

4. Identify five important components of client outcomes:

   a. _____

   b. _____

   c. _____

   d. _____

   e. _____

5. List four types of information that nursing interventions must contain:

   a. _____

   b. _____

   c. _____

   d. _____

6. Explain the difference between a measurable and a nonmeasurable verb and give an example of each: _____

   _____

   _____

7. When does discharge planning begin?

   _____

   _____

8. How is the plan of care documented?

_____

_____

9. In the following vignette, identify two additional needs (human responses of concern) facing Michelle; then set a goal with one outcome and two interventions for each need.

_____

_____

VIGNETTE: Michelle, the 14-year-old female with compound fractures of the right lower leg and a mild concussion, has other problems in addition to acute pain, as was previously discussed. Her wound was contaminated by dirt and she had significant blood loss before paramedics arrived. Although the wound was flushed with sterile saline and antibiotic solution before being packed and dressed, a cast was not applied because of tissue swelling and concerns about the wound and bone. Instead, an external fixation device (a metal frame with pins extending through the skin and bone) is currently being used for immobilization of the tibia and fibula. The device is too heavy and awkward for Michelle to move without causing increased pain, and she is to remain on bedrest for 24 hours. In addition, IV antibiotics are to be administered every 4 hours.

1. Need: _____

_____

Goal: _____

Outcome: _____

Interventions: _____

    1. _____

    2. _____

2. Need: _____

_____

Goal: _____

Outcome: _____

Interventions: _____

    1. _____

    2. _____

_____

BIBLIOGRAPHY

Bulechek, G. M., & McCloskey, J. C. (1989). Nursing interventions: Treatments for potential diagnoses. In R. M. Carrol-Johnson (Ed.). *Proceedings of Eighth Conference, North American Nursing Diagnosis Association.* Philadelphia: J. B. Lippincott.

Johnson, M., & Maas, M. (Eds.). (2000). *Iowa Outcomes Project: Nursing Outcomes Classification (NOC)*, ed 2. St. Louis: Mosby.

Kalish, R. (1983). *The Psychology of Human Behavior*, ed 5. Monterey, CA: Brooks/Cole.

Maslow, A. H. (1970). *Motivation and Personality*, ed 2. New York: Harper & Row.

McCloskey, J. C., & Bulechek, G. M. (Eds.). (2000). *Nursing Interventions Classification (NIC)*, ed 3. St. Louis: Mosby.

Mueller, A, Johnston, M. & Bligh, D. (2002). Joining mind mapping and care planning to enhance student critical thinking and achieve holistic nursing care. *Nursing Diagnosis 13*(1):24–27, January–March.

SUGGESTED READINGS

Nursing Outcomes

Booten, D., & Naylor, M. D. (1995). Nurse's effect on changing patient outcomes. *Image J Nurs Schol, 27*:95–99.

Cox, R. A. (1998). Implementing nursing sensitive outcomes into care planning at a long-term facility. *J Nurs Care Qual, 12*(5):41–51.

Denehey, J. (1998). Integrating Nursing Outcomes Classification into education. *J Nurs Care Qual, 12*(5):73–83.

Head, B., et al. (1997). Outcomes for home and community nursing in integrated delivery systems. *Caring, 16*(1):50–56.

Hajewski, C., Maupin, J. M., Rapp, D. A., & Pappas, J. (1998). Implementation and evaluation of Nursing Outcomes Classification in a patient education plan. *J Nurs Care Qual, 12*(5):30–40.

Johnson, M., & Maas, M. (1998). The Nursing Outcomes Classification. *J Nurs Care Qual, 12*(5):9–20.

Lang, N. M., & Marek, K. D. (1990). The classification of patient outcomes. *J Prof Nurs, 6*(3):158–163.

Maas, M., et al. (1996). Classifying nursing-sensitive outcomes. *Image J Nurs Schol, 28*:295–301.

Moorhead, S., Clarke, M., Willitis, M., & Tomsha, K. A. (1998). Nursing Outcomes Classification implementation projects across care continuum. *J Nurs Care Qual, 12*(5):51–63.

Pierce, S. L. (1997). Nurse-sensitive health care outcomes in acute care settings: An integrative analysis of the literature. *J Nurs Care Qual, 11*(4):60–72.

Prophet, C. M., & Delaney, C. W. (1998). Nursing Outcomes Classification: Implications for nursing information systems and the computer-based patient record. *J Nurs Care Qual, 12*(5):21–29.

Timm, J. A., & Behrenbech, J. G. (1998). Implementing the Nursing Outcomes Classification in clinical information system in a tertiary care setting. *J Nurs Care Qual, 12*(5):65–72.

Nursing Interventions

Daley, J., et al. (1995). Use of standardized nursing diagnoses and interventions in long-term care. *Journal of Gerontological Nursing, 21*(8):29–36.

McCloskey, J. C., & Bulechek, G. M. (1993). The NIC taxonomy structure: Iowa Intervention Project. *Image J Nurs Schol, 25*:178–192. St. Louis: Mosby

McCloskey, J. C., & Bulechek, G. M. (1994). Standardizing the language of nursing treatments: An overview of the issues. *Nurs Outlook, 42*(10):56–63.

Wakefield, B., et al. (1995). Nursing Interventions Classification: A standardized language for nursing care. *Journal of Health Care Quality, 17*:26–33.

Authors' Note: For an extensive listing of NIC-related publications, see Appendix C in McCloskey, J. C., & Bulechek, G. M. (Eds.). (2000). *Iowa Interventions Project: Nursing Interventions Classification (NIC)*, ed 3.

Nursing Language

Delaney, C., et al. (1992). Standardized nursing language for health care information systems. *J Med Syst,* *16*:145–159.

McCloskey, J. C., & Bulechek, G. M. (1994). Standardizing the language of nursing treatments: An overview of the issues. *Nurs Outlook, 42*(10):56–63.

Werley, H., & Lang, N. (Eds.). (1988). *Identification of Nursing Minimum Data Set.* New York: Springer.

Chapter 5

The Implementation Step: Putting the Plan of Care into Action

Identifying Caregiving Priorities

Ethical and Legal Concerns

Delivering Nursing Care

Ongoing Data Collection
Documentation
Verbal Communication with the Healthcare Team

Summary

■ **ANA Standard 5:** Implementation: The nurse implements the interventions identified in the plan of care.

At this point in the nursing process, you are ready to perform the interventions and activities recorded in the client's plan of care. In order to **IMPLEMENT** this plan in a timely and cost-effective manner, you first identify the priorities for providing client care. Then, as care is provided, you monitor and document the client's response to each of the interventions and communicate this information to other healthcare providers as appropriate. Then, using the data, you evaluate and revise the plan of care in the following step of the nursing process (see Chapter 6).

IMPLEMENT/ IMPLEMENTATION: fourth step of nursing process, in which the plan of care is put into action; performing identified interventions/ activities.

Identifying Caregiving Priorities

Regardless of how well a plan of care has been constructed, it cannot predict everything that will occur with a particular client on a daily basis. Your individual knowledge base, expertise, and recognition of agency routines allow you to exhibit the flexibility necessary to adapt to the changing needs of the client. While listening closely to the change-of-shift report, you will get the first clues about where to begin. On a worksheet such as the one shown in Figure 5–1 or a form supplied by the agency/facility, you record specific information, interventions, and activities that are sequential or time related.

Also, you review the plan of care for outcomes that are to be evaluated during the shift and for routine procedures/treatments and medication administration. Complete Practice Activity 5–1 at this time.

After completion of the shift report, a baseline assessment of each client can provide clues about general physical status, equipment/supply needs, and safety concerns (e.g., patency of invasive lines [catheters/tubes] and intravenous [IV] flow rate). At this time, you may recognize a change in the significance or severity of a client need that could affect the plan of care.

FOR EXAMPLE: Robert, who is being treated for pneumonia, appears dyspneic at 7:30 AM. You will need to do a more thorough focused assessment now to determine his immediate needs. This could include obtaining pulse oximetry/arterial blood gases (ABGs) and restarting supplemental oxygen. In addition, you may decide against getting Robert up in a chair to eat his breakfast. Thus, interventions previously identified are not appropriate at this time, and new or alternate interventions are needed.

This is also the time to review the plan of care with the client/significant other to schedule activities and verify the client's responsibilities.

FOR EXAMPLE: Donald, admitted 48 hours ago for depression and alcohol withdrawal, displays coarse tremors of his hands and an unsteady gait and requires assistance with self-care. It is 7:30 AM and breakfast trays have just arrived. Donald is required to attend the Community Meeting at 8:15 AM before

Client	7	8	9	10	11	12	1	2	3	Comments
Rbt		Vital signs Chair	Med	Bed bath	IV	V.S. Chair	Med	I & O		

FIGURE 5–1. Sample worksheet for the 7:00 AM to 3:00 PM shift. While listening to the change-of-shift report, you review the plan of care and begin to plan how you will implement specific interventions. You notice that Robert is to eat meals sitting up in a chair; therefore, he should be helped out of bed before the meal trays arrive on the unit. You identify times for medications, times for expected change of the IV bottle, and the routine times for calculating the intake and output for the shift. In addition, you are aware that Robert's family usually visits at lunchtime, so you schedule hygiene needs appropriately while allowing Robert rest periods between activities.

PRACTICE ACTIVITY 5–1
Setting Your Work Schedule for Implementing the Plan of Care

VIGNETTE: Michelle incurred a compound fracture of the right lower leg 2 days ago. In reviewing the plan of care, you take note of the following:

- Assist with bed bath
- Calculate input and output (I&O) every 8 hours (2 PM)
- Change dressing twice a day and prn (9 AM)
- Assess vital signs every 4 hours (8 AM, 12 noon)
- Monitor circulation/nerve function R lower leg every hour × 24 hours, then every 4 hours (8 AM, 12 noon) and prn
- IV medications (8 AM, 2 PM)
- Up in chair with meals (7:30 AM, 12 noon)
- Walk in halls three times a day after instructed in crutch walking

1. Organize the above interventions and activities on the worksheet below:

Worksheet

Pt.	7	8	9	10	11	12	1	2	3	Comments

2. During nursing rounds, just after the change-of-shift report on 6/13, you find that Michelle is crying and she reports sudden throbbing pain in her right lower leg. How will this affect your work plan? _____

_____

proceeding to individually prescribed activities. Donald is ambivalent about his morning care, but in reviewing the scheduled activities, he decides that he will postpone his shower until his 10:30 AM break.

Ethical and Legal Concerns

Legal and ethical concerns related to the interventions also need to be considered. The wishes of the client and family/significant others regarding what is being done need to be discussed and respected.

FOR EXAMPLE: Robert has decided that if he should suffer respiratory failure, he is not to be placed on a mechanical ventilator. This does not negate the need for intervention when you notice that he is developing problems. You still need to act promptly to prevent or limit further deterioration. Therefore, in addition to providing oxygen and assessing breath sounds and airway patency, you could elevate the head of Robert's bed, encourage Robert to deep-breathe and cough regularly, and notify other healthcare providers (e.g., physician and respiratory therapist) as appropriate, as well as the identified family member or contact person.

Take a few minutes to consider the legal and ethical concerns of Robert's decision and work through Practice Activity 5–2 before continuing with the next section.

It is beyond the scope of this text to discuss these critical issues in detail. To assist you in your studies, an extensive bibliography on advance directives, ethics, and legal issues is included in the Suggested Readings. Also see Appendix E, ANA's Code of Ethics for Nurses.

Delivering Nursing Care

Interventions may be composed of many activities ranging from simple tasks to complex procedures. These activities may require direct "hands-on" care (such as a

---

PRACTICE ACTIVITY 5-2
Legal and Ethical Concerns of Care

As noted, Robert had completed a form directing healthcare providers to withhold advanced life-support measures, including the use of a mechanical ventilator.

1. Have you and your family members completed advance directives stating specific healthcare

   desires? _____

   If not, why? _____

   _____

2. As a nurse, how do you feel about adhering to advance directives as stipulated by an elderly

   client? _____

   For a premature infant as stipulated by the parents? _____

   _____

3. Review the Code of Ethics for Nurses (see Appendix E) and choose two principles you believe
   may address your responsibility to clients/guardians in regard to their decisions limiting care.

   _____

   _____

complete bed bath), or they may merely require that the healthcare provider assist a client by setting up a basin of water and washing his back. Other frequent activities include instructing a client and/or significant other regarding the management of care and then supervising these efforts. The client and/or significant others may need to be counseled regarding psychosocial concerns, treatment regimens, or alternative ways to manage healthcare needs. Throughout these activities, you also monitor the client and such resources as diagnostic studies and/or progress reports from other healthcare providers for changes in health status/development of complications.

Before implementing the interventions listed in the plan of care, you need to be sure that you:

- **Understand the reason for doing the intervention, its expected effect, and any potential hazards that can occur.** Without this knowledge, the nurse cannot be sure that the intervention will be beneficial. In addition, it will be difficult to determine if the desired effect is being achieved or if adaptations are required to provide for specific client needs/safety concerns.

  FOR EXAMPLE: You realize that a pulse oximetry/ABG study will provide information about Robert's current oxygenation status/needs, and also that he requires supplemental oxygen to increase his oxygen level. That means you will implement these interventions in a slightly different sequence; that is, the diagnostic study (pulse oximetry/ABG) should be obtained before the supplemental oxygen is begun, so that test results are not affected by the additional oxygen.

- **Provide an environment or milieu conducive to carrying out the planned interventions.** What is happening in the environment (e.g., noise, temperature, activities) is known to affect the client's physical and psychological self.

  FOR EXAMPLE: Exposing Robert for a bed bath when the room is cold can cause him physical discomfort and affect his psychological response. *Or,* Michelle has difficulty focusing on your instructions for administering medications when the volume of her roommate's TV is turned up and visitors are talking loudly.

- **Consider which interventions can be combined to allow you to accomplish the activities within your time constraints.** In some cases, shortcuts may be chosen or activities combined, which is acceptable as long as consideration is given to the successful accomplishment of the outcome.

  FOR EXAMPLE: While administering Serax to Donald at 8:00 AM, you can review the drug's actions, side effects, and adverse reactions. *Or,* while assisting Sally with her sitz bath, you may choose to discuss her concerns about caring for herself and the new babies once she has been discharged.

As noted in Box 5–1, one "simple" intervention such as providing a bedpan for a client actually encompasses multiple nursing activities that, when listed individually, may appear to take considerable time and energy to perform. However, by carefully prioritizing interventions and sequencing related activities you can accomplish these tasks quickly.

BOX 5–1

The Truth About Bedpans

Even the simplest of nursing tasks is really a complex series of actions and judgments, requiring professional knowledge and experience in order to provide optimal patient care. Read through the short article reprinted below.* You will be surprised to see just how complicated supplying a patient with a bedpan can be.

There are many nursing activities interwoven in the "simple" act of providing a bedpan. As a nurse, you assess the patient's:

Level of consciousness and mood, including self-image while dependent with these bodily functions

Skin color, temperature, and suppleness

Respiratory pattern and rate, breath sounds, and dyspnea with or without activity

Comfort level with voiding or with stool

Range of motion, strength, and any pain with movement

Urine for color, amount, odor, and by-products such as mucus or blood

Stool for color, consistency, amount, and by-products such as mucus, undigested food, or blood

You also determine:

If urine assessment relates to medications (Lasix, Pyridium, aminoglycosides), fluid intake, disease process (diabetes, dehydration, renal failure), or infection

If stool assessment relates to medication (antibiotics, barium enema, narcotics), food or fluid intake, disease process (cholelithiasis, Crohn's disease, bleeding ulcers), infection, activity or inactivity

If assessment demands any action and whether the doctor needs to be notified

You then go on to teach:

Symptoms to watch for, comfort measures, and ways to maintain or achieve normal functioning

Disease process and how it affects the individual

On top of all that, you:

Promote self-esteem by using proper technique, including disposal of waste material.

Obtain necessary specimens using correct procedure and send to lab.

Make sure patient is clean and dry to promote good skin integrity.

Model good handwashing technique on completion.

* "The Truth about Bedpans" by Karen Tolin, RN, Joplin, MO, printed by *RN* Magazine.

Ongoing Data Collection

Once you have formulated the plan of care and put it into action, you should monitor the client to collect additional data. As you talk to the client, note changes in tone of voice and expression; when you reposition the client or provide a back rub, be aware of such abnormalities as a reddened area on the coccyx. All of these data need to be noted, and their meaning validated. This information will be used in decision making regarding the need for new goals, outcomes, and interventions, and in re-prioritizing the plan of care during the evaluation process.

DOCUMENTATION

It is legally required that professionals in all healthcare settings document nursing observations, the care provided, and the client's response. This record serves as a communication tool and a resource to aid in determining the effectiveness of care and to assist in setting priorities for ongoing care. In order to simplify record keeping and to promote timely and accurate charting, many agencies use flow sheets to document routine activities, monitoring, and ongoing client care (Fig. 5–2). Flow sheets reduce the need for writing detailed progress notes. Instead, only variations from the recorded baseline and any exceptions requiring additional explanation are written in the progress note. Additional discussion about documentation and the use of progress notes will be presented in Chapter 7.

VERBAL COMMUNICATION WITH THE HEALTHCARE TEAM

In addition to the written record, client information is shared verbally with other healthcare providers. Whether reporting to another nurse, reviewing with a physician, or discussing with professionals providing other resources (e.g., social worker, dietitian, or physical therapist), the manner in which information is conveyed, as well as the content itself, can affect the way in which this information is heard. This, in turn, can have an impact on the quality of the health care provided. For this reason, it is important to avoid judgmental language and to be conscious of tone of voice and body language. Presenting information in an objective and accurate manner reduces the likelihood of being misunderstood or of negatively influencing the client's care.

FOR EXAMPLE: When Sally talked to the nurse, she tearfully expressed concern about going home. The nurse reported this information to the oncoming shift personnel and to the doctor by saying: "I think Sally is trying to manipulate us. She says she's not ready to go home, and she thinks if she 'acts weak,' she won't have to leave the hospital."

After listening to this judgmental report, the oncoming nurse's response might be one of defensiveness and the nurse might be inclined to "show" Sally that she is indeed ready to go home. The nurse may also subconsciously stop listening and is likely to be less receptive to what Sally is saying. Contrast the previous example with the one that appears below.

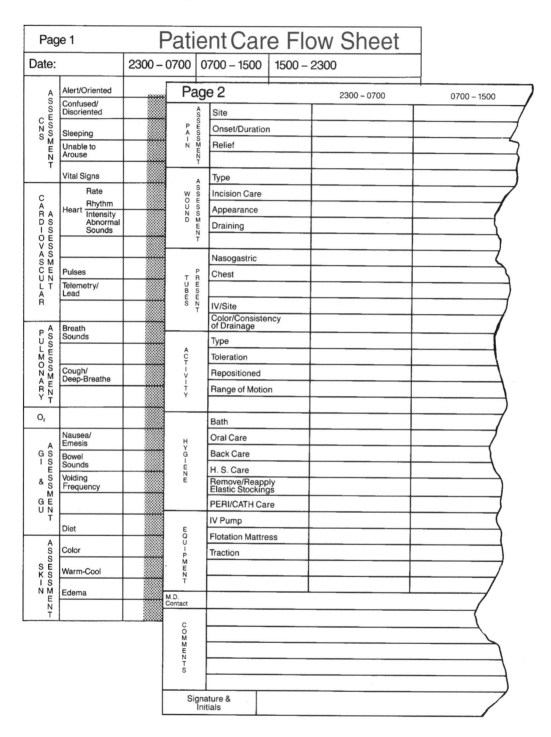

FIGURE 5–2. Sample flow sheet.

FOR EXAMPLE: If the nurse reports: "Sally has expressed concern about her ability to manage at home. She was weak when we got her up this morning, requiring assistance with walking. Then she spent the afternoon talking on the telephone, at one point ignoring the cries of Baby B until I responded to the room. We need information about her situation at home and her need for assistance with newborn care of twins."

In this report, the nurse expresses a need in terms that challenge colleagues to find a solution. This need is approached with an open mind as additional data are gathered and appropriate resources are identified. Maintaining an open mind and actively problem solving provide opportunities for creating solutions instead of additional problems, thus promoting a positive client/nurse experience.

The primary format for communicating the client's current situation and needs in the acute care setting is the nursing change-of-shift report. This type of report may be done either in person or via tape recorder. Because time for this activity is usually limited, it is necessary for staff members to be brief and organized while still providing pertinent data. After basic client data (e.g., room number, name, age, diagnosis, and physician) are supplied, reporting may be done "by exception." This means that only occurrences that are out of the ordinary are reported. You report:

- **Abnormalities/changes in assessment findings**
    "Robert became short of breath during AM rounds and required supplemental oxygen at 2 L/min by nasal cannula." *or* "Michelle's right lower leg edema is resolving."

- **Diagnostic procedures and results**
    "Robert's oxygen saturation is 92% on 2 L of oxygen; chest x-ray report is pending."

- **Variations from usual routine**
    "Robert was not out of bed this AM but was up for lunch and tolerated sitting up in a chair for 45 minutes without difficulty."

- **Activities not completed on your shift**
    "The crutches are in Michelle's room, a physical therapist will return at 4 PM to instruct her in their use; then we can begin getting her out of bed."

- **Status of invasive treatments**
    "Sally's IV of lactated Ringer's with 2 amps of Pitocin is infusing in the left forearm at 60 ml/hr with 300 ml remaining."

- **Additions or changes to the plan of care** (this includes evaluation of outcomes and the status of client needs)
    "Robert's Airway Clearance need has recurred, requiring aggressive pulmonary toilet every 2 hours and use of incentive spirometer."

Change-of-shift reports may include nursing rounds, with each client being visited by the offgoing and oncoming nurse together. Nursing rounds are beneficial in verifying the status of invasive treatments, the appearance of wounds/dressings, and the current condition of the client (e.g., degree of jaundice, level of coolness of an extremity, etc.). It is imperative for nurses to maintain the confidentiality of client

PRACTICE ACTIVITY 5–3
Communicating Nursing Information to Other Caregivers

Work through the questions below.

1. Two methods of communicating your observations about client care and activities to other nurses are by:

   a. _____

   b. _____

2. Discuss the benefits of nursing rounds. _____
   _____

3. Underline the information listed below that you would include in your change-of-shift report:
   Sally Ate well Age 20 Dr. Jefferson
   Weak and unsteady while up in hall
   Episiotomy reddened, slight edema, no drainage second day postpartum
   Scheduled for discharge tomorrow
   Received oral pain medication at 11 AM with reported relief
   Does not want to go home
   Sister in to visit at lunchtime
   Coordination for home care services in progress with the Discharge Planner
   Spent afternoon talking on phone
   Has not named Baby B and at times has ignored infant cues

4. The wife of a prominent local politician is admitted for treatment of alcoholism. You could discuss her admission and course of therapy with which of the following people?

   _____ attending/primary physician

   _____ the nursing supervisor

   _____ a pediatric nurse (her best friend)

   _____ your husband

   _____ the client's son

   _____ an interested newspaper reporter

   _____ other nurses on your unit

information, and usually it is preferable to review the change-of-shift information before leaving the report room and going to the client's bedside.

Client confidentiality is an ethical/moral concern that must be respected by each professional at all times. These concerns are extended to conversations at the nursing station, on the telephone, or wherever client information is discussed. This includes refraining from discussions with those not directly involved in the client's care (e.g., staff on other units, your own family, friends and acquaintances of the client).

Before concluding this chapter, take a moment to complete Practice Activity 5–3.

Summary

In putting the plan of care into action and providing effective client care, you review resources to determine priorities, consulting with and considering the desires of the client during this **IMPLEMENTATION** step of the nursing process. You identify who is responsible for the actions to be taken and set realistic timeframes for carrying out actions. Changes in the client's needs must be continually monitored because client care takes place in a dynamic environment. The relevance of new data collected in each interaction with the client is determined according to what is already known. This newly gathered information is documented and shared with other healthcare providers as appropriate. Throughout these activities, flexibility is important to allow for changed circumstances, interruptions, and so forth.

Before we begin the next chapter, let us return to the fifth standard of the ANA Standard of Clinical Nursing Practice and review the measurement criteria necessary to achieve and ensure compliance with the standard. The knowledge and skill required to meet the criteria listed in Box 5–2 were described in this chapter on the **IMPLEMENTATION** step of the nursing process.

Chapter 6 will enable you to see how continuous evaluation of nursing actions helps you determine whether or not specific interventions are leading to achievement of the desired outcomes. In addition, evaluation of client plans of care serves as a mechanism for review of the care provided on a unit or within an agency. This review process addresses professional issues of overall quality of care and also provides a means by which outside agencies can evaluate the institution.

BOX 5–2

Measurement Criteria for ANA Standard V

ANA Standard V: Implementation: The nurse implements the interventions identified in the plan of care.

1. Interventions are consistent with the established plan of care.
2. Interventions are implemented in a safe and appropriate manner.
3. Interventions are documented.

1. Identify three activities involved in implementing the plan of care:

   a. _____

   b. _____

   c. _____

2. Discuss the importance of understanding the expected effect and potential hazards of the interventions you will implement: _____

   _____

3. Explain the purpose for ongoing data collection throughout the **IMPLEMENTATION** step of the nursing process: _____

   _____

4. List two reasons why documentation of the care provided is important:

   a. _____

   b. _____

5. Name three activities you might use to carry out interventions for planned client care:

   a. _____ b. _____ c. _____

6. What is the advantage of reporting "by exception"? _____

   _____

7. When and where is client confidentiality important? _____

   _____

8. Flexibility in providing client care is important because: _____

   _____

9.

> **VIGNETTE:** Robert signed Advance Directives asking that no extraordinary means (e.g., intubation and mechanical ventilation) be used to prolong his life. When his condition changed, his daughter was notified as required. While visiting with her father, she is surprised to learn of his decision. She is very upset and a confrontation develops. Robert tells her, "it is none of your business," and refuses to enter into further conversation.

   a. What can you do now? _____

   _____

   _____

SUGGESTED READINGS

Doenges, M. E., Moorhouse, M. F., & Geissler-Murr, A. C. (2002). *Nurse's Pocket Guide: Nursing Diagnoses with Interventions*, ed. 9. Philadelphia: F. A. Davis.

McCloskey, J. C., & Grace, H. L. (Eds.). (2001). *Current Issues in Nursing*, ed 6. St. Louis: Mosby.

Advance Directives, Ethics, and Legal Aspects

Aiken, T. D., & Catalano, J. T. (1994). *Legal, Ethical, and Political Issues in Nursing*. Philadelphia: F. A. Davis.

American Nurses' Association. (1998). *Legal Aspects of Standards and Guidelines for Clinical Nursing Practice*. Washington, DC: American Nurses' Association.

Arras, J. D. (1995). (Ed.). *Bringing the Hospital Home: Ethical and Social Implications of High-tech Home Care*. Baltimore: Johns Hopkins University.

Bandman, E. L., & Bandman, B. (1995). *Nursing Ethics Through the Life Span*, ed 3. Norwalk, CT: Appleton & Lange.

Beckmann, J. P. (1996). *Nursing Negligence: Analyzing Malpractice in the Hospital Setting*. Thousand Oaks, CA: Sage Publications.

Benner, P. A., Tanner, C. A., & Chesla, C. A. (1998). *Expertise in Nursing Practice: Caring, Clinical Judgment, and Ethics*. New York: Springer.

Berger, A. S. (1995). *When Life Ends: Legal Overviews, Medicolegal Forms, and Hospital Policies*. Westport, CN: Praeger.

Bishop, A. H., & Scudder, J. R. (1996). *Nursing Ethics: Therapeutic Caring*. Boston: Jones & Bartlett.

Brent, N. J. (2000). *Nurses and the Law: A Guide to Principles and Applications*, ed 2. Philadelphia: Saunders.

Burkhardt, M. A., & Nathaniel, A. K. (2002). *Ethics & Issues in Contemporary Nursing*, ed 2. Albany, NY: Delmar.

Cantor, N. L. (1993). *Advance Directives and the Pursuit of Death with Dignity*. Bloomington: Indiana University Press.

Catalano, J. T. (1995). *Ethical and Legal Aspects of Nursing*, ed 2. Springhouse, PA: Springhouse.

Concern for Dying. (1991). *Advance Directive Protocols and the Patient Self-Determination Act*. New York: Author.

Davis, A. J., Arosker, M. A., & Liaschinko, J. (1997). *Ethical Dilemmas and Nursing Practice*, ed 4. Stamford, CT: Prentice Hall.

Dougas, D. J., & McCullough, L. B. (1991). The values history: The evaluation of the patient's values and advanced directives. *J Fam Prac*, 32:145–153.

Doukas, D. J., & Reichel, W. (1993). *Planning for Uncertainty: A Guide to Living Wills and Other Advance Directives for Health Care*. Baltimore: Johns Hopkins University.

English, D. D. (1994). *Bioethics: A Clinical Guide for Medical Students*. New York: W. W. Norton.

Fiesta, J. (1997). *Legal Implications in Long-term Care*. Albany: Delmar.

Guido, G. W. (1997). *Legal Issues in Nursing*, ed 2. Stamford, CT: Appleton & Lange.

Hall, J. K. (1996). *Nursing Ethics and Law*. Philadelphia: W. B. Saunders.

Husted, G. L., & Husted, J. H. (2001). *Ethical Decision Making in Nursing and Healthcare*, ed 3. St. Louis: Mosby.

Kapp, M. B. (1994). (Ed.). *Patient Self-determination in Long-term Care: Implementing the PSDA in Medical Decisions*. New York: Springer.

Kikuchi, H., & Simmons, D. R. (1996). (Eds.). *Truth in Nursing Inquiry*. Thousand Oaks, CA: Sage Publications.

King, N. M. P. (1996). *Making Sense of Advance Directives*. Washington, DC: Georgetown University Press.

Lashley, F. R. (Ed.). (1997). *The Genetics Revolution: Implications for Nursing*. Washington, DC: American Academy of Nursing.

Martin, S., & Vitello, J. M. (1992). Making a critical decision before it becomes critical. *Heart Lung*, 21:15A–18A.

Reigle, J. (1992). Preserving patient self-determination through advance directives. *Heart Lung*, 21:196–198.

Salipante, D. M. (1998). Cultural diversity. Refusal of blood by a critically ill patient: A healthcare challenge. *Critical Care Nurse*, 18(2):68–76.

Scanlon, C., & Fibison, W. (1995). *Managing Genetic Information: Implications of Nursing Practice*. Washington, DC: American Nurses Publishing.

Silverman, H. J., Fry, S. T., & Armistead, N. (1994). Nurses' perspective on implementation of the Patient Self-Determination Act. *J Clin Ethics*, 5:30–37.

Silverman, H. J., Vinicky, J. K., & Gasner, M. R. (1992). Advance directives: Implications for critical care. *Crit Care Med*, 20:1027–1031.

Singleton, K. A., Dever, R., & Donner, T. A. (1992). Durable power of attorney: Nursing implications. *Dimensions of Critical Care Nursing*, 11:41–46.

Snider, G. L. (1995). Withholding and withdrawing life-sustaining therapy: All systems are not yet "go." *Am J Crit Care Med*, 151:279–281.

Sullivan, G. H., & Mattera, M. D. (1997). *RN's Legally Speaking: How to Protect Your Patients and Your License*. Montvale, NJ: Medical Economics.

Trandel-Korenchuk, D. M., & Trandel-Korenchuk, K. M. (1997). Nursing and the Law, ed 5. Gaithersburg, MD: Aspen.

Veins, D. C. (1989). A history of nursing's code of ethics. *Nursing Outlook*, 37(1): 43–49.

White, G. B. (1992). *Ethical Dilemmas in Contemporary Nursing Practice*. Washington, DC: American Nurses Publishing.

White, P. D. (1997). The role of the critical care nurse in counseling families about advance directives. *Critical Care Nursing Clinics of North America*, 9:53–61.

Zucker, M. B., & Zucker, H. D. (1997). (Eds.). *Medical Futility and the Evaluation of Life-sustaining Interventions*. Cambridge, NY: Cambridge University Press.

Change-of -Shift Report

Barbera, M. L. (1994). Giving report: How to sidestep common pitfalls. *Nursing*, 24(9):41.

Bosek, M. S. D., & Fugate, K. (1994). Intershift report: a quality improvement project. *MEDSURG Nursing*, 3(2):128–132.

Coleman, S., & Henneman, E. A. (1991). Comprehensive patient care and documentation through unit-based nursing rounds. *Clinical Nurse Specialist*, 5(2): 117–120.

Copp, L. A. (1998). Change of shift report. *J Prof Nurs*, 14(2):63–64.

Cox, S. S. (1994). Taping report tips to record by. *Nursing*, 24(3):64.

Fraser, L. E., O'Brien, K., Tobar, I., & Waller, D. M. (1991). Patient care plans for intershift report. *Journal of Pediatric Nursing: Nursing Care of Children and Families*, 6(5):310–316.

Guido, G. W. (1988). Legal commentary: Shift reports. *Dimensions Critical Care Nursing* Nov–Dec; 7:380.

Howell, M. (1994). Confidentiality during staff reports at the bedside. *Nursing Times*, 90(34):44–45.

Liukkonen, A. (1993). The content of nurses' oral shift reports in homes for elderly people. *J Adv Nurs*, 18(7):1095–1100.

McMahon, R. (1990). What are we saying? *Nursing Times*, 86(30):38–40.

Monahan, M. L., et al. (1998). Change of shift report: A time for communication with patients. *Nursing Management*, 19(2):80.

Mosher, C., & Bontomasi, R. (1996). How to improve your shift report. *Am J Nurs*, 96(8):32–43.

Patterson, P. K., Blehm, R., Foster, J., Fuglee, K., & Moore, J. (1995). Nurse information needs for efficient care continuity across patient units. *J Nurs Adm*, 25(10):28–36.

Reiley, P. J., & Stengrevics, S. S. (1989). Change-of-shift report: Put it in writing! *Nursing Management*, 20(9):54–56.

Taylor, C. (1993). Intershift report: Oral communication using a quality assurance approach. *J Clin Nurs*, 2(5):266–267.

Wolf, Z. R. Learning the professional jargon of nursing during change of shift report. *Holistic Nursing Practice*, 4(1):78–83.

Chapter 6

The Evaluation Step: Determining Whether Desired Outcomes Have Been Met

Reassessment

Modification of the Plan of Care

Termination of Services

Enhancing Delivery of Quality Care

Summary

■ **ANA Standard 6:** Evaluation: The nurse evaluates the client's progress toward attainment of outcomes.

The final step of the nursing process is evaluating the client's response to the care delivered, to make sure the desired outcomes developed in the PLANNING step and documented in the plan of care have been achieved. EVALUATION, which is an ongoing process, is necessary for determining how well the plan of care is working. As the client's condition changes, information is added to the client database, requiring revision and updating of the plan of care; this is an essential component of the EVALUATION step.

Although the process of evaluation may seem similar to the activity of assessment, there are important differences. Instead of identifying the client's general status and needs, the evaluation focuses on the appropriateness of the care provided and the

EVALUATION: final step of the nursing process. A continuous process essential to assuring the quality and appropriateness of the care provided that is done by reviewing client responses, to determine effectiveness of the plan of care in meeting client needs.

119

client's progress or lack of progress toward the desired outcomes. Evaluation is an interactive, continuous process. As each nursing action is performed, the client's response is noted and evaluated in relation to the identified outcomes. Then, based on the client's response, appropriate revisions of nursing interventions and/or client outcomes may be necessary.

Although it is frequently viewed simplistically as a pass-or-fail judgment, evaluation should actually be seen as a constructive opportunity to provide positive feedback to both the client and caregivers for their efforts, and to encourage them to continue to strive for a higher level of functioning or wellness. It is an opportunity for problem solving and personal growth. The EVALUATION step has three components: reassessment, modification of the plan of care, and finally, termination of services. The first two components form a continuous loop of recurring assessment and reaction, which eventually leads to the third component. This "termination of services" may sound rather abrupt, but this final part of the EVALUATION step is in reality the next step for the client in looking toward the future and "moving on." Termination in part includes completion of discharge planning; it addresses those client nursing diagnoses or client needs that were not fully attained during the timeframe when nursing care was provided. Further description of this part of the EVALUATION step is presented later in this chapter.

Reassessment

Reassessment is a constant "measuring and monitoring" of the client's status that looks at the client's response to nursing interventions and progress toward attaining the desired outcome. This evaluation process is ongoing; it does not occur only when an outcome is to be reviewed or a determination of the client's readiness for discharge is to be made. Data collected as the plan of care was implemented in step 4 of the nursing process are now evaluated or reassessed. Evaluation of the data determines:

- **The appropriateness of the nursing actions**

    FOR EXAMPLE: Robert's dyspnea has resolved with the provision of oxygen and attention to pulmonary toilet (i.e., periodic deep-breathing exercises, effective cough, position changes, and use of the incentive spirometer). *Or,* Donald's tremors have lessened since he received his AM dose of Serax.

- **The need to revise the interventions**

    FOR EXAMPLE: Robert was kept in bed for breakfast but should be able to be out of bed for lunch. *Or,* while you were assisting Michelle to walk the length of the hall, you noted that she is unsteady on her crutches and will initially require the assistance of two individuals to provide for client and employee safety.

- **The development of new client needs**

    FOR EXAMPLE: Sally is scheduled for discharge tomorrow. Her current weakness and lack of attention to her infant's cues raise concerns about her current coping abilities and the potential for parenting/attachment problems, as well as issues of self-care.

- **The need for referral to other resources**

  FOR EXAMPLE: Sally's physician is notified of your observations, and possible solutions are discussed. A family meeting may be requested, to clarify roles/responsibilities and availability of assistance. The home health nurse is to be contacted to arrange self-care and homemaker assistance and to supervise Sally's situation after discharge. Referrals to community support groups (such as Mothers of Twins) may be made to provide additional assistance and problem-solving options.

- **The need to rearrange priorities to meet the changing demands of care**

  FOR EXAMPLE: You had planned to get Robert up in the chair for breakfast, but the focused assessment revealed a change in his respiratory status requiring new interventions and revision of the plan. Or, external factors may occur, such as the emergency department calling to say that they have a new client requiring admission. You need to review and reschedule the activities planned for Robert in order to accommodate these additional and unplanned responsibilities.

While evaluating the client's response to care, you note progress toward the specified outcomes. In addition, because each outcome has an identified timeframe, achievement of the outcomes is periodically reviewed. You must now determine whether the outcomes have been met completely, partially, or not at all; and whether or not the plan of care needs to be revised. Outcome(s) may be evaluated by:

- **Direct observation**

  FOR EXAMPLE: Did the client ambulate the length of the hall without developing dyspnea? Did the client demonstrate proper technique for the administration of insulin? Is the client free of skin breakdown?

- **Client interview**

  FOR EXAMPLE: Does the client report decreased level of pain after administration of oral pain medication? Can the client list available community resources? Is the client able to verbalize the signs/symptoms that require medical evaluation or follow-up?

- **Review of records** (e.g., progress notes, flow sheets, medication record)

  FOR EXAMPLE: Has the client's temperature remained within normal range? Are the intake and output balanced? Has the client gained weight? Has a laxative been required for constipation?

An important aspect of this process is the involvement of the client. How does the client believe he or she is doing? Inclusion of the client's point of view can reveal important insights that may provide additional data for evaluating and revising the plan of care.

As mentioned in Chapter 4, the Omaha System's Problem Rating Scale for Outcomes provides three levels of evaluation. Box 6–1 lists the three system concepts of knowledge, behavior, and status. Also, review Appendix K to see an example of one of the many evaluation tools available in the Nursing Outcomes

BOX 6–1

Omaha Problem-Rating Scale for Outcomes

CONCEPT	1	2	3	4	5
Knowledge	No knowledge	Minimal knowledge	Basic knowledge	Adequate knowledge	Superior knowledge
Behavior	Not appropriate	Rarely appropriate	Inconsistently appropriate	Usually appropriate	Consistently appropriate
Status	Extreme signs/ symptoms	Severe signs/ symptoms	Moderate signs/ symptoms	Minimal signs/ symptoms	No signs/ symptoms

Source: Martin, K. S., & Scheet, N. J. (1992). *The Omaha System: A Pocket Guide for Community Health Nursing.* Philadelphia: W. B. Saunders.

Classification. (Similar five-point scales are also used by NOC to evaluate the outcome indicators.)

If the outcomes were completely met, ask yourself the following questions: "Do any interventions need to be continued, or which interventions can be terminated?" "How easily were the outcomes achieved?" "Can the timeframe be shortened?" In determining why a desired outcome was not met completely, the following questions may help provide clarification:

- Were the outcomes realistic and appropriate?
- Was the client involved in setting the outcomes?
- Does the client believe the outcomes were important?
- Does the client know why the outcomes have not been met?
- Have all the interventions that were identified been carried out and in the timeframe specified? If not, why not? Were they too vague or misinterpreted?
- What variables may have affected achievement of the outcomes?
- Were new needs/adverse client responses detected early enough to allow appropriate changes to be made in the plan of care?

In addition, you review the orders and progress notes of all healthcare providers and identify factors that helped or hindered achievement of outcomes. The findings are then documented on the plan of care and/or progress notes as appropriate and shared with the client.

Modification of the Plan of Care

When you have completely evaluated the outcomes and the plan of care, you may find that the client's condition has changed in a direction that was or was not anticipated, regardless of your nursing interventions and the client's desire to achieve the stated outcomes. At this point, a change in treatment approach is indicated, and the plan of care must be modified to reflect these changes.

PLAN OF CARE: MICHELLE

Client: Michelle   Age: 14—3/2/88   Gender: F   Admission: 6/11/02 5:30 PM   Dx: Compound Fx R tibia/fibula, closed head injury/mild concussion

Date	Client Diagnostic Statement	Goal	Interventions	Outcomes	Status
	Acute Pain: related to movement of bone fragments, soft tissue injury/edema, and use of external fixator, as evidenced by verbal reports, guarding, muscle tension, narrowed focus, and tachycardia	Pain-free or controlled by discharge	1. Maintain limb rest R leg × 24 hr to 5 PM 6/12. 2. Elevate lower leg with folded blanket. 3. Apply ice to area as tolerated × 48 hr to 5 PM 6/13. 4. Place cradle over foot of bed. 5. Document reports and characteristics of pain. 6. Medicate with Demerol 75 mg and Phenergan 25 mg IM q4h prn, or Vicodin 5 mg PO q4h prn. 7. Demonstrate/encourage use of progressive relaxation techniques, deep-breathing exercises, visualization. 8. Provide alternate comfort measures, position change, backrub. 9. Encourage use of diversional activities.	Verbalizes relief of pain within 30–60 min of administration of medication Identifies methods that provide relief by 9 AM, 6/12 Uses relaxation skills to reduce level of pain by 9 AM, 6/12	
	Risk for Infection: risk factors of broken skin, traumatized tissues, decreased hemoglobin levels, invasive procedures, environmental exposure	Free of infection	1. Monitor temp, VS q4h. 2. Aseptic dressing change bid 9 AM, 9 PM, and prm. 3. Pin care per protocol bid 9 AM, 9 PM. 4. Routine IV site care daily. 5. Document condition of wound, IV, and pin sites q4h. 6. Review ways client can reduce risk of infection. 7. Administer cefoxitin 2 g IV piggyback q8h (8 AM, 4 PM, 12 AM).	Identifies and practices interventions to reduce risk of infection by 5 PM, 6/12 Identifies signs/symptoms requiring medical evaluation by 9 AM, 6/13 Displays initial wound healing free of purulent drainage/signs of infection by discharge	

(Continued)

PLAN OF CARE: MICHELLE (Continued)

Client: Michelle **Age:** 14—3/2/88 **Gender:** F **Admission:** 6/11/02 5:30 PM **Dx:** Compound Fx R tibia/fibula, closed head injury/ mild concussion

Date	Client Diagnostic Statement	Goal	Interventions	Outcomes	Status
	Impaired Physical Mobility: related to musculoskeletal impairment and pain, and restrictive therapy (external fixator), as evidenced by reluctance to attempt movement and imposed restrictions of movement	Ambulates safely with assistive device	1. Monitor circulation/nerve function R leg q1h × 24 hr to 5 PM, 6/12, then q4h and prn. 2. Support R leg fixator during movement. 3. Support feet with footboard. 4. Encourage use of side rails/overhead trapeze for position change. 5. Demonstrate/assist with ROM exercises to unaffected limbs q2h. 6. Assist out of bed, non-weight-bearing R leg 6 PM, 6/12. 7. Instruct in/monitor use of crutches 6/13. 5 PM, 6/12.	Participates in activities to maintain muscle strength by 9 AM, 6/12 Increases level of activity beginning 6 PM, 6/12 and ongoing Demonstrates techniques/behaviors that enable resumption of activities by 6 PM, 6/13 Maintains position of function R leg, free of foot drop—ongoing	

As basic physiological needs such as air, water, food, and safety are met, nursing care can progress to such higher-level concerns as self-esteem. Alternatively, higher-level needs may be put "on hold" while those associated with newly emerging basic needs are addressed. At any time, the nurse may identify or activate additional client diagnostic statements, goals, and/or desired outcomes and corresponding interventions. An earlier chapter discussed the difficulty of dealing with more than three to five client problems at one time. The actual number varies from client to client and the complexity of the nursing diagnoses present, but the point is, there may simply be too many client needs to be addressed in the initial plan of care. Priority setting is required when this situation exists, with progression to higher-level needs as the client's condition permits.

When the desired outcomes are evaluated and found to be unmet, the reasons need to be identified and documented, and the outcomes then revised or new ones written. When revising client outcomes, keep in mind that they may simply need to be restated or their timeframes lengthened, so the client can successfully achieve them.

FOR EXAMPLE: When Donald was first admitted for acute alcoholism and depression, initial concerns focused on issues of client safety/potential for injury, changes in sensory interpretation, anxiety, and general nutrition. When Donald completed his initial withdrawal from alcohol and his physical condition stabilized, nursing attention became focused on previously identified problems concerning individual coping and role performance.

As the plan of care is modified, remember to address the changing needs of the client/significant others and the changes in the client's health status, environment, and therapeutic regimen. To assist in this process, a client care conference may be scheduled, or a consultation with a colleague or other resource people with special knowledge may be necessary to gain additional insight and to problem-solve solutions.

Practice Activity 6–1 provides an opportunity for you to review and evaluate the plan of care for Michelle. Read the narrative accompanying Michelle's plan of care, and follow the directions for evaluating whether Michelle has attained the stated outcomes. Write your evaluations in the STATUS column of the plan of care. Once you have completed Practice Activity 6–1, turn to Practice Activity 6–2 and add your modifications to Michelle's plan of care in the space provided.

Termination of Services

When the desired outcomes have been achieved and the broader goals met, termination of care is planned. The focus at this point is on how the client will manage on his or her own. Although termination of care occurs when all goals/outcomes are met, it is possible that some will not be met before discharge. The goals/outcomes that have not been met need to be reviewed, and the reasons why they were not met should be documented. Some nursing diagnoses, such as Anxiety or imbalanced Nutrition, may require months or years to be completely resolved. Because the hospitalization is only one point along the client's health continuum, it is realistic that not all outcomes will be achieved or all nursing diagnoses resolved.

PRACTICE ACTIVITY 6–1
Evaluating Client Outcomes

Read over the following case study information. It has been used to develop a plan of care for Michelle.

When Michelle was admitted to the hospital the evening of 6/11, a physiological (Maslow's) or survival (Kalish) need of pain avoidance was identified (i.e., Acute Pain). A higher-level need of safety or stimulation was noted (i.e., Impaired Physical Mobility), as was a safety need of protection (i.e., Risk for Infection).

The following morning (6/12) during the 8 AM assessment, Michelle indicated that she was successful in obtaining relief of pain after periodic injection of analgesics. Michelle also found that deep-breathing exercises and focusing her attention on the scenic picture at the foot of her bed helped minimize the severity of recurrent muscle spasms in her right leg. In addition, frequent weight shifts using the overhead trapeze and range-of-motion exercises reduced general aches and joint stiffness, and meditation enhanced general relaxation.

The nurse noticed that most of Michelle's breakfast tray was untouched. Michelle reported she wasn't very hungry but did want fruit juice and other fluids. After the morning bed bath, the dressings were changed and the right leg wound was evaluated. Skin edges were pink, and serous drainage was odorless. Pin sites were also cleaned and no signs of inflammation noted. At lunch, Michelle's intake was poor. She indicated that she was having difficulty opening her mouth and chewing, and she had an aching sensation located in her right temple and ear.

During the afternoon assessment at 4:30 PM, Michelle's nurse verified that Michelle understood and was using infection control techniques of proper handwashing and avoidance of contact with wound and pin sites.

When Michelle was set up on the side of the bed before her dinner, she reported dizziness and sharp pain in her right leg, and she became pale and diaphoretic. She was returned to the supine position, and a focused assessment was performed, revealing a blood pressure of 92/60. Within 20 minutes, Michelle's color had improved, the dizziness was gone, blood pressure had improved to 110/72, and the pain was relieved with medication.

In reviewing the excerpts from Michelle's plan of care, complete the status column denoting whether the outcomes have been met (m), partially met (pm), or not met (nm) appropriately for the timeframes indicated.

PRACTICE ACTIVITY 6–2
Modification of the Plan of Care

Based on your evaluation, how would you alter Michelle's plan of care from Practice Activity 6–1?

_____

_____

_____

_____

The discharge plans that began at the time of admission and were periodically updated are finalized and put into action. It must be verified that the client or significant other has received written and verbal instructions regarding treatments, medications, and activities to be followed/referred to at home. Signs and symptoms indicating the need for continued contact with the healthcare providers are reviewed. When necessary, referral/contact phone numbers and other information about resources (including appropriate web sites) are given to the client/significant other. It must also be determined whether contact has been made with appropriate providers (e.g., social worker, home health nurse, or equipment suppliers) for follow-up care as indicated.

Concerns regarding unmet needs, the importance of follow-up monitoring, and progress toward long-term goals after discharge were discussed in Chapter 4. Depending on how your facility or agency has decided to deal with these issues, you may choose to document your findings and client instructions in a discharge summary, which also identifies additional suggestions for the client and family to resolve unmet needs and achieve long-range outcomes/goals. A copy of this nursing discharge summary may then be given to the client. Box 6–2 shows how client teaching information can be organized and conveyed to the client/significant other.

Even though the client has been discharged, it is important for the client and family to know what has been accomplished and how they can continue to enhance the client's future health status. In addition, the discharge summary may be shared with the home care nurse or the nurse practitioner/primary physician for inclusion in the office record to promote continuity of care with continued work toward goals and monitoring of progress/changing needs.

Enhancing Delivery of Quality Care

Evaluation is an important step for determining the success of the plan of care because it involves a review of all the steps of the nursing process. Although client care is evaluated on an individual basis, unit and/or general agency-based nursing audit committees focus attention on selected groups of clients, such as those receiving chemotherapy or those with longer than normal lengths of stay. Comparing overall outcomes and noting the effectiveness of specific interventions are the clinical components of evaluation that can become the bases of research for validating the nursing process. This external evaluation process is the key for refining standards of care and determining the protocols, policies, and procedures necessary for the provision of quality nursing care in a particular agency.

Summary

During the **EVALUATION** step of the nursing process, the nurse monitors and reports on the current status of the identified client needs according to the outcomes that were developed in the **PLANNING** step. The evaluation process includes the client, significant others, and whoever else is involved in the care of the client. This process is a positive one in which the client's responses to the nursing interventions are evaluated to determine whether or not the desired outcomes were achieved. When the

BOX 6–2

Example of Client Teaching Information for Client Going Home on Antidysrhythmic Medication

Dear Client:
This drug has been prescribed for you. This is what you should know about your drug to get the most from your therapy.

1. Antidysrhythmics are taken to regulate your heart rhythm.
2. Antidysrhythmic drugs may have to be taken for the rest of your life.
3. Quinidine, procainamide hydrochloride (Pronestyl), propranolol (Inderal), and phenytoin (Dilantin) are taken with meals.
4. Do not take your antidysrhythmics concurrently with [fill in appropriate drugs].
5. Always check with your doctor or pharmacist before taking other drugs because interactions may occur. Drugs known to cause interactions include over-the-counter products for nasal congestion, allergy, pain, or obesity. Drugs of abuse such as marijuana may raise blood pressure and stimulate heart activity and thus increase abnormal heart rhythm.
6. If you forget to take your antidysrhythmic, do not take the forgotten dose. **Do not** try to catch up by taking two doses at the same time.
7. Do not stop taking your drug unless directed by your doctor.
8. If you have any side effects from your drug, call your doctor. Side effects from taking antidysrhythmics include low blood pressure, light headedness, gastrointestinal distress, changes in rate or rhythm of the heart, and often blurred vision. Keep a written log of the effects that are noted and the time of day, such as in the morning upon awaking, with meals, or with activity.
9. Weigh yourself weekly. A gain of 1–2 lb a week may be a sign of increased water retention. Call your doctor if this occurs.
10. Check your feet and ankles for swelling. If this occurs, call your doctor.
11. Limit your coffee, tea, or cola drinks because caffeine may cause an increase in abnormal heart rhythm.
12. Store these drugs in a tight, light-resistant bottle to prevent breakdown of drug.

Source: Kuhn, M. A. (1998). *Pharmacotherapeutics: A Nursing Process Approach*, ed 4. Philadelphia: F. A. Davis.

findings are analyzed and it is determined that the outcomes have been met, termination of services is begun and discharge planning is completed. However, if the outcomes have not been met (totally or in part), reassessment is required to determine why this is the case. Consideration must be given to factors such as new information, unexpected complications, or the choice of the wrong nursing diagnosis as possible reasons when a desired client outcome is not achieved. At this point, the nursing process should be reinitiated and the plan of care modified to include the newly identified nursing diagnoses, outcomes, and/or interventions. This modification, in turn, will be re-evaluated at an appropriate time.

The evaluation process can also be more broadly applied at an institutional level to measure the overall quality of care. It is increasingly used to set standards and to supply client information about many facets of the care provided by healthcare agencies. The EVALUATION step needs to be viewed positively as an opportunity for growth, both for individuals and for the profession as a whole. It is essential for the effective delivery of client care, and so is a process to be valued rather than avoided and/or glossed over quickly.

Now, let us return to the sixth and last standard of the ANA Standard of Clinical Nursing Practice and review the measurement criteria necessary to achieve and ensure compliance. The knowledge and skill required to meet the criteria listed in Box 6–3 were described in this chapter. The measurement criteria for this standard, combined with the previous standards, provides a valuable tool for evaluating your understanding and application of the nursing process.

Accurate documentation of the findings of the EVALUATION step is essential for ensuring the continuity of care described in the plan of care. This topic is discussed in Chapter 7.

BOX 6–3

Measurement Criteria for ANA Standard VI

ANA STANDARD VI EVALUATION: The nurse evaluates the client's progress toward attainment of outcomes.

Measurement Criteria
1. Evaluation is systematic, ongoing, and criterion-based.
2. The client, family, and other healthcare providers are involved in the evaluation process, as appropriate.
3. Ongoing assessment data are used to revise diagnoses, outcomes, and the plan of care, as needed.
4. Revisions in diagnoses, outcomes, and the plan of care are documented.
5. The effectiveness of interventions is evaluated in relation to outcomes.
6. The client's responses to interventions are documented.

1. What is the difference between assessment and evaluation? _____

_____

_____

2. What is the primary purpose of the evaluation process? _____

_____

3. The evaluation process provides what three opportunities for the client and nurse?

   a. _____

   b. _____

   c. _____

4. List the three methods in which client outcomes may be evaluated, and give an example for each:

   Method of Evaluation   **Example**

   a. _____   _____

   b. _____   _____

   c. _____   _____

5. Because it is advisable to deal with only three to five nursing diagnoses at a time, how are needs prioritized? _____

_____

6. When is consideration of discharge planning begun? _____

_____

7.

VIGNETTE: Today is Donald's fifth hospital day. At the start of the shift, you have completed a focused assessment to evaluate progress/changes in status of the identified client needs. Donald's initial nausea has resolved and his intake yesterday was approximately 3,000 calories. During rounds, you notice he has eaten all of the food on his breakfast tray. He fills out the next day's menu, neglecting to include any vegetables and selecting only one fruit.

Later, during group, Donald talks about his options for employment and says he knows an employment agency and a business where he can check about possible jobs. He also mentions a friend who he believes might be willing to help him. He says he is realizing that he is really OK, even though the loss of his job was a devastating event for him following so soon after his divorce. He acknowledges that his feelings of anxiety led to an increase in his drinking. He further says he still has feelings of sadness and occasionally feels a sense of despair but believes he will feel better as he begins to get his life back together again. He seems tentative about accepting his need to be involved in AA, saying he doesn't know "where they meet, or anyone who attends the meetings."

a. *Evaluation*: Based on the previous information, evaluate Donald's progress regarding his problems of imbalanced Nutrition: less than body requirements, ineffective Coping, and ineffective Role Performance, as outlined in the Plan of Care.

b. *Modification:* How would you change Donald's plan of care? _____

_____

_____

c. *Termination:* How might new concerns regarding the client affect your discharge plans?

_____

_____

_____

BIBLIOGRAPHY

Kuhn, M. A. (1998). *Pharmacotherapeutics: A Nursing Process Approach*, ed 4. Philadelphia: F. A. Davis.

Martin, K. S., & Scheet, N. J. (1992). *The Omaha System: A Pocket Guide for Community Health Nursing*. Philadelphia: W. B. Saunders.

SUGGESTED READINGS

Carpenito, L. J. (1999). *Nursing Care Plans and Documentation*, ed 3. Philadelphia: J. B. Lippincott.

Cox, H., et al. (2002). *Clinical Applications of Nursing Diagnosis: Adult, Child, Women's, Psychiatric, and Home Health Considerations*, ed 4. Philadelphia: F. A. Davis.

Craft-Rosenberg, M. J., & Denehy, J. A. (2000) (Eds.). *Nursing Interventions for Infants, Children, and Families*. Philadelphia: W. B. Saunders.

Doenges, M. E., Moorhouse, M. F., & Geissler-Murr, A. C. (2002). *Nurse's Pocket Guide: Nursing Diagnoses with Interventions*, ed 8. Philadelphia: F. A. Davis.

Doenges, M. E., Moorhouse, M. F., & Geissler-Murr, A. C. (2002). *Nursing Care Plans: Guidelines for Planning and Documenting Client Care*, ed 6. Philadelphia: F. A. Davis.

Holloway, N. M. (1998). *Medical-Surgical Care Planning*, ed 3. Springhouse, PA: Springhouse.

Joint Commission on Accreditation of Healthcare Organizations. (1997). *Nursing Practice and Nursing Outcomes Measurement*. Oakbrook Terrace, IL: Author.

Leuner, J. D., Manton, A. K., Kelliher, D. B., Sullivan, S. P., & Doherty, M. (1990). *Mastering the Nursing Process: A Case Study Approach*. Philadelphia: F. A. Davis.

Maas, M., Buckwalter, K. C., & Hardy, M. (1991). *Nursing Diagnosis and Interventions for the Elderly*. Menlo Park, CA: Addison-Wesley

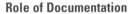

Chapter 7

Documenting the Nursing Process

Role of Documentation

Progress Notes
Staff Communication
Evaluation
Relationship Monitoring
Reimbursement
Legal Documentation
Accreditation
Training and Supervision

Techniques for Descriptive Note Writing
Judgmental Language
Descriptive Language
Content of Note/Entry
Format of Note/Entry

Summary

■ **JCAHO STANDARD:** Patient-Specific Data/Information
IM.7.1. A medical record is initiated and maintained for every individual assessed or treated. The medical record incorporates information from subsequent contacts between the patient and the organization.
IM.7.2. The medical record contains sufficient information to identify the patient, support the diagnosis, justify the treatment, document the course and results accurately, and facilitate continuity of care among healthcare providers.

Role of Documentation

Documentation not only is a requirement for accreditation; it also is a legal require-ment in any healthcare setting. From a nursing focus, documentation provides a record of the use of the nursing process for the delivery of individualized client care. The initial ASSESSMENT is recorded in the client history or database.

The IDENTIFICATION of client needs and the PLANNING of client care are recorded in the plan of care. The IMPLEMENTATION of the plan is recorded in the progress notes and/or flow sheets. Finally, the EVALUATION of care may be docu-mented in the progress notes and/or plan of care.

The goals of the documentation system are to:

- Facilitate the delivery of quality client care.
- Ensure documentation of progress with regard to client-focused outcomes.
- Facilitate interdisciplinary consistency and the communication of treatment goals and progress.

Progress Notes

The plan of care that has been developed for a particular client serves as a framework or outline for the charting of administered care. As noted, this information may be recorded on flow sheets and/or progress notes. Progress notes are an integral compo-nent of the overall medical record and should include all significant events that occur during the client's hospitalization/treatment program. The notes should be written in a clear and objective fashion and in a manner that reflects progress toward desired measurable outcomes with the use of planned staff interventions. Progress notes have seven major functions, and any given note may be written to address one function more than the others. Thus it is important to recognize the seven major functions of progress notes:

1. Staff communication
2. Evaluation
3. Relationship monitoring
4. Reimbursement
5. Legal documentation
6. Accreditation
7. Training and supervision

STAFF COMMUNICATION

Clearly, staff arriving for the next and subsequent shifts need to know what has occurred during the current shift so they can make appropriate judgments regarding client management. Colleague-to-colleague communication is the most obvious function of the progress note, yet it is only a piece of the communication picture. Nursing staff members are in the unique position of being in contact with the client for extended periods and in a variety of situations. As a nurse, your observations of your client's behavior and response to therapy provide invaluable information to the physician or other providers who may see the client for only a few minutes each day. Whether the client's current desired outcomes and interventions are discontinued or revised, or new ones developed, depends on the information gathered.

EVALUATION

Periodic review of the client's progress and the effectiveness of the treatment plan is performed by the nurse and/or the treatment team. An evaluation of the client's progress may be documented on the plan of care and/or in the progress notes.

For the purposes of review (e.g., nursing audit committees and state, federal, and private agencies such as the Board of Health, Medicare, Joint Committee on the Accreditation of Healthcare Organizations [JCAHO]), the medical record should be written to facilitate an assessment of the care given the client. Progress notes need to be written to reflect the client's progress toward measurable outcomes and the interventions used. Someone not associated with the healthcare facility should be able to read the notes, determine if the plan of care is being implemented, and assess whether progress is being made toward the measurable outcomes. The medical record should serve as a method of tracking the client's response to treatment and, consequently, as a means for evaluating the quality of care provided.

RELATIONSHIP MONITORING

The therapeutic relationship between staff and client is an important aspect of treatment in any setting. The **NURSE/CLIENT RELATIONSHIP** is the tool used by the nurse to help the client make the most of his or her own abilities. In the psychiatric setting, many of the client's pathologies are manifested in these relationships, and indications of progress are first identified through the client's ability to relate more positively and openly with staff, as well as with peers and family. Therefore, monitoring the client's relationships is essential, and notes detailing observations of these relationships (how the client interacts in group situations, in competitive settings, in one-on-one interactions, etc.) have important clinical implications in any setting.

NURSE/CLIENT RELATIONSHIP: a therapeutic relationship built on a series of interactions, developing over time and meeting the needs of the client.

Finally, regardless of the setting, the client's relationship with significant other(s) can have an impact on general well-being, progress toward recovery, independence in self-care, and (ultimately) a successful transition to the home setting. Thus, observation and monitoring of these interactions are important components of nursing care.

REIMBURSEMENT

Third-party payors are insistent that the why, when, where, how, what, and who of services be clearly documented. An absence of such documentation may result in termination of funding for individual clients and, therefore, termination of treatment. The medical record is a primary site for maintaining information about the client's treatment and associated revenues; it provides proof of services. Therefore, progress notes must document any significant observations about what is happening to the client during illness, treatment, and recovery. Data about medications, details about equipment used, and any other pertinent information must be recorded as well.

LEGAL DOCUMENTATION

Nurses have a legal and moral duty to do no harm to clients. Harm can result from a nurse's action or inaction. Careful attention to all the steps of the nursing process reduces the possibility that harm will result from errors of omission (failing to take appropriate action as a result of missing an actual nursing diagnosis) or errors of commission (taking inappropriate action because of misdiagnosis or overdiagnosis).

In our litigious society, with its pervasive threat of malpractice lawsuits, all aspects of the medical record (including the information contained in daily progress notes) may be important for legal documentation. Both the implementation of interventions and progress toward the measurable outcomes should be documented in the progress notes of the client's medical record. Progress notes and flow sheets need to document that appropriate actions have been carried out and precautions have been taken, as required to implement the treatment plan. These notations must be specific about date and time and must be signed by the person who makes the entry. In addition, the time an entry is written needs to be noted, along with the time the activity actually occurred (when charting is delayed). Errors in the document must be crossed out with one line so that it is still legible; they must be identified by the author as an "error," and then initialed. White-outs or cross-outs that make the information unreadable are not acceptable because they could be construed to mean that the individual or facility is trying to alter the facts. When charting by computer, remember that additions or changes made to the record can be tracked as to actual date/time of the entry and the author.

ACCREDITATION

One of the essential requirements for healthcare facilities (as determined by JCAHO and/or other accreditation and licensing agencies) is maintenance of a medical record. JCAHO standards state that the medical record must be documented accurately and in a timely manner. Therefore, the importance of completing notes on schedule and in a manner that facilitates retrieval of data should be emphasized. In addition, the JCAHO standards specify that, "Nursing care data related to patient assessments, nursing diagnoses and/or patient needs, nursing interventions, and patient outcomes are permanently integrated into the medical record."

TRAINING AND SUPERVISION

An often underestimated aspect of note writing is the value of notes for training and supervision purposes. An experienced nurse's description of how a complicated situation was handled, a supervisor's analysis of the problems presented by a new admission, and a description of patterns noted in a particular client's response to care are all examples of notes that provide models for the remainder of the staff. Supervisors also gain insight into an employee's abilities by reading her or his progress notes and may be able to isolate areas in which additional supervision or training/education would be beneficial.

At this point, complete Practice Activity 7–1 before proceeding to the next section.

PRACTICE ACTIVITY 7–1
Elements of Progress Notes

Give a brief explanation of how progress notes provide for the following elements of the nurse/client relationship.

1. Staff communication: _____

   _____

   _____

2. Evaluation: _____

   _____

   _____

3. Relationship monitoring: _____

   _____

   _____

4. Reimbursement: _____

   _____

   _____

5. Legal documentation: _____

   _____

   _____

6. Accreditation: _____

   _____

   _____

7. Training/Supervision: _____

   _____

   _____

Techniques for Descriptive Note Writing

Potential readership for notes written in the medical record might include coworkers, clinical nurse specialists, nurse practitioners, physicians, therapists, psychiatrists, psychologists, social workers, nurse reviewers, lawyers, judges, utilization reviewers, insurance personnel, surveyors, agency representatives, and parents or guardians, as well as the client. Because of the number of possible readers, the need for clarity and accuracy in the progress notes is a priority.

From the notes, the reader should be able to form a clear picture of what occurred with the client. The best way to ensure the clarity of progress notes is through the use of descriptive (or observational) statements. The following guideline for writing observation-based notes compares and contrasts judgmental and descriptive language.

JUDGMENTAL LANGUAGE

We are all aware of the possibilities for miscommunication that exist in ordinary conversation. The dangers of miscommunication may be even greater when information is written, and the opportunities for clarification that are available in face-to-face communication are absent in the written word. We are accustomed to speaking and writing in a judgmental (and therefore ambiguous) manner without even being aware of it. Judgmental statements include phrases that:

- Make reference to undefined periods of time
- Refer to undefined quantities
- Refer to unsupported qualities
- Fail to specify any objective basis for the judgment made

For examples, consider the following statements:

- "S/he asks for pain medication *too often*."
- "He is *uncooperative* today."
- "She did a *good job* on her incentive spirometer today."
- "He is a *manipulative* client."
- "The new client is really *difficult*."
- "He has a *poor* outlook."
- "She had a *bad attitude* about doing her physical therapy this morning."

The italicized words in each of the previous statements represent judgments (or conclusions), not facts. Without any elaboration or basis for comparison, each of the statements is a statement of opinion, open to varying interpretations. Contrast these with the statements in Box 7–1.

Undefined Periods of Time

Statements that refer to undefined periods of time may contain words or phrases such as the following:

often	almost always	most of the time
rarely	frequently	now and then
seldom	occasionally	every so often

BOX 7–1

Comparison of Judgmental and Behavioral Notes

The important thing to know about judgmental statements is that they can be translated into more precise terms. For example:

Judgmental: The client did pretty well today.

Behavioral: The client followed directions for drawing up and administering his insulin without any mistakes.

Judgmental: The meeting with the physical therapist did not go very well.

Behavioral: The client stated she "could not do the exercises which were to be started today."

Judgmental: The client had a bad attitude all day.

Behavioral: The client argued with staff five times during the shift.

Judgmental: The client became aggressive.

Behavioral: The client clenched his fists and yelled at the nurse, "I'd like to hit you." He then hit the wall twice with his right fist.

Judgmental: The client would not follow directions.

Behavioral: The client drank a glass of water 30 minutes before his scheduled surgery in spite of reminders to remain NPO.

Judgmental: The client ate poorly.

Behavioral: The client ate one third of her lunch (all of the broccoli and corn; no meat, potatoes, or bread) and drank 50 ml of apple juice.

As you can see from the previous examples, it often takes a bit more thought to write a note that is objectively descriptive. However, the benefits in clarity of communication make the effort essential for the many purposes of progress notes.

Use of these and similar phrases without clarification may leave the statement unclear and judgmental. How often, for example, is "every so often"? Is it every 5 minutes, once an hour, or three times per shift? This is not to say that the staff member must time each and every interaction or occurrence. Rather, be aware of the potential for confusion in these words. Ask yourself: Do I need to be more specific about the time of the event mentioned in this note? If you are documenting for potential legal purposes (an injury, for example), specificity is essential; however, for routine communication purposes, this may not be the case. For example, if you note, "The client was quiet for most of the shift today," it is not necessary to record the exact number of minutes during which he or she was quiet or not quiet for reasonably accurate communication to occur.

Undefined Quantities

Statements that refer to undefined quantities may use such words or phrases as the following:

some	enough	a great deal	too much
a lot	many	very little	large amount

As with the previous statements, each of these terms is open to interpretation. "A lot" of complaints to one person, for example, might mean 5; to another it might mean 20. Or, "a moderate amount of bloody drainage" could be 200 ml, or only 50 ml of fluid. It is generally advisable to avoid undefined quantities.

Unsupported Qualities

All descriptive adjectives applied to clients have the potential to fall under this category because they may involve making subjective judgments beforehand. Of most concern, however, are words that could be called "semitechnical" in nature such as:

passive	irritating	incompetent
nervous	manipulative	overprotective
demanding	alcoholic	disturbed

Because these kinds of words have connotations in the health field beyond the scope of their ordinary definitions, more common adjectives may pose less of a problem and may have less potential for misunderstanding. However, observed behaviors may call for conclusions that are influenced by your own biases and cultural background. It is best to verify the connotations of the following terms with others, and particularly with the client, before you use them:

friendly	unhappy	enthusiastic	proud
attentive	excited	bored	observant
aloof	apathetic	cheerful	happy

Finally, slang words, which are used informally and mostly by small subcultural groups, are unclear and should not be included in a professionally written note in any case. For example:

hyped-up	spaced-out	bummed	crazy
loose	pushy cool	tanked-up	

Objective Basis for Judgments

Some statements clearly express a judgment on the part of the observer and are offered without any objective basis. Such statements may cause the reader to ask "How do you know this client ..."

- is improving?
- has a good attitude?
- enjoys reading?
- hates his roommate?

Recording your observations and providing an objective basis for your judgment reduces the possibility of miscommunication or misinterpretation, and the reader will not have to look elsewhere for clarification. Consider the following statements. Although the italicized words represent a judgment or conclusion, objective facts or behavioral observations are provided to support or substantiate the judgment.

- Michelle is *improving*; she walked the length of the hall using her crutches unassisted.

- Robert has a *good attitude*, expressing optimism that he will be able to prevent a recurrence of pneumonia.
- Sally *enjoys reading*, spending 1 to 2 hours a day in this activity.
- Donald *expresses anger* toward his roommate's smoking, loud conversations with visitors, and commandeering of the TV. (**Note:** Making the inference that Donald hates his roommate because of his expression of anger results in an unclear or unsupported judgment.)

DESCRIPTIVE LANGUAGE

As noted previously, descriptive language includes observations only and avoids statements that are evaluative or judgmental, unless observational evidence can be presented to back up the judgment. You will remember that being able to actually observe the client doing something was the criterion of a well-written outcome. The situation is similar for observation-based progress notes; properly written objective statements refer to specific observable or measurable events. Descriptive statements:

- **Contain measurable periods of time**

  FOR EXAMPLE:

10 times in 1 hour	every half-hour	15 minutes
48 hours	four times a day	once

- **Contain measurable quantities**

  FOR EXAMPLE:

20 percent of the diet	all of the clients
six out of eight	completely saturated
none	5 ml

- **Provide a basis or rationale for qualities named in the note**

  FOR EXAMPLE:

  Sally's lochia flow is moderate to heavy, saturating one peripad in approximately 1 hour on two separate occasions.

  Donald's intake at lunch was poor, consisting of 1/2 cup of soup, 2 bites of sandwich, and 1/2 glass of milk.

You may have gotten the impression in the preceding section that you can never use adjectives in your notes. This is far from the case. In fact, you should give your impressions of the client.

Statements in which you note that the client "seemed" or "appeared" to be exhibiting a certain physical/emotional state are inferential statements. These include a subset of descriptive statements in which you infer the client's state based on your observations of the client's behavior and interactions, your knowledge of the client's patterns, and the connections you make between behavior/affect and what has been happening during the illness. Such statements are often of great value.

However, you do not allow your subjective impressions to stand alone, particularly if your observation involves some of the more "semitechnical" qualities noted earlier. You also need to provide some reasons why you believed the client was "improving," "demanding," "manipulative," or whatever.

FOR EXAMPLE:

Robert was upset by his daughter's objections to his Advance Directive choices, cutting off the discussion and instructing her to "mind her own business."

Donald is passive, responding to the nurse's questions regarding scheduling of his care by replying: "whatever you want to do."

Sally appears distressed, expressing concern about how she will manage two newborns when she already has two children at home, needs to return to work, and has no energy to do anything.

Michelle's mother is oversolicitous, refusing to leave her daughter's bedside and performing care activities that Michelle is capable of doing herself.

When comparisons or judgments are made, a descriptive statement should state the source or basis of judgment.

FOR EXAMPLE:

According to the client's laboratory reports, ...
Psychological testing showed that ...
The other client stated that ...
Judging by the fact that ...

Also note that whenever the source of a judgment is specified, the statement becomes a behavioral report. Because such a report can be observed, this type of statement is an observation and is therefore descriptive. Consider the differences between the following two statements:

The client is stronger today.
The physical therapist reports, "Michelle is stronger today."

The first statement is clearly judgmental because of the undefined phrase, "stronger today." The second, however, is an observable event. Obviously (although the physical therapist may be wrong), it is an objective fact that the physical therapist said that the client is stronger today. It may help to think of such statements as quotations. What the physical therapist said does not influence our ability to observe him or her saying it, and then objectively reporting that observation. However, physical therapy notes should reflect measurable descriptions of the client situation.

Finally, you can chart observations in a nonjudgmental manner: "Michelle displayed increased endurance, walked the length of the hall without assistance, appeared more confident with crutch use." In Box 7–1, additional examples further illustrate how judgmental statements may be interpreted and restated more objectively. To further assist you in your understanding of how to document descriptive progress notes, take a moment to complete Practice Activity 7–2.

CONTENT OF NOTE/ENTRY

The term *progress note* indicates that the client's progress is to be documented, along with the implementation of the treatment plan. Contents should be as specific and accurate as possible.

PRACTICE ACTIVITY 7–2
Writing Nonjudgmental Statements

*Circle either **J** or **O/B** for each of the following statements to identify either judgmental (**J**) or observational/behavioral (**O/B**) documented statements. If the statement is judgmental, rewrite to reflect observational/behavioral language.*

1. Mrs. Jewel has a poor body image since undergoing a mastectomy. **J O/B** _____

   _____

2. Mr. Dunn needs to be evaluated regarding his competence to manage his household affairs because of his left-sided weakness since his stroke. **J O/B** _____

   _____

   _____

3. Miss Janus does a good job of breast self-examination. **J O/B** _____

   _____

4. Mary Bird does not eat enough for her current level of activity. **J O/B** _____

   _____

5. Mr. Lambert stops taking his medication; then when he has a seizure, he presents at the doctor's office for treatment. **J O/B** _____

   _____

6. It has been a long time since Mr. Babbitt had his medication evaluated. **J O/B** _____

   _____

   _____

For communication purposes, it is important to record in the progress notes any information that is of importance to oncoming shifts, as well as observations you have made that may be significant for other healthcare providers. Box 7–2 profiles the information that should be included. Remember, you are actually charting for the future. You know what is happening today. However, the reader of tomorrow, next week, or next year must rely on your written words to share your understanding of the client's situation at a given moment.

For example, when applying restraints, which constitutes a major event with both therapeutic and legal ramifications, you need to document the exact time the procedure was initiated, whether any injuries resulted, and so forth. It is also necessary to document what led up to the situation, how staff and other participants reacted, what less restrictive measures were tried, and any significant observations

---

BOX 7–2

Content of Successful Progress Notes

Examples of the kind of information important to record in the progress notes include:

- **Unsettled or unclear problems or "issues"** that need to be dealt with, including attempts to contact other healthcare providers
- **Noteworthy incidents or interviews** involving the client that would benefit from a more detailed recording
- **Other pertinent data,** such as notes on phone calls, home visits, and family interactions
- **Additional critical incident data,** such as seemingly significant or revealing statements made by the client, an insight you have into a client's patterns of behavior, client injuries, the use of any special treatment procedure, or other major events such as episodes of pain, respiratory distress, panic attacks, medication reactions, suicidal comments
- **Administered care activities or observations,** if not recorded elsewhere on flow sheets (physician visits, completion of ordered tests, nonroutine medications, etc.)

---

regarding the incident. An example of how to document a therapeutic event is presented in Box 7–3.

Other tools that promote accurate communication include the use of correct grammar and spelling, legible handwriting, and nonerasable ink. To promote clarity, avoid repeating data when possible. Because this is "the client's record," it is not necessary to use the term "the client"; however, periodically using the client's name can help the reader to identify the proper chart and prevent problems of charting on the wrong record, especially when you chart on several clients' records at a time. Use abbreviations with caution, or avoid them in most instances. Although some institutions provide a list of approved abbreviations that identifies the correct meaning (such as those included in Appendix I), abbreviations can be misleading or easily misinterpreted, resulting in misunderstandings and errors with serious consequences. For example, a client reading his record might not realize that "SOB" stands for short of breath.

Last, but not least, remember to be brief. Entries need to be concise, short, succinct sentences or phrases that provide enough information to communicate your observations, thoughts, and plans. The entries must be consistent in style and format to avoid confusion and to comply with agency policies. Avoid repetition/ redundancy. Do not rewrite what is already recorded on flow sheets, but do use the progress note to expand on the flow sheet as appropriate and to note the client's response. For example: when documenting your repeat assessment of a wound, you may chart "no change" (if that is the case) if your baseline or previous observations are recorded.

> **BOX 7–3**
>
> ## *Documenting a Therapeutic Event*
>
> Twenty-four hours after Donald was admitted to the unit with a diagnosis of acute alcoholism, he became disoriented to time, place, and person; was extremely agitated; and was "picking in the air", saying he was trying to "catch the bugs." He was given medication and placed in restraints in a seclusion room with the door open. This was charted as follows:
>
> **4:00 PM:** Suddenly became agitated. Medicated with Valium, reoriented to place/events in quiet tones as staff paced with him, and reinforced that he would be kept safe. Agitation escalated, unable to remain in one place for longer than 60 seconds, expressed fear of the "things" he was seeing. Agreed to use of restraints to help keep him safe until he could regain control and/or medication becomes effective.
>
> **4:15 PM:** Procedure explained as Donald was put in seclusion room C and placed in 4-point wrist/ankle restraints without incident or injury. He was informed that door would remain open and a staff member would check on him every 10 minutes, or more frequently as needed. Vital signs: B/P 150/90, P 120. Respirations 32.
>
> **4:20 PM:** Dr. Carter notified of current events.
>
> **4:30 PM:** Level of agitation reassessed. Donald reports feeling less anxious, but still "jumpy" inside. Remains restless. Restraints continued.

FORMAT OF NOTE/ENTRY

Several charting formats have been used for documentation. These include block notes, with a single entry covering an entire shift (e.g., 7 AM–3 PM); narrative timed notes (e.g., 8:30 AM, Ate all of breakfast); and the problem-oriented medical record system (**POMR** or **PORS**) using the **SOAP/SOAPIER** approach (Box 7–4), to name a few. The last format can provide thorough documentation, but it was designed by physicians for episodic care and requires that entries be tied to a client problem identified from a problem list.

A system format created by nurses for documentation of frequent/repetitive care is FOCUS CHARTING™. It was designed to encourage looking at the client from a positive rather than a negative (or problem-oriented) perspective by using precise documentation to record the nursing process. Recording assessment, interventions, and evaluation information in a DAR (Data, Action, and Response) format (Box 7–5) facilitates tracking and following what is happening to the client at any given moment. Charting focuses on client and nursing concerns. The focal point is client status and the associated nursing care. The "Focus" is always stated to reflect the client's concern/need rather than a nursing task or medical diagnosis. Box 7–6 highlights some of the distinguishing features of a Focus.

Whatever documentation system you use, an organized format is a method of identifying, working through, and solving the client's needs. **SOAP** and **DAR** help

POMR OR PORS: Problem-Oriented Medical Record—a method of recording data about the health status of a client by focusing on the client's problems.

SOAP/SOAPIER: format for documentation—subjective, objective, analysis, plan; implementation, evaluation, revision.

DAR: format for documentation—data, action, response.

BOX 7-4

Components of the SOAP/SOAPIER Charting Format

The **SOAP** format is generally used for the initial assessment of the client. Once the plan of care is implemented and the evaluation process begun, the **SOAPIER** format becomes more appropriate.

Subjective: Statements from client/others
Objective: Measurable or observable data
Analysis: Interpretations/conclusions based on the subjective and/or objective data
Plan: What is to be done about the identified problem(s)
Implementation: How plan is carried out
Evaluation: Client's response to the interventions
Revision: How the plan of care will be changed

---

organize your thinking and provide structure, which can promote creative problem solving. Structured communication facilitates consistency between various services and healthcare providers. Compare the charts in Tables 7–1 and 7–2 for a client with type 2 diabetes (non–insulin-dependent diabetes mellitus) who has an ulceration of the left foot.

A copy of the back page of the interactive plan-of-care worksheet is included in Figure 7–1. It is an example of one method of documenting by focusing on certain aspects of the nursing process. The DOCUMENTATION section of the interactive plan-of-care worksheet is divided into three possible areas for which documentation is appropriate and may be required in certain agencies. The first section is reassessment data. In this area, you will review the client's initial assessment data to note any changes. Also, data derived from MONITORING-focused nursing interventions ("monitor vital signs every shift" or "monitor serum potassium level every 8 hours") are documented in this section. The second documentation area directs attention to the nursing interventions implemented to assist clients in attaining their stated

---

BOX 7-5

Components of the FOCUS CHARTING™ Format

Focus: Nursing diagnosis, client need/concern, sign/symptom, event
Data: Subjective/objective information describing and/or supporting the focus
Action: Immediate/future nursing actions based on assessment and consistent with/complementary to the goals and nursing action recorded in the client plan of care
Response: Describes the effects of interventions and whether or not the goal/outcome was met

---

BOX 7–6

What Is a Focus?

The nurse often speaks of "a focus" for her assessment, diagnosis, and planning of care.

- A client need/concern or nursing diagnosis

  FOR EXAMPLE:

  Airway   Nutrition   Fluid excess

Deficient Knowledge regarding wound care

The "stem" or diagnostic label is taken from the plan of care. You do not need to use time and space to repeat the entire diagnostic statement.

- Signs/symptoms of potential importance

  FOR EXAMPLE:

  Fever   Confusion
  Hypotension   Nausea
  Dysrhythmia   Edema

These require monitoring or limited intervention, but if the signs and symptoms persist, a client need will be identified and added to the plan of care. **FOR EXAMPLE:** Continued nausea can affect fluid volume; sustained dysrhythmias and hypotension may develop into a cardiac output concern.

- Significant event or change in status

  FOR EXAMPLE:

  Admission/transfer   Seizure activity
  Fall out of bed   Respiratory arrest

- A single incident may evolve into a client need for inclusion in the plan of care

  FOR EXAMPLE: A fall raises concerns about Risk for Injury, or, possibly, Disturbed Thought Processes, if client is disoriented; or a respiratory arrest may be related to Ineffective Airway Clearance or Ineffective Breathing Pattern.

- Specific standards of care/hospital policy

  FOR EXAMPLE:

  Admission/discharge   Preoperative visit
  Summary   Discharge planning
  Routine shift assessment

TABLE 7–1. Sample SOAP/IER Charting Format for Richard

Date	Time	Number/Problem*	SOAP Format†
6/30/02	1400	1 (Skin Integrity)	**S:** "That hurts" (when tissue surrounding wound palpated).
			O: Scant amount serous drainage on dressing. Wound borders pink. No odor present.
			A: Wound shows early signs of healing, free of infection.
			P: Continue skin care per plan of care.

In order to document more of the nursing process, some institutions have added the following: Implementation, Evaluation, and Review (if plan was altered)

Date	Time	Number/Problem*	SOAP Format†
			I: NS irrigation as ordered. Applied wet sterile dressing with paper tape.
			E: Wound clean, no drainage present.
			Signed: *E. Moore RN*
6/30/02	2100	2 (Pain)	**S:** "Dull, throbbing pain (in left foot), no radiation to other areas."
			O: Muscles tense. Moving about bed, appears uncomfortable.
			A: Persistent pain.
			P: Foot cradle placed on bed.
			Darvon 65 mg given PO.
			Signed: *M. Liskin, LPN.*
	2130		**E:** Reports pain relieved. Appears relaxed.
			Signed: *B. Marsh RN*
6/30/02	1100	3 (Deficient Knowledge, diabetic teaching)	**S:** Listed questions/concerns of self and wife. (Copy attached to teaching plan.)
			O: Attended group teaching session with wife and read Understanding Your Diabetes.
			A: Richard and wife need review of information and practice for insulin administration.
			P: Review questions/concerns and meet with dietitian.
			I: He demonstrated insulin administration technique for wife to observe. Procedure handout sheet for future reference provided to couple. Scheduled meeting for them with dietitian at 1300 today to discuss remaining questions.
			E: Richard more confident in demonstration, performed activity without hesitation, correctly and without hand tremors. Richard explained steps of procedure and reasons for actions to wife. Couple identified resources to contact if questions/problems arise.
			Signed: *B. Briner, RN*

* As noted on Plan of Care.
†S = Subjective: Statements from client/others.
O = Objective: Measurable or observable data.
A = Analysis: Interpretations/conclusions based on the subjective and/or objective data.
P = Plan: What is to be done about the identified problem(s).
I = Implementation: How plan is carried out.
E = Evaluation: Client's response to the interventions.
R = Revision: How the plan of care will be changed.

TABLE 7–2. **Sample of DAR for Richard**

Date	Time	Focus	DAR Format*
6/30/02	1400	Skin integrity L foot	**D:** Scant amount serous drainage on dressing, wound borders pink, no odor present, denies discomfort except with direct palpation of surrounding tissue **A:** NS irrigation as ordered. Sterile wet dressing applied with paper tape **R:** Wound clean—no drainage present. Signed: *E. Moore RN*
6/30/02	2100	Pain L foot	**D:** Reports dull/throbbing ache L foot—no radiation. Muscles tense, restless in bed. **A:** Foot cradle placed on bed. Darvon 65 mg given PO. Signed: *M. Liskin L.P.N.*
6/30/02	2200	Pain L foot	**R:** Reports pain relieved. Appears relaxed. Signed: *B. Marsh RN*
	1100	Deficient Knowledge, diabetic teaching	**D:** Attended group teaching session with wife. Both have read ***Understanding Your Diabetes.*** **A:** Reviewed list of questions/concerns from Richard and wife. (Copy attached to teaching plan.) Richard demonstrated insulin administration technique for wife to observe. Procedure handout sheet for future reference provided to couple. Scheduled meeting for them with dietitian at 1300 today to discuss remaining questions. **R:** Richard more confident in demonstration, performed activity without hesitation, correctly and without hand tremors. He explained steps of procedure and reasons for actions to wife. Couple identified resources to contact if questions/problems arise. Signed: *B. Briner, RN*

The following is an example of documentation of a client need/concern that currently does not require identification as a client problem (nursing diagnosis) or inclusion in the plan of care and therefore is not easily documented in the SOAP format:

Date	Time	Focus	DAR Format*
6/29/02	2320	Gastric distress	**D:** Awakened, from light sleep by "indigestion/burning sensation." Places hand over epigastric area. Skin warm/dry, color pink, vital signs unchanged. **A:** Given Mylanta 30 ml PO. Head of bed elevated approximately 15 degrees. **R:** Reports pain relieved. Appears relaxed, resting quietly. Signed: *E Moore, RN*

* D = Data: Subjective/objective information describing and/or supporting the focus.
A = Action: Immediate or future nursing actions that address the focus, any changes required for the plan of care.
R = Response: Description of client responses to care provided and whether goals/outcomes are met.
Source: Lampe, S. S. (1997). *FOCUS CHARTING*™. Minneapolis: Creative Nursing Management.

Desired Outcome and Client Criteria: The Client will:

PLANNING

TIME OUT!

The desired outcome must meet criteria to be accurate. The outcome must be specific, realistic, measurable, and include a time frame for completion. Does the action verb describe the client's behavior to be evaluated? Can the outcome be used in the evaluation step of the nursing process to measure the client's response to the nursing interventions listed below?

Interventions	Rationale for Selected Intervention and References

EVALUATION

TIME OUT!

Do your interventions assist in achieving the desired outcome? Do your interventions address further monitoring of the client's response to your interventions and to the achievement of the desired outcome? Are qualifiers: when, how, amount, time, and frequency used? Is the focus of the action's verb on the nurse's actions and not on the client? Do your rationales provide sufficient reason and directions?

What was your client's response to the interventions?

Was the desired outcome achieved?   If no, what revisions to either the desired outcome or interventions would you make?

☐ Yes   ☐ No

Documentation Focus: Now that you have completed the evaluation, the next step is to document your care and the client's response. Use the areas below to enter your progress note information.

Reassessment Data:

DOCUMENTATION

Interventions Implemented:

Client's Response:

INSTRUCTOR'S COMMENTS:

FIGURE 7–1. Reverse side of the interaction plan worksheet previously introduced, providing documentation of the nursing process.

desired outcomes. Examples may include, "Assisted client with ambulation bid," or "Instructed in proper use of a walker." Finally, the third section is the client's response to your interventions: How well did the client tolerate his assisted ambulation? Or, did the client use the walker in the correct manner as demonstrated?

Summary

Documentation of client care information communicates and reflects the individualization of care you provide. Documentation promotes continuity of client care among the varied healthcare providers and serves as a basis for evaluation of the care provided. Finally, the documentation process continually reinforces your accountability and responsibility to implement and evaluate the nursing process. As your documentation skills improve, you will save time by consistently using a documentation system that focuses on specific issues. Accurate documentation can also help the clinician in meeting legal and accreditation requirements.

The last chapter in this text includes a client case study to help you bring all the steps of the nursing process together. The case study provides information about a new client, Mr. R. Simmons. His completed client database and the physician's admitting orders are provided, to assist you in identifying possible nursing diagnoses, developing appropriate desired outcomes for Mr. Simmons, and selecting nursing interventions that will assist him in attaining the desired outcomes.

The final chapter also presents an evaluation checklist that was developed to include the important aspects of all the American Nurses' Association's Standards of Clinical Nursing Practice detailed throughout this text. This comprehensive evaluation checklist serves as a helpful tool for your self-evaluation and ensures that your assigned written care-planning tasks are correctly accomplished.

1. You are writing a paper regarding documentation. Identify three goals of the documentation process that you will include:

   a. _____

   b. _____

   c. _____

2. Steps of the nursing process are documented on which form?

   Steps   **Form**

   _____ Assessment   a. Plan of care

   _____ Diagnosis/Need Identification   b. Progress notes

   _____ Planning   c. Client database

   _____ Implementation   d. Flow sheets

   _____ Evaluation

3. List five functions of progress notes:

   a. _____

   b. _____

   c. _____

   d. _____

   e. _____

4. Complete the following statements describing the JCAHO's standards for documentation.

   a. A medical record is _____ and _____ for every individual assessed or treated. The medical record incorporates information from subsequent contacts between the _____ and the _____.

   b. The medical record contains _____ to _____ the client, support the _____, justify the _____, document the course and results accurately, and facilitate _____ of care among healthcare providers.

5. When the healthcare provider is documenting for reimbursement, five factors need to be included. These are: _____

   _____

6. Two ways in which the plan of care can be used for supervision are: _____

   _____

7. The best way to ensure clarity of the progress notes is: _____

   _____

8. Rewrite the following judgmental statements to make them nonjudgmental:

a. He is uncooperative today. _____

_____

b. He is a manipulative client. _____

_____

c. She had a bad attitude about taking her medication this morning. _____

_____

d. The new client is really difficult. _____

_____

9. List three types of judgmental statements:

a. _____

b. _____

c. _____

10. Name three types of data that are important to record in the progress notes:

a. _____

b. _____

c. _____

11. List five additional factors that can enhance accurate communication:

a. _____

b. _____

c. _____

d. _____

e. _____

12. What actions can be taken to correct an error in charting? _____

_____

13. Name three charting formats:

a. _____ b. _____ c. _____

14. Read the following Vignette and record the client data using the SOAP and DAR formats, as well as the format used in your facility/agency, if different.

VIGNETTE: Sally was discharged home with the twins on the evening of her third postpartal day. On the morning of day 5, she is visited by the public health nurse, who specializes in maternal/newborn care.

Sally is dressed in a robe and slippers, her hair is uncombed, her color is pale, and she has dark circles under her eyes. She is sitting in a recliner, bottlefeeding Baby A. Her mother is sitting on the couch, feeding Baby B. The living area is noted to be clean and neat with comfortable ambient temperature. The two older children are reported to be at preschool from 9:00 AM to 2:30 PM daily.

The postpartal assessment form is completed, with physical findings within normal limits. Sally reports that her bowels are working "slowly" (small, firm BM this AM), with fluid intake of approximately 2 liters per day and moderate appetite—"just too tired to really eat or do anything else." Sally's mother indicates that she is providing household assistance—cooking, cleaning, and child care. Sally and her mother agree that fatigue is a major concern for Sally. Both Sally and her mother are up twice during the night to feed the twins. Sally does take short naps during the day. Sally is observed to display usual attachment behaviors toward Baby A (Laura); however, her interaction with Baby B (unnamed) is of short duration, appears to lack warmth, and is restricted to care-taking activities.

You provide Sally with a teaching sheet that describes postpartal fatigue and discusses dietary needs/supplements, energy conservation techniques, and the importance of balanced activity/exercise and rest. You suggest that Sally's husband might get up for one feeding during the night to allow her a longer period of uninterrupted sleep and provide him with additional opportunity for interaction with his daughters.

Next, you ask Sally how she feels about being the mother of twins. Sally becomes tearful and states, "I just don't know what I'm going to do when Mom goes home." You ask if she would like to have a visit from a member of the Mothers of Multiples group. You also suggest that she hold a family meeting to problem-solve her concerns. You then discuss your observation that Sally appears more comfortable with Laura than with her twin, asking Sally to describe her perceptions of and feelings for Baby B. After reflecting on the question, Sally says she has felt so overwhelmed that she hasn't truly accepted the reality of having twins. She is visibly upset, berating herself for being a "poor mother." You tell her that it is not unusual to be overwhelmed by the reality of a multiple birth, even when it is planned for in advance of delivery.

You ask Sally to think about what she needs to help her resolve this situation. Sally states that she needs to spend more time getting to know Baby B, allowing other family members to care for and interact with Laura. Following a discussion about the individual characteristics of her other children, Sally says Baby B is unique in her level of alertness and her "acceptance" of anyone who cares for her. "She deserves a name reflecting family ties and thanksgiving for the special gift of twins." You encourage Sally to read the literature about twins provided before her discharge and to apply techniques she has previously found successful in dealing with stressful situations. You schedule a follow-up visit for 1 week later and leave a contact number in case Sally should have any questions or need assistance before your next visit. When you depart, Sally appears focused on ways to improve her current situation—smiling, displaying a lighter mood, and giving a firm handshake.

15.

POMR/SOAP FORMAT: Problem: _____

   S: _____

_____

   O: _____

_____

   A: _____

_____

   P: _____

_____

   I: _____

_____

   E: _____

_____

   R: _____

_____

DAR FORMAT: Focus:

   D: _____

_____

_____

   A: _____

_____

_____

   R: _____

_____

_____

FORMAT USED IN YOUR INSTITUTION/AGENCY, if different: _____

_____

_____

_____

_____

BIBLIOGRAPHY

Lampe, S. S. (1997). *Focus Charting™*. Minneapolis: Creative Nursing Management.

SUGGESTED READINGS

Burke, L. J. (1995). *Charting by Exception Applications: Making It Work in Clinical Settings*. Albany: Delmar.

Burke, L. J. (1998). *Charting Made Incredibly Easy*. Springhouse, PA: Springhouse.

Eggland, E. T., & Eggland, N. H. (1994). *Nursing Documentation: Charting, Recording, and Reporting*. Philadelphia: Lippincott Williams & Wilkins.

Fischbach, F. T. (1991). *Documenting Care: Communication, the Nursing Process and Documentation Standards*. Philadelphia: F. A. Davis.

Iyer, P. W., & Camp, N. H. (1999). *Nursing Documentation: A Nursing Process Approach*, ed 3. St. Louis: Mosby.

Kerr, S. D. (1992). A comparison of four nursing documentation systems. *Journal of Nursing Staff Development*, 8(1):26–31.

(1999). *Mastering Documentation*, ed 2. Springhouse, PA: Springhouse.

Meiner, S. (1999). *Nursing Documentation: Legal Focus Across Practice Settings*. Thousand Oaks, CA: Sage Publications.

Yocum, F. (1993). *Documentation Skills for Quality Patient Care*. Tipp City, OH: Awareness Productions.

Chapter 8

Interactive Care Planning: From Assessment to Client Response

This final chapter provides you with the opportunity to apply and evaluate the steps of the nursing process presented in the previous chapters. A case study based on simulated assessment data gathered on your client, Mr. Simmons, and the inclusion of physician admission orders add to the realism of this nursing process exercise. The objective and subjective data are organized within the Doenges and Moorhouse 13 diagnostic divisions assessment tool, which was described earlier in Chapter 2. (A copy of the complete assessment tool is available for your future use in Appendix C.)

Instructions for Case Study

First, read over the admitting physician's orders and reflect on how your implementation of these orders will assist you in structuring Mr. Simmons' plan of care. After reviewing the physician's orders, review the extensive client database gathered on Mr. Simmons. As you study the database, start to record or highlight those subjective and objective cues that suggest a client need (or problem) and that may be similar to the defining characteristics of possible nursing diagnoses for Mr. Simmons. One purpose of this exercise is for you to identify two accurate nursing diagnoses. The accuracy of your nursing diagnoses depends on the availability of the subjective and objective data gathered during the admission history and physical examination and the subsequent matching of these data with the defining characteristics of the nursing diagnoses described by NANDA. Remember, all the NANDA nursing diagnoses, their related risk factors, and their defining characteristics are included in Appendix A.

To further assist you in comparing Mr. Simmons' assessment data with the defining characteristics of possible nursing diagnoses, Table 8–1 presents the 13 diagnostic divisions, with selected associated NANDA nursing diagnoses. By reviewing this information, you will be able to better visualize the relationship between the varied nursing diagnoses and the focused assessments of the different diagnostic divisions.

For example, when the client's assessment data gathered in the **ELIMINATION** diagnostic division are analyzed, if abnormal subjective and/or objective data are present, your next step would be to direct your attention to Table 8–1. Review the 12 NANDA nursing diagnoses associated with the **ELIMINATION** diagnostic division. Once you have identified a possible nursing diagnosis from the **ELIMINATION** division, your next task is to review the defining characteristics of that nursing diagnosis (Appendix A) and determine if there is an accurate match with your data. Box 8–1 provides an abbreviated checklist to assist you as you begin diagnosing and constructing plans of care.

Case Study Care Planning Worksheet

Use the case study care planning worksheets on pages 174–181 to enter your two client diagnostic statements (NANDA nursing diagnosis label, the related factors [etiologies], and evidence of signs/symptoms you used in making the diagnosis) for Mr. Simmons. Then, use the worksheets to list two outcome statements for each of the diagnostic statements you have identified for Mr. Simmons. Next, select at least three nursing interventions that will assist Mr. Simmons in achieving the two measurable outcome statements you have listed, and record them in the space provided on the worksheets.

The two-page Interactive Care Plan Worksheet described can also assist you during this care-planning and evaluation exercise. Review the TIME OUT sections; information provided here will further assist you in accurately complying with the criteria required for developing accurate diagnostic statements, constructing client outcome statements, and selecting appropriate nursing interventions.

Care-Planning Evaluation Checklist

The evaluation checklist (Fig. 8–1) is included in this chapter to provide a workable guide for constructing Mr. Simmons' plan of care, as well as for future use in care-planning assignments. The evaluation checklist was designed to include the criteria

TABLE 8–1. **Nursing Diagnoses Organized According to Diagnostic Divisions**

After data have been collected and areas of concern/need have been identified, consult the Diagnostic Divisions framework to review the list of nursing diagnoses that fall within the individual categories. This will assist you with the choice of the specific diagnostic labels to accurately describe the data from the client database. Then, with the addition of etiology (when known) and signs and symptoms, the client diagnostic statement emerges.

Diagnostic Division: Activity/Rest: Ability to engage in necessary/desired activities of life (work and leisure) and to obtain adequate sleep/rest

Diagnoses

Activity Intolerance

Activity Intolerance, risk for

Disuse Syndrome, risk for

Diversional Activity, deficient

Fatigue

Mobility, impaired bed

Mobility, impaired wheelchair

Sleep Deprivation

Sleep Pattern, disturbed

Transfer Ability, impaired

Walking, impaired

CIRCULATION—Ability to transport oxygen and nutrients necessary to meet cellular needs

Diagnoses

Autonomic Dysreflexia

Autonomic Dysreflexia, risk for

Cardiac Output, decreased

Intracranial, decreased adaptive capacity

Tissue Perfusion, ineffective (specify type: renal, cerebral, cardiopulmonary, gastrointestinal, peripheral)

EGO INTEGRITY—Ability to develop and use skills and behaviors to integrate and manage life experiences

Diagnoses

Adjustment, impaired

Anxiety [specify level]

Anxiety, death

Body Image, disturbed

Conflict, decisional (specify)

Coping, defensive

Coping, ineffective

Denial, ineffective

Energy Field, disturbed

Fear

Grieving, anticipatory

Grieving, dysfunctional

Hopelessness

(Continued)

TABLE 8–1. Nursing Diagnoses Organized According to Diagnostic Divisions (Continued)

Personal Identity, disturbed
Post-Trauma Syndrome
Post-Trauma Syndrome, risk for
Powerlessness
Powerlessness, risk for
Rape-Trauma Syndrome
Rape-Trauma Syndrome: compound reaction
Rape-Trauma Syndrome: silent reaction
Relocation Stress Syndrome
Relocation Stress Syndrome, risk for
Self-Esteem, chronic low
Self-Esteem, situational low
Self-Esteem, risk for situational low
Sorrow, chronic
Spiritual Distress
Spiritual Distress, risk for
Spiritual Well-being, readiness for enhanced

ELIMINATION—Ability to excrete waste products

Diagnoses
Bowel Incontinence
Constipation
Constipation, perceived
Constipation, risk for
Diarrhea
Urinary Elimination, impaired
Urinary Incontinence, functional
Urinary Incontinence, reflex
Urinary Incontinence, stress
Urinary Incontinence, total
Urinary Incontinence, urge
Urinary Incontinence, risk for urge
Urinary Retention [acute/chronic]

FOOD/FLUID—Ability to maintain intake of and utilize nutrients and liquids to meet physiological needs

Diagnoses
Breastfeeding, effective
Breastfeeding, ineffective
Breastfeeding, interrupted
Dentition, impaired
Failure to Thrive, adult
[Fluid Volume, deficient (hyper/hypotonic)]

TABLE 8–1. **Nursing Diagnoses Organized According to Diagnostic Divisions** (Continued)

Fluid Volume, deficient [isotonic]

Fluid Volume, excess

Fluid Volume, risk for deficient

Fluid Volume, risk for imbalanced

Infant Feeding Pattern, ineffective

Nausea

Nutrition: imbalanced, less than body requirements

Nutrition: imbalanced, more than body requirements

Nutrition: imbalanced, risk for more than body requirements

Oral Mucous Membrane, impaired

Swallowing, impaired

HYGIENE—Ability to perform basic activities of daily living

Diagnoses

Self-Care Deficit: bathing/hygiene

Self-Care Deficit: dressing/grooming

Self-Care Deficit: feeding

Self-Care Deficit: toileting

NEUROSENSORY—Ability to perceive, integrate, and respond to internal and external cues

Diagnoses

Confusion, acute

Confusion, chronic

Infant Behavior, disorganized

Infant Behavior, risk for disorganized

Infant Behavior, readiness for enhanced, organized

Memory, impaired

Peripheral Neurovascular, dysfunction, risk for

Sensory Perception, disturbed (specify: visual, auditory, kinesthetic, gustatory, tactile, olfactory)

Thought Processes, disturbed

Unilateral Neglect

PAIN/DISCOMFORT—Ability to control internal/external environment to maintain comfort

Diagnoses

Pain, acute

Pain, chronic

RESPIRATION—Ability to provide and use oxygen to meet physiological needs

Diagnoses

Airway Clearance, ineffective

Aspiration, risk for

Breathing Pattern, ineffective

Gas Exchange, impaired

Ventilation, impaired spontaneous

(Continued)

TABLE 8–1. **Nursing Diagnoses Organized According to Diagnostic Divisions** (Continued)

Ventilatory Weaning Response, dysfunctional
SAFETY—Ability to provide safe, growth-promoting environment
Allergy Response, latex
Allergy Response, risk for latex
Body Temperature, risk for imbalanced
Environmental Interpretation Syndrome, impaired
Falls, risk for
Health Maintenance, ineffective
Home Maintenance, impaired
Hyperthermia
Hypothermia
Infection, risk for
Injury, risk for
Injury, risk for perioperative positioning
Mobility, impaired physical
Poisoning, risk for
Protection, ineffective
Self-Mutilation
Self-Mutilation, risk for
Skin Integrity, impaired
Skin Integrity, risk for impaired
Suffocation, risk for
Suicide, risk for
Surgical Recovery, delayed
Thermoregulation, ineffective
Tissue Integrity, impaired
Trauma, risk for
Violence, [actual/]risk for other-directed
Violence, [actual/]risk for self-directed
Wandering [specify sporadic or continual]
SEXUALITY—[Component of Ego Integrity and Social Interaction]

Diagnoses
Ability to meet requirements/characteristics of male/female role
Sexual Dysfunction
Sexuality Patterns, ineffective
SOCIAL INTERACTION—Ability to establish and maintain relationships

Diagnoses
Attachment, risk for impaired parent/infant/child
Caregiver Role Strain
Caregiver Role Strain, risk for
Communication, impaired verbal
Coping, community, ineffective

TABLE 8–1. **Nursing Diagnoses Organized According to Diagnostic Divisions** (Continued)

Coping, community, readiness for enhanced
Coping, family: compromised
Coping, family: disabled
Coping, family: readiness for enhanced
Family Processes, dysfunctional: alcoholism
Family Processes, interrupted
Loneliness, risk for
Parental Role Conflict
Parenting, impaired
Parenting, risk for impaired
Role Performance, ineffective
Social Interaction, impaired
Social Isolation

TEACHING/LEARNING—Ability to incorporate and use information to achieve healthy
   lifestyle/optimal wellness

Diagnoses
Development, risk for delayed
Growth, risk for disproportionate
Growth and Development, delayed
Health-Seeking Behaviors (specify)
Noncompliance [Adherence, ineffective] (specify)
Therapeutic Regimen: Community, ineffective management
Therapeutic Regimen: Family, ineffective management
Therapeutic Regimen: effective management
Therapeutic Regimen: ineffective management

---

presented in the TIME OUT sections of the Interactive Care Plan Worksheets, the requirements of the ANA's Standards of Clinical Nursing Practice presented in the previous chapters, and the current standards for JCAHO Management of Information. An additional copy of the checklist is included so that you'll be able to take it with you to your assigned nursing unit and use it to help construct plans of care and evaluate your implementation of the steps of the nursing process.

Use the evaluation checklist after you have documented your first attempts at identifying Mr. Simmons' two nursing diagnoses, his two measurable outcome statements, and the appropriate nursing interventions for each outcome statement. Review the checklist's criteria against your completed case study care plan worksheet for feedback on how well your plan of care for Mr. Simmons is being accomplished.

Practicing Critical Thinking

Once you have worked through the exercise and completed your plan of care for Mr. Simmons, take a few moments to stimulate the right side of your brain and construct a mind map that demonstrates any linkages you have identified.

BOX 8–1

Diagnostic Decision Making

1. Read the physician's admitting orders.
2. Review all of the data included in the 13 diagnostic divisions. Pay particular attention to Mr. Simmons' subjective data, which describe his perception of his illness and his responses to the various healthcare problems described.
3. Review the discharge considerations section at the end of the assessment tool. Can this information assist you in accurately identifying his nursing diagnoses?
4. Record or highlight any abnormal responses or observations identified while reviewing Mr. Simmons' assessment data.
5. Review the assessment tool's individual diagnostic divisions where you recorded or highlighted abnormal data.
6. In those divisions where abnormal data were highlighted, review the nursing diagnoses associated with the Diagnostic Division (see Table 8–1).
7. Select a possible nursing diagnosis from the diagnostic division.
8. Review the defining characteristics of your selected possible nursing diagnosis (see Appendix A).
9. Compare the recorded or highlighted data with the selected nursing diagnosis' defining characteristics. Is there sufficient match? (Refer to Appendix F, Lunney's Scale.) "Yes": Move to step 10. "No": Return to the assessment tool and ensure you have reviewed all the appropriate data. If your review is sufficient, then return to step 6 because another possible nursing diagnosis may be appropriate for consideration.
10. Once you have decided on an accurate nursing diagnosis, complete the client diagnostic statement by adding the related factor(s) specific to Mr. Simmons' situation (refer again to Appendix A).
11. Now develop a client outcome statement for Mr. Simmons' identified nursing diagnosis. Two options are available for this step.
    a. Look at the nursing diagnosis and define how Mr. Simmons could resolve this identified response to his healthcare problem. For example, if his nursing diagnosis is Anxiety, an appropriate path in the development of an outcome statement would include "a reduction or elimination of his identified anxiety."
    b. A second strategy in outcome statement development is to review the *related factor(s)* and develop an outcome reflecting either elimination or reduction of the related factor(s). For example, if the Anxiety is determined to be related to a change in health status, then his outcome statement could reflect a correction in health status or return to premorbid state, or in this case, more appropriately, an increase in Mr. Simmons' control of his condition.

Diagnostic Decision Making

---

12. Once you have developed the outcome statements for Mr. Simmons, your attention must now turn to selecting appropriate nursing interventions to assist him in achieving the desired outcome. Several methods can be employed to assist you in selecting nursing interventions.

FOR EXAMPLE: Your assigned medical-surgical or fundamentals texts are excellent resources for nursing interventions and their rationales. Other resources include care planning guides (such as Doenges, Moorhouse, and Geissler-Murr's *Nursing Care Plans*, ed 6, 2002) or nursing diagnosis handbooks (such as Doenges, Moorhouse, and Geissler-Murr's *Nurse's Pocket Guide*, ed 8, 2002) that provide outcome statements and nursing interventions for each NANDA nursing diagnosis.

13. Repeat steps 6–12 for your second nursing diagnosis.

Conclusion

The nursing process steps described in this text are an integral part of the day-to-day science and practice of nursing. Regardless of the nursing practice setting you choose, the steps of the nursing process are universal in their application.

It is our hope that this interactive approach has been helpful in stimulating critical thinking and providing instruction on how to use the steps of the nursing process. The several interactive approaches were all designed to assist you in developing the necessary cognitive, affective, and psychomotor learning skills required to successfully apply the decision-making steps in the nursing process. We extend our best wishes to you as you begin your nursing career.

Putting Together What You Have Learned About the Nursing Process

Review the following vignette and nursing history. Then, create a plan of care for your client, Mr. Simmons. Identify two client needs and write the client diagnostic statement and two outcomes. Choose three interventions for each client diagnostic statement.

VIGNETTE: Mr. R. Simmons, who has had type 2 diabetes for 10 years, presented to his physician's office with a nonhealing ulcer on his left foot, of 3 weeks' duration. Screening studies done in the doctor's office revealed blood glucose (BG) of 356 per fingerstick and Chemstix of 2%. Because of distance from a medical provider and lack of local community services, he is admitted to the hospital.

CRITERIA	Yes	No	Instructor's Comments

1. Client assessment data include areas of biophysical, psychosocial, environmental, self-care, and/or discharge planning.
2. Appropriate assessment techniques used (interviewing, questioning).
3. Assessment data are documented in appropriate manner (nursing history form, progress note, flow sheet).
4. Client diagnostic statement is accurately derived from assessment data.
5. Client diagnostic statement is verified against NANDA defining characteristics and related factors.
6. Client diagnostic statement is verified with client, significant other(s), and/or other healthcare providers.
7. Client's desired outcome is derived from the identified diagnostic statement.
8. Outcome is specific to the identified diagnostic statement.
9. Outcome is realistic in relation to the client's current and potential resources and capabilities.
10. Outcome is attainable in relation to the client's current and potential resources and capabilities.
11. Outcome includes a realistic timeframe for attainment.
12. Outcome is mutually formulated with client and/or significant other(s).
13. Plan of care includes nursing interventions based on the identified client diagnostic statement and the desired outcome.
14. Selected nursing interventions assist the client in attaining the desired outcome.
15. Interventions include monitoring the client's response to the implemented nursing interventions.
16. Interventions include monitoring the client's response toward the attainment of the outcome.
17. Interventions include the qualifiers of who, what, how, amount, time, and frequency.
18. The action verb describing the nursing intervention focuses on the nurse's behavior, not the client's.
19. Interventions are implemented in a safe manner.
20. Rationale included for a selected nursing intervention thoroughly explains the reason for selection and the desired effect of implementation.
21. Reassessment is used to revise client diagnostic statements, desired outcomes, and/or nursing interventions.
22. Evaluation includes the client's response to implemented nursing interventions.
23. Evaluation includes the client's progress toward desired outcome attainment.
24. Documentation of client care includes reassessment data.
25. Documentation of client care includes reference to nursing interventions implemented.
26. Documentation of client care includes reference to the client's response to nursing interventions.

FIGURE 8–1. Evaluation checklist for Interactive Care Plan Worksheets. (Adapted in part from ANA Standards of Clinical Nursing Practice and the Joint Commission Standards for Management of Information.)

ADMITTING PHYSICIAN'S ORDERS

Culture/sensitivity and Gram stain of foot ulcer
Random blood glucose on admission and fingerstick BG qid
CBC, electrolytes, serum lipid profile, glycosylated Hb in AM
Chest x-ray and ECG in AM
Diabeta 10 mg PO bid
Glucophage 500 mg PO qd to start—will increase gradually
Humulin N insulin 10 U q AM and hs. Begin insulin instruction for postdis-
    charge self-care if necessary
Dicloxacillin 500 mg PO q6h; start after culture obtained
Darvocet-N 100 mg q4h prn for pain
Diet—2,400 calories/three meals with two snacks
Arrange consultation with dietitian
Up in chair ad lib with feet elevated
Foot cradle for bed
Irrigate lesion L foot with NS tid, then cover with wet-to-dry sterile dressing
Vital signs bid

CLIENT ASSESSMENT DATABASE

Name: R. Simmons   **Informant:** Client
Reliability (Scale 1–4): 3
Age: 69   **DOB:** 5/3/33   **Race:** Caucasian   **Gender:** M
Adm. date: 6/28/02   **Time:** 7 PM   **From:** Home

ACTIVITY/REST

Reports (Subjective)

Occupation: Farmer
Usual activities/hobbies: Reading, playing cards. "Don't have time to do much. Anyway, I'm too tired most of the time to do anything after the chores."
Limitations imposed by illness: "I have to watch what I order if I eat out."
Sleep: Hours: 6–8 hr/night   **Naps:** No   **Aids:** No
Insomnia: "Not unless I drink coffee after supper." Usually feels rested when awakens at 4:30 AM, but has been feeling fatigued last several weeks. Up 1 or 2 times at night to void.

Exhibits (Objective)

Observed response to activity: Limps, favors L foot when walking
Mental status: Alert/active
Neuro/muscular assessment: Muscle mass/tone: Bilaterally equal/firm
Posture: Erect   **ROM:** Full all extremities
Strength: Equal three extremities/favors L leg/foot currently

CIRCULATION

Reports (Subjective)

Slow healing: Lesion L foot, 3 weeks' duration
Extremities: Numbness/tingling: "My feet feel cold and tingling like sharp pins poking the bottom of my feet when I walk the quarter mile to the mailbox."
Cough/character of sputum: Occ./white
Change in frequency/amount of urine: Yes/voiding more lately

Exhibits (Objective)

Peripheral pulses: Radials 3+; popliteal, dorsalis, postibial/pedal, all 1+
B/P: R: Lying: 146/90 **Sit:** 140/86 **Stand:** 138/90
         L: Lying: 142/88 **Sit:** 138/88 **Stand:** 138/84
Pulse: Apical: 86 **Radial:** 86 **Quality:** Strong **Rhythm:** Regular
Chest auscultations: Few wheezes clear with cough, no murmurs/rubs
Jugular vein distention: -0-
Extremities:
   Temperature: Feet cool bilat./legs warm
   Color: Skin: Legs pale
   Capillary refill: Slow both feet (approx 5 sec)
   Homans' sign: -0- **Varicosities:** Few enlarged superficial veins both calves
   Nails: Toenails thickened, yellow, brittle
   Distribution and quality of hair: Coarse hair to midcalf, none on ankles/toes
Color: General: Ruddy face/arms **Mucous membranes/lips:** Pink
Nailbeds: Blanch well **Conjunctiva and sclera:** White

EGO INTEGRITY

Reports (Subjective)

Stress factors: "Normal farmer's problems: weather, pests, bankers, etc."
Ways of handling stress: "I get busy with the chores and talk things over with my livestock, they listen pretty good."
Financial concerns: Has Medicare but no supplemental or disability insurance, needs to hire someone to do chores while here.
Relationship status: Married
Cultural factors: Rural/agrarian, eastern European descent, "American, no ethnic ties."
Religion: Protestant/practicing
Lifestyle: Middle class/self-sufficient farmer
Recent changes: No
Feelings: "I'm in control of most things, except the weather and this diabetes." Concerned re possible therapy change "from pills to shots."

Exhibits (Objective)

Emotional status: Generally calm; appears frustrated at times
Observed physiological response(s): Occasionally sighs deeply/frowns, shrugs shoulders/throws up hands, shoulders tense, fidgeting with coin

ELIMINATION

Reports (Subjective)

Usual bowel pattern: Most every PM
Last BM: Last night   **Character of stool:** Firm/brown
Bleeding: -0-   **Hemorrhoids:** -0-   **Constipation:** Occ.
Laxative used: Hot prune juice
Urinary: No problems, has been voiding more frequently/gets up 1 or 2 times to void during night
Character of urine: Pale yellow

Exhibits (Objective)

Abd. tender: No   **Soft/firm:** Soft   **Palpable mass:** None
Bowel sounds: Active all four quads

FOOD/FLUID

Reports (Subjective)

Usual diet (type): 2400 ADA (occ. "cheats" with dessert, "My wife watches it pretty closely.")
No. of meals daily: 3/1 snack
Dietary pattern:
B: Fruit juice/toast/ham/decaf coffee
L: Meat/potatoes/veg/fruit/milk
D: Meat sandwich/soup/fruit/decaf coffee
Snack: Milk/crackers at hs.   **Usual beverage:** skim milk, 2–3 cups decaf coffee, and drinks "a lot of water—several qts"
Last meal/intake: Dinner: Hot roast beef sandwich, vegetable soup, pear with cheese, decaf coffee
Loss of appetite: "Never, but lately I don't feel as hungry as usual."
Nausea/vomiting: -0-   **Food allergies:** None
Heartburn/food intolerance: Cabbage causes gas, coffee after supper causes heartburn
Mastication/swallowing probs: No   **Dentures:** Partial upper plate
Usual weight: 175   **Recent changes:** Has lost about 4 lb this month
Diuretic therapy: No

Exhibits (Objective)

Wt: 170 lb   **Ht:** 5′10″   **Build:** Stocky   **Skin turgor:** Good/leathery
Appearance of tongue: Midline, pink   **Mucous membranes:** Pink, intact
Condition of teeth/gums: Good, no irritation/bleeding noted
Breath sounds: Few wheezes cleared with cough
Bowel sounds: Active all four quads
Urine Chemstix 2%/Fingerstick 356 (Dr office) random BG drawn on adm

HYGIENE

Reports (Subjective)

Activities of daily living: Independent in all areas
Preferred time of bath: PM

Exhibits (Objective)

General appearance: Clean, shaven, short cut hair, hands rough and dry, skin on feet dry, cracked and scaly, no body odor
Scalp & eyebrows: Scaly white patches

NEUROSENSORY

Reports (Subjective)

Headache: "Occasionally behind my eyes when I worry too much."
Tingling/Numbness: Feet, once or twice a week (as noted)
Eyes: Vision loss; far-sighted, "seems a little blurry now"
Exam: 2 yr ago
Ears: Hearing loss **R:** "Some" **L:** No (has not been tested)
Nose: Epistaxis: -0- **Sense of smell:** "No problem"

Exhibits (Objective)

Mental status: Alert; oriented to time, place, person, situation
Affect: Concerned **Memory: Remote/Recent:** Clear and intact
Speech: Clear/coherent, appropriate
Pupil reaction: PERLA/small **Glasses:** Reading **Hearing Aid:** No
Handgrip/release: Strong/equal

PAIN/DISCOMFORT

Reports (Subjective)

Primary focus: Medial aspect, heel of L foot
Intensity (0–10): 4–5 **Quality:** Dull ache with occ. sharp stabbing sensation
Frequency/duration: "Seems like all the time." **Radiation:** No
Precipitating factors: Shoes, walking **How relieved:** ASA, not helping
Additional concerns: Sometimes has back pain following chores/heavy lifting, relieved by ASA/liniment rubdown; knees ache at times, uses topical heat ointment

Exhibits (Objective)

Facial grimacing: When lesion border palpated
Guarding affected area: Pulls foot away **Narrowed focus:** No
Emotional response: Tense, irritated

RESPIRATION

Reports (Subjective)

Dyspnea: -0- **Cough:** occ. morning cough, white sputum
Emphysema: -0- **Bronchitis:** -0- **Asthma:** -0- **Tuberculosis:** -0-
Smoker: Filters **Pack/day:** 1/2 **No. of pack years:** 25+
Use of respiratory aids: -0-

Exhibits (Objective)

Respiratory rate: 22 **Depth:** Good **Symmetry:** Equal, bilateral
Auscultation: Few wheezes, clear with cough

Cyanosis: -0-   **Clubbing of fingers:** -0-
Sputum characteristics: None to observe
Mentation/restlessness: Alert/oriented/relaxed

SAFETY

Reports (Subjective)

Allergies: -0-   **Blood transfusions:** -0-
Sexually transmitted disease: None
Fractures/dislocations: L clavicle, 1967, fell getting off tractor
Arthritis/unstable joints: "I think I've got some in my knees."
Back problems: Occ. lower back pain
Vision impaired: Requires glasses for reading
Hearing impaired: Slightly (R), compensates by turning "good ear" toward speaker

Exhibits (Objective)

Temperature: 99.4°F tympanic
Skin integrity: Impaired L foot   **Scars:** R inguinal, surgical
Rashes: -0-   **Bruises:** -0-   **Lacerations:** -0-   **Blisters:** -0-
Ulcerations: Medial aspect L heel, 2.5 cm diameter, approx. 3 mm deep, draining sm. amt. cream color/pink-tinged matter, no odor noted
Strength (general): Equal all extremities   **Muscle tone:** firm
ROM: Good   **Gait:** Favors L foot   **Paresthesia/Paralysis:** -0-

SEXUALITY: MALE

Reports (Subjective)

Sexually active: Yes   **Use of condoms:** No (monogamous)
Recent changes in frequency/interest: "I've been too tired lately."
Penile discharge: -0-   **Prostate disorder:** -0-   **Vasectomy:** -0-
Last proctoscopic exam: 2 yr ago   **Prostate exam:** 1 yr ago
Practice self-exam: Breast/testicles: No
Problems/concerns: "I don't have any problems, but you'd have to ask my wife if there are any complaints."

Exhibits (Objective)

Exam: Breast: no masses   **Testicles:** deferred   **Prostate:** deferred

SOCIAL INTERACTIONS

Reports (Subjective)

Marital status: Married 45 yr   **Living with:** Wife
Report of problems: None
Extended family: One daughter lives in town (30 miles away); one daughter married/grandson, living out of state
Other: Several couples, he and wife play cards/socialize 2–3 times/month
Role: Works farm alone; husband/father/grandfather
Report of concerns related to illness/condition: None until now

Coping behaviors: "My wife and I have always talked things out. You know the 11th commandment is 'Thou shalt not go to bed angry.'"

Exhibits (Objective)

Speech: Clear, intelligible
Verbal/nonverbal communication with family/SO(s): Speaks quietly with wife, looking her in the eye; relaxed posture
Family interaction patterns: Wife sitting at bedside, relaxed, both reading paper, making occasional comments to each other

TEACHING/LEARNING

Reports (Subjective)

Dominant language: English   **Second language:** no   **Literate:** Yes
Education level: 2 years of college
Health and illness beliefs/practices/customs: "I take care of the minor problems and only see the doctor when something's broken."
Advance directives: In chart
Familial risk factors/relationship:
Diabetes: Maternal uncle   **Tuberculosis:** Brother died, age 27
Heart disease: Father died, age 78, heart attack
Strokes: Mother died, age 81   **High B/P:** Mother
Prescribed medications: Drug: Diabeta **Dose:** 10 mg **Schedule:** 8 AM/6 PM. Last dose 6 PM today **Purpose:** Control diabetes
Does client take medications regularly? Yes
Home glucose monitoring: Urine: "Stopped several months ago when I ran out of TesTape. It was always negative anyway."
Nonprescription (OTC) drugs: Occ. ASA
Use of alcohol (amount/frequency): Socially, occ. beer
Tobacco: Smokes 1/2 pack/day
Admitting diagnosis (physician): Hyperglycemia with nonhealing lesion L foot
Reason for hospitalization (client): "Sore on foot and the doctor is concerned about my blood sugar, and says I'm supposed to learn this fingerstick test now."
History of current concern: "Three weeks ago I got a blister on my foot from breaking in my new boots. It got sore so I lanced it, but it isn't getting any better."
Client's expectations of this hospitalization: "Clear up this infection and control my diabetes."
Other relevant illness and/or previous hospitalizations/surgeries: 1969 R inguinal hernia repair
Evidence of failure to improve: Lesion L foot, 3 wk
Last physical exam: Complete 1 yr ago, office follow-up 6 mo ago

DISCHARGE CONSIDERATIONS (AS OF 6/28)
Anticipated discharge: 7/1/02 (3 days)
Resources: Self; wife   **Financial:** "If this doesn't take too long to heal, we got some savings to cover things."
Community supports: Diabetic Support Group (has not participated)

Anticipated lifestyle changes: Become more involved in management of condition
Assistance needed: May require farm help for several days
Teaching: Learn new medication regimen and wound care; review diet, encourage smoking cessation
Referral: Supplies: Downtown Pharmacy or AARP
Equipment: Glucometer—AARP
Follow-up: Primary care provider 1 wk after discharge to evaluate wound healing and potential need for additional changes in diabetic regimen

INTERACTIVE CARE PLAN WORKSHEET

Student Name:

NURSING DIAGNOSIS	Client's Medical Diagnosis:
DEFINITION:	
DEFINITION: CHARACTERISTICS:	
RELATED FACTORS:	
STUDENT INSTRUCTIONS:	In the space below, enter the subjective and objective data gathered during your client assessment.

A S S E S S M E N T	Subjective Data Entry	Objective Data Entry
TIME OUT!	**Student Instructions:** To be sure your client diagnostic statement written below is accurate you need to review the defining characteristics and related factors associated with the nursing diagnosis and see how your client data match. Do you have an accurate match or are additional data required, or does another nursing diagnosis need to be investigated?	
D I A G N O S I S	**CLIENT DIAGNOSTIC STATEMENT:**	Nursing Diagnosis (specify) _____ _____ **Related to** _____ _____

	Desired Outcome and Client Criteria:	The Client will:	
P L A N N I N G	**TIME OUT!**	The desired outcome must meet criteria to be accurate. The outcome must be specific, realistic, measurable, and include a time frame for completion. Does the action verb describe the client's behavior to be evaluated? Can the outcome be used in the evaluation step of the nursing process to measure the client's response to the nursing interventions listed below?	
	Interventions	Rationale for Selected Intervention and References	
E V A L U A T I O N	**TIME OUT!**	Do your interventions assist in achieving the desired outcome? Do your interventions address further monitoring of the client's response to your interventions and to the achievement of the desired outcome? Are qualifiers: when, how, amount, time, and frequency used? Is the focus of the action's verb on the nurse's actions and not on the client? Do your rationales provide sufficient reason and directions?	
	What was your client's response to the interventions?		
	Was the desired outcome achieved? ☐ Yes ☐ No	If no, what revisions to either the desired outcome or interventions would you make?	
D O C U M E N T A T I O N	Documentation Focus: Now that you have completed the evaluation, the next step is to document your care and the client's response. Use the areas below to enter your progress note information.		
	Reassessment Data:		
	Interventions Implemented:		
	Client's Response:		

INSTRUCTOR'S COMMENTS:

Worksheets for Students' Use

INTERACTIVE CARE PLAN WORKSHEET

Client's Medical Diagnosis:

NURSING DIAGNOSIS

DEFINITION:

DEFINITION: CHARACTERISTICS:

RELATED FACTORS:

STUDENT INSTRUCTIONS:

In the space below, enter the subjective and objective data gathered during your client assessment.

Subjective Data Entry

Objective Data Entry

A S S E S S M E N T

TIME OUT!

Student Instructions: To be sure your client diagnostic statement written below is accurate you need to review the defining characteristics and related factors associated with the nursing diagnosis and see how your client data match. Do you have an accurate match or are additional data required, or does another nursing diagnosis need to be investigated?

CLIENT DIAGNOSTIC STATEMENT:

Nursing Diagnosis (specify) _____

Related to _____

D I A G N O S I S

P L A N N I N G	**Desired Outcome and Client Criteria:** The Client will: **TIME OUT!** The desired outcome must meet criteria to be accurate. The outcome must be specific, realistic, measurable, and include a time frame for completion. Does the action verb describe the client's behavior to be evaluated? Can the outcome be used in the evaluation step of the nursing process to measure the client's response to the nursing interventions listed below?	**Rationale for Selected Intervention and References** **Interventions**
E V A L U A T I O N	**TIME OUT!** Do your interventions assist in achieving the desired outcome? Do your interventions address further monitoring of the client's response to your interventions and to the achievement of the desired outcome? Are qualifiers: when, how, amount, time, and frequency used? Is the focus of the action's verb on the nurse's actions and not on the client? Do your rationales provide sufficient reason and directions? **What was your client's response to the interventions?** **Was the desired outcome achieved?** If no, what revisions to either the desired outcome or interventions would you make? ☐ Yes ☐ No	
D O C U M E N T A T I O N	**Documentation Focus:** Now that you have completed the evaluation, the next step is to document your care and the client's response. Use the areas below to enter your progress note information. **Reassessment Data:** **Interventions Implemented:** **Client's Response:**	

INSTRUCTOR'S COMMENTS:

INTERACTIVE CARE PLAN WORKSHEET

Student Name:

NURSING DIAGNOSIS

Client's Medical Diagnosis:

DEFINITION:

DEFINITION: CHARACTERISTICS:

RELATED FACTORS:

STUDENT INSTRUCTIONS:

In the space below, enter the subjective and objective data gathered during your client assessment.

Subjective Data Entry

Objective Data Entry

A S S E S S M E N T

TIME OUT!

Student Instructions: To be sure your client diagnostic statement written below is accurate you need to review the defining characteristics and related factors associated with the nursing diagnosis and see how your client data match. Do you have an accurate match or are additional data required, or does another nursing diagnosis need to be investigated?

CLIENT DIAGNOSTIC STATEMENT:

D I A G N O S I S

Nursing Diagnosis (specify) _____

_____

Related to _____

_____

	Desired Outcome and Client Criteria:	The Client will:
P L A N N I N G	**TIME OUT!** The desired outcome must meet criteria to be accurate. The outcome must be specific, realistic, measurable, and include a time frame for completion. Does the action verb describe the client's behavior to be evaluated? Can the outcome be used in the evaluation step of the nursing process to measure the client's response to the nursing interventions listed below?	
	Interventions	Rationale for Selected Intervention and References
E V A L U A T I O N	**TIME OUT!** Do your interventions assist in achieving the desired outcome? Do your interventions address further monitoring of the client's response to your interventions and to the achievement of the desired outcome? Are qualifiers: when, how, amount, time, and frequency used? Is the focus of the action's verb on the nurse's actions and not on the client? Do your rationales provide sufficient reason and directions?	
	What was your client's response to the interventions?	
	Was the desired outcome achieved? ☐ Yes ☐ No If no, what revisions to either the desired outcome or interventions would you make?	
D O C U M E N T A T I O N	**Documentation Focus:** Now that you have completed the evaluation, the next step is to document your care and the client's response. Use the areas below to enter your progress note information.	
	Reassessment Data:	
	Interventions Implemented:	
	Client's Response:	

INSTRUCTOR'S COMMENTS:

INTERACTIVE CARE PLAN WORKSHEET

Student Name:

NURSING DIAGNOSIS				Client's Medical Diagnosis:
DEFINITION:				
DEFINITION: CHARACTERISTICS:				
RELATED FACTORS:				
STUDENT INSTRUCTIONS:			In the space below, enter the subjective and objective data gathered during your client assessment.	

A S S E S S M E N T

Subjective Data Entry	Objective Data Entry

TIME OUT!

Student Instructions: To be sure your client diagnostic statement written below is accurate you need to review the defining characteristics and related factors associated with the nursing diagnosis and see how your client data match. Do you have an accurate match or are additional data required, or does another nursing diagnosis need to be investigated?

D I A G N O S I S

CLIENT DIAGNOSTIC STATEMENT:	Nursing Diagnosis (specify) _____ _____ Related to _____ _____

	Desired Outcome and Client Criteria: The Client will:	**Rationale for Selected Intervention and References**
P L A N N I N G	**TIME OUT!** The desired outcome must meet criteria to be accurate. The outcome must be specific, realistic, measurable, and include a time frame for completion. Does the action verb describe the client's behavior to be evaluated? Can the outcome be used in the evaluation step of the nursing process to measure the client's response to the nursing interventions listed below?	
	Interventions	
E V A L U A T I O N	**TIME OUT!** Do your interventions assist in achieving the desired outcome? Do your interventions address further monitoring of the client's response to your interventions and to the achievement of the desired outcome? Are qualifiers: when, how, amount, time, and frequency used? Is the focus of the action's verb on the nurse's actions and not on the client? Do your rationales provide sufficient reason and directions?	
	What was your client's response to the interventions?	
	Was the desired outcome achieved? ☐ Yes ☐ No If no, what revisions to either the desired outcome or interventions would you make?	
D O C U M E N T A T I O N	**Documentation Focus:** Now that you have completed the evaluation, the next step is to document your care and the client's response. Use the areas below to enter your progress note information.	
	Reassessment Data:	
	Interventions Implemented:	
	Client's Response:	

INSTRUCTOR'S COMMENTS:

North American Nursing Diagnosis Association (NANDA) Nursing Diagnoses with Definitions, Related/Risk Factors, and Defining Characteristics

Activity Intolerance

DEFINITION: Insufficient physiological or psychological energy to endure or complete required or desired daily activities

RELATED FACTORS: ° Generalized weakness ° Sedentary lifestyle ° Bedrest or immobility ° Imbalance between oxygen supply and demand ° [Cognitive deficits/emotional status; secondary to underlying disease process/depression] ° [Pain, vertigo, extreme stress]

DEFINING CHARACTERISTICS

Subjective: ° Report of fatigue or weakness ° Exertional discomfort or dyspnea ° [Verbalizes no desire and/or lack of interest in activity]

Objective: ° Abnormal heart rate or blood pressure response to activity ° Electrocardiographic changes reflecting dysrhythmias or ischemia ° [Pallor, cyanosis]

Functional Level Classification (Gordon, 1987):

Level I: Walk, regular pace, on level indefinitely; one flight or more but more short of breath than normally

Level II: Walk one city block [or] 500 ft on level; climb one flight slowly without stopping

Level III: Walk no more than 50 ft on level without stopping; unable to climb one flight of stairs without stopping

Level IV: Dyspnea and fatigue at rest

NOTE: Information appearing in [ ] has been added by the authors to clarify and facilitate the use of nursing diagnoses.

Activity Intolerance, risk for*

DEFINITION: At risk of experiencing insufficient physiological or psychological energy to endure or complete required or desired daily activities

RISK FACTORS: ◦ History of previous intolerance ◦ Presence of circulatory/respiratory problems ◦ Deconditioned status ◦ Inexperience with the activity ◦ [Diagnosis of progressive disease state/debilitating condition such as cancer, multiple sclerosis—MS; extensive surgical procedures] ◦ [Verbalized reluctance/inability to perform expected activity]

Adjustment, impaired

DEFINITION: Inability to modify lifestyle/behavior in a manner consistent with a change in health status

RELATED FACTORS: ◦ Disability or health status requiring change in lifestyle ◦ Multiple stressors; intense emotional state ◦ Low state of optimism; negative attitudes toward health behavior; lack of motivation to change behaviors ◦ Failure to intend to change behavior ◦ Absence of social support for changed beliefs and practices ◦ [Physical and/or learning disability]

DEFINING CHARACTERISTICS

SUBJECTIVE: ◦ Denial of health status change ◦ Failure to achieve optimal sense of control

OBJECTIVE: ◦ Failure to take actions that would prevent further health problems ◦ Demonstration of nonacceptance of health status change

Airway Clearance, ineffective

DEFINITION: Inability to clear secretions or obstructions from the respiratory tract to maintain a clear airway

RELATED FACTORS:

Environmental: ◦ Smoking ◦ Second-hand smoke ◦ Smoke inhalation

Obstructed airway: ◦ Retained secretions ◦ Secretions in the bronchi ◦ Exudate in the alveoli ◦ Excessive mucus ◦ Airway spasm ◦ Foreign body in airway ◦ Presence of artificial airway

Physiological: ◦ Chronic obstructive pulmonary disease (COPD) ◦ Asthma ◦ Allergic airways ◦ Hyperplasia of the bronchial walls ◦ Neuromuscular dysfunction ◦ Infection

DEFINING CHARACTERISTICS

Subjective: ◦ Dyspnea

Objective: ◦ Diminished or adventitious breath sounds (rales, crackles, rhonchi, wheezes) ◦ Cough, ineffective or absent ◦ Sputum production ◦ Changes in respiratory rate and rhythm ◦ Difficulty vocalizing ◦ Wide-eyed ◦ Restlessness ◦ Orthopnea ◦ Cyanosis

Allergy Response, latex

DEFINITION: An allergic response to natural latex rubber products

RELATED FACTORS: ◦ No immune mechanism response [although this is true of irritant and allergic contact dermatitis, type I/immediate reaction is a true allergic response]

DEFINING CHARACTERISTICS

Type I reactions [hypersensitivity; IgE-mediated reaction]: ◦ Immediate reaction (< 1 hour) to latex proteins (can be life threatening) ◦ Contact urticaria progressing to generalized symptoms ◦ Edema of the lips, tongue, uvula, and/or throat ◦ Shortness of breath, tightness in chest, wheezing, bronchospasm leading to respira-

---

NOTE: Information appearing in [ ] has been added by the authors to clarify and facilitate the use of nursing diagnoses.

*[Note: A risk diagnosis is not evidenced by signs and symptoms because the problem has not yet occurred, and nursing interventions are directed at prevention. Therefore, risk factors present are noted instead.]

tory arrest; hypotension, syncope, cardiac arrest ○ May also include: ○ *Orofacial characteristics—* edema of sclera or eyelids; erythema and/or itching of the eyes; tearing of the eyes; nasal congestion, itching, and/or erythema; rhinorrhea; facial erythema; facial itching; oral itching; ○ *Gastrointestinal characteristics—*abdominal pain; nausea; ○ *Generalized characteristics—*flushing; general discomfort; generalized edema; increasing complaint of total body warmth; restlessness

Type IV reactions [chemical and delayed-type hypersensitivity]: ○ Delayed onset (hours) ○ Eczema ○ Irritation ○ Reaction to additives (e.g., thiurams, carbamates) causes discomfort ○ Redness

IRRITANT [CONTACT DERMATITIS] REACTIONS: ○ Erythema; [dry, crusty, hard bumps] ○ Chapped or cracked skin ○ Blisters

Allergy Response, latex, risk for

DEFINITION: At risk for allergic response to natural latex rubber products

RISK FACTORS: ○ History of reactions to latex (e.g., balloons, condoms, gloves) ○ Allergies to bananas, avocados, tropical fruits, kiwi, chestnuts, poinsettia plants ○ History of allergies and asthma ○ Professions with daily exposure to latex (e.g., medicine, nursing, dentistry) ○ Conditions associated with continuous or intermittent catheterization ○ Multiple surgical procedures, especially from infancy (e.g., spina bifida)

Anxiety [mild, moderate, severe, panic]

DEFINITION: Vague uneasy feeling of discomfort or dread accompanied by an autonomic response (the source often nonspecific or unknown to the individual); a feeling of apprehension caused by

anticipation of danger. It is an altering signal that warns of impending danger and enables the individual to take measures to deal with threat

RELATED FACTORS: ○ Unconscious conflict about essential [beliefs]/goals and values of life ○ Situational/maturational crises ○ Stress ○ Familial association/heredity ○ Interpersonal transmission/contagion ○ Threat to self-concept [perceived or actual] ○ [Unconscious conflict] ○ Threat of death [perceived or actual] ○ Threat to or change in health status [progressive/debilitating disease, terminal illness], interaction patterns, role function/status, environment [safety], economic status ○ Unmet needs ○ Exposure to toxins ○ Substance abuse ○ [Positive or negative self-talk] ○ [Physiological factors, such as hyperthyroidism, pheochromocytoma, drug therapy including steroids, and so on]

DEFINING CHARACTERISTICS

Subjective: Behavioral: ○ Expressed concerns due to change in life events

Objective: Behavioral: ○ Poor eye contact ○ Glancing about ○ Scanning and vigilance ○ Extraneous movement (e.g., foot shuffling, hand/arm movements) ○ Fidgeting ○ Restless-ness ○ Diminished productivity ○ [Crying/tearfulness] ○ [Pacing/purposeless activity] ○ [Immobility]

Subjective: Affective: ○ Regretful ○ Scared ○ Rattled ○ Distressed ○ Apprehension ○ Uncertainty ○ Fearful; feelings of inadequacy ○ Anxious ○ Jittery ○ [Sense of impending doom] ○ [Hopelessness]

Objective: Affective: ○ Increased wariness ○ Focus on self ○ Irritability ○ Overexcited ○ Anguish ○ Painful and persistent increased helplessness

Subjective: Cognitive: ○ Fear of unspecific consequences ○ Awareness of physiological symptoms

---

NOTE: Information appearing in [ ] has been added by the authors to clarify and facilitate the use of nursing diagnoses.

Objective: Cognitive: ○ Preoccupation ○ Impaired attention ○ Difficulty concentrating ○ Forgetfulness ○ Diminished ability to problem-solve ○ Diminished learning ability ○ Rumination ○ Tendency to blame others ○ Blocking of thought ○ Confusion ○ Decreased perceptual field

Subjective: Physiological: ○ Shakiness ○ Worried ○ Regretful ○ Dry mouth (s) ○ Tingling in extremities (p) ○ Heart pounding (s) ○ Nausea (p) ○ Abdominal pain (p) ○ Diarrhea (p) ○ Urinary hesitancy (p) ○ Urinary frequency (p) ○ Faintness (p) ○ Weakness (s) ○ Decreased pulse (p) ○ Respiratory difficulties (s) ○ Fatigue (p) ○ Sleep disturbance (p) ○ [Chest, back, neck pain]

Objective: Physiological: ○ Voice quivering; trembling/hand tremors ○ Increased tension ○ Facial tension ○ Increased pulse ○ Increased perspiration ○ Cardiovascular excitation (s) ○ Facial flushing (s) ○ Superficial vasoconstriction (s) ○ Increased blood pressure (s) ○ Twitching (s) ○ Increased reflexes (s) ○ Urinary urgency (p) ○ Decreased blood pressure (p) ○ Insomnia ○ Anorexia (s) ○ Increased respiration (s)

Anxiety, death

DEFINITION: Apprehension, worry, or fear related to death or dying

RELATED FACTORS: To be developed by NANDA

DEFINING CHARACTERISTICS

Subjective: ○ *Fear of:* Developing a terminal illness ○ The process of dying ○ Loss of physical and/or mental abilities when dying ○ Premature death because it prevents the accomplishment of important life goals ○ Leaving family alone after death ○ Delayed demise ○ Negative death images or unpleasant thought about any event related to death or dying ○ Anticipated pain related to dying ○ Powerlessness over issues related to dying ○ Total loss of control over any aspect of one's own death ○ *Worrying about:* The impact of one's own death on SOs; being the cause of other's grief and suffering ○ Concerns of overworking the caregiver as terminal illness incapacitates self ○ Concern about meeting one's creator or feeling doubtful about the existence of God or higher being ○ Denial of one's own mortality or impending death

Objective: ○ Deep sadness

Aspiration, risk for

DEFINITION: At risk for entry of gastrointestinal secretions, oropharyngeal secretions, or [exogenous food] solids or fluids into tracheobronchial passages [due to dysfunction or absence of normal protective mechanisms]

RISK FACTORS: ○ Reduced level of consciousness ○ Depressed cough and gag reflexes ○ Impaired swallowing [owing to inability of the epiglottis and true vocal cords to move to close off trachea] ○ Facial/oral/neck surgery or trauma ○ Wired jaws ○ Situation hindering elevation of upper body [weakness, paralysis] ○ Incomplete lower esophageal sphincter [hiatal hernia or other esophageal disease affecting stomach valve function] ○ Delayed gastric emptying ○ Decreased gastrointestinal motility ○ Increased intragastric pressure ○ Increased gastric residual ○ Presence of tracheostomy or endotracheal (ET) tube; [inadequate (or over-) inflation of tracheostomy/ET tube cuff] ○ [Presence of] gastrointestinal tubes ○ Tube feedings/medication administration

---

NOTE: Information appearing in [ ] has been added by the authors to clarify and facilitate the use of nursing diagnoses.
(s) - sympathetic; (p) = parasympathetic

Attachment, risk for impaired parent/infant/child

DEFINITION: Disruption of the interactive process between parent/significant other and infant that fosters the development of a protective and nurturing reciprocal relationship

RISK FACTORS: ○ Inability of parents to meet personal needs ○ Anxiety associated with the parent role ○ Substance abuse ○ Premature infant ○ Ill infant/child who is unable to effectively initiate parental contact due to altered behavioral organization ○ Separation ○ Physical barriers ○ Lack of privacy ○ [Parents who themselves experienced altered attachment] ○ [Uncertainty of paternity; conception as a result of rape/sexual abuse] ○ [Difficult pregnancy and/or birth (actual or perceived)]

Autonomic Dysreflexia

DEFINITION: Life-threatening, uninhibited sympathetic response of the nervous system to a noxious stimulus after a spinal cord injury [SCI] at T7 or above

RELATED FACTORS: ○ Bladder or bowel distention ○ [Catheter insertion, obstruction, irrigation] ○ Skin irritation ○ Lack of patient and caregiver knowledge ○ [Sexual excitation] ○ [Environmental temperature extremes]

DEFINING CHARACTERISTICS

Subjective: ○ Headache (a diffuse pain in different portions of the head and not confined to any nerve distribution area) ○ Paresthesia ○ Chilling ○ Blurred vision ○ Chest pain ○ Metallic taste in mouth ○ Nasal congestion

Objective: ○ Paroxysmal hypertension (sudden periodic elevated blood pressure in which systolic pressure >140 mm Hg and diastolic >90 mm Hg) ○ Bradycardia or tachycardia (heart rate <60 or >100 beats per minute, respectively) ○ Diaphoresis (above the injury) ○ Red splotches on skin (above the injury) ○ Pallor (below the injury) ○ Horner's syndrome (contraction of the pupil, partial ptosis of the eyelid ○ enophthalmos and sometimes loss of sweating over the affected side of the face) ○ Conjunctival congestion ○ Pilomotor reflex (gooseflesh formation when skin is cooled)

Autonomic Dysreflexia, risk for

DEFINITION: At risk for life-threatening, uninhibited response of the sympathetic nervous system post spinal shock, in an individual with a spinal cord injury [SCI] or lesion at T6 or above (has been demonstrated in patients with injuries at T7 and T8)

RISK FACTORS:

Musculoskeletal—Integumentary Stimuli: ○ Cutaneous stimulations (e.g., pressure ulcer, ingrown toenail, dressing, burns, rash) ○ Sunburns ○ Wounds ○ Pressure over bony prominences or genitalia ○ Range of motion exercises ○ Spasms ○ Fractures ○ Heterotrophic bone

Gastrointestinal Stimuli: ○ Constipation ○ Difficult passage of feces ○ Fecal impaction ○ Bowel distention ○ Hemorrhoids ○ Digital stimulation ○ Suppositories ○ Enemas ○ Gastrointestinal system pathology ○ Esophageal reflux ○ Gastric ulcers ○ Gallstones

Urologic Stimuli: ○ Bladder distention/spasm ○ Detrusor sphincter dyssynergia ○ Instrumentation or surgery; calculi ○ Urinary tract infection ○ Cystitis ○ Urethritis ○ Epididymitis

Regulatory Stimuli: ○ Temperature fluctuations ○ Extreme environmental temperatures

Situational Stimuli: ○ Positioning ○ Surgical procedure ○ Constrictive clothing (e.g., straps,

NOTE: Information appearing in [ ] has been added by the authors to clarify and facilitate the use of nursing diagnoses.

stockings, shoes) ○ Drug reactions (e.g., decongestants, sympathomimetics, vasoconstrictors, narcotic withdrawal)

Neurological Stumuli: ○ Painful or irritating stimuli below the level of injury ○ Cardiac/pulmonary problems ○ Pulmonary emboli ○ Deep vein thrombosis

Reproductive [and Sexuality] Stimuli: ○ Sexual intercourse ○ Ejaculation ○ Menstruation ○ Pregnancy ○ Labor and delivery ○ Ovarian cyst

Body Image, disturbed

DEFINITION: Confusion in mental picture of one's physical self

RELATED FACTORS: ○ Biophysical illness ○ Trauma or injury ○ Surgery ○ [Mutilation, pregnancy] ○ Illness treatment [change caused by biochemical agents (drugs), dependence on machine] ○ Psychosocial ○ Cultural or spiritual ○ Cognitive/perceptual ○ Developmental changes ○ [Significance of body part or functioning with regard to age, sex, developmental level, or basic human needs] ○ [Maturational changes]

DEFINING CHARACTERISTICS

Subjective: ○ Verbalization of feelings/perceptions that reflect an altered view of one's body in appearance, structure, or function ○ Change in lifestyle ○ Fear of rejection or of reaction by others ○ Focus on past strength, function, or appearance ○ Negative feelings about body (e.g., feelings of helplessness, hopelessness, or powerlessness) ○ [Depersonalization/grandiosity] ○ Preoccupation with change or loss ○ Refusal to verify actual change ○ Emphasis on remaining strengths ○ Heightened achievement ○ Personalization of part or loss by name ○ Depersonalization of part or loss by impersonal pronouns

Objective: ○ Missing body part ○ Actual change in structure and/or function ○ Nonverbal response to actual or perceived change in structure and/or function ○ Behaviors of avoidance, monitoring, or acknowledgment of one's body ○ Not looking at/not touching body part ○ Trauma to nonfunctioning part ○ Change in ability to estimate spatial relationship of body to environment ○ Extension of body boundary to incorporate environmental objects ○ Hiding or overexposing body part (intentional or unintentional) ○ Change in social involvement ○ [Aggression; low frustration tolerance level]

Body Temperature, risk for imbalanced

DEFINITION: At risk for failure to maintain body temperature within normal range

RISK FACTORS: ○ Extremes of age, weight ○ Exposure to cold/cool or warm/hot environments ○ Dehydration ○ Inactivity or vigorous activity ○ Medications causing vasoconstriction/vasodilation ○ Altered metabolic rate ○ Sedation ○ [Use or overdose of certain drugs or exposure to anesthesia] ○ Inappropriate clothing for environmental temperature ○ Illness or trauma affecting temperature regulation [e.g., infections, systemic or localized; neoplasms, tumors; collagen/ vascular disease]

Bowel Incontinence

DEFINITION: Change in normal bowel habits characterized by involuntary passage of stool

RELATED FACTORS: ○ Self-care deficit—toileting ○ Impaired cognition ○ Immobility ○ Environmental factors (e.g., inaccessible bathroom) ○ Dietary habits ○ Medications ○ Laxative abuse ○ Stress ○ Colorectal lesions ○ Incomplete emptying of bowel ○ Impaction ○ Chronic diarrhea ○ General decline in muscle

---

NOTE: Information appearing in [ ] has been added by the authors to clarify and facilitate the use of nursing diagnoses.

tone ∘ Abnormally high abdominal or intestinal pressure ∘ Impaired reservoir capacity ∘ Rectal sphincter abnormality ∘ Loss of rectal sphincter control ∘ Lower/upper motor nerve damage

DEFINING CHARACTERISTICS

Subjective: ∘ Recognizes rectal fullness but reports inability to expel formed stool ∘ Urgency ∘ Inability to delay defecation ∘ Self-report of inability to feel rectal fullness

Objective: ∘ Constant dribbling of soft stool ∘ Fecal staining of clothing and/or bedding ∘ Fecal odor ∘ Red perianal skin ∘ Inability to recognize inattention to urge to defecate

Breastfeeding, effective

DEFINITION: Mother-infant dyad/ family exhibits adequate proficiency and satisfaction with breast-feeding process

RELATED FACTORS: ∘ Basic breastfeeding knowledge ∘ Normal breast structure ∘ Normal infant oral structure ∘ Infant gestational age greater than 34 weeks ∘ Support sources [available] ∘ Maternal confidence

DEFINING CHARACTERISTICS

Subjective: ∘ Maternal verbalization of satisfaction with the breastfeeding process

Objective: ∘ Mother able to position infant at breast to promote a successful latch-on response ∘ Infant is content after feedings ∘ Regular and sustained suckling/swallowing at the breast [e.g., 8–10 times/24 h] ∘ Appropriate infant weight patterns for age ∘ Effective mother/infant communication pattern (infant cues, maternal interpretation and response) ∘ Signs and/or symptoms of oxytocin release (letdown or milk ejection reflex) ∘ Adequate infant elimination patterns for age; [stools soft; more than 6 wet diapers/day of unconcentrated urine] ∘ Eagerness of infant to nurse

Breastfeeding, ineffective

DEFINITION: Dissatisfaction or difficulty a mother, infant, or child experiences with the breastfeeding process

RELATED FACTORS: ∘ Prematurity ∘ Infant anomaly ∘ Poor infant sucking reflex ∘ Infant receiving [numerous or repeated] supplemental feedings with artificial nipple ∘ Maternal anxiety or ambivalence ∘ Knowledge deficit ∘ Previous history of breastfeeding failure ∘ Interruption in breastfeeding ∘ Nonsupportive partner/family ∘ Maternal breast anomaly ∘ Previous breast surgery ∘ [Painful nipples/breast engorgement]

DEFINING CHARACTERISTICS

Subjective: ∘ Unsatisfactory breastfeeding process ∘ Persistence of sore nipples beyond the first week of breastfeeding ∘ Insufficient emptying of each breast per feeding ∘ Actual or perceived inadequate milk supply

Objective: ∘ Observable signs of inadequate infant intake [decrease in number of wet diapers, inappropriate weight loss or inadequate gain] ∘ Nonsustained or insufficient opportunity for suckling at the breast ∘ Infant inability [failure] to attach onto maternal breast correctly ∘ Infant arching and crying at the breast ∘ Resistant latching on ∘ Infant exhibiting fussiness and crying within the first hour after breastfeeding ∘ Unresponsive to other comfort measures ∘ No observable signs of oxytocin release

Breastfeeding, interrupted

DEFINITION: Break in the continuity of the breastfeeding process as a result of inability or inadvisability to put baby to breast for feeding

RELATED FACTORS: ∘ Maternal or infant illness ∘ Prematurity ∘ Maternal employment ∘ Contraindications to breastfeeding (e.g., drugs, true breast milk jaundice) ∘ Need to abruptly wean infant

---

NOTE: Information appearing in [ ] has been added by the authors to clarify and facilitate the use of nursing diagnoses.

DEFINING CHARACTERISTICS

Subjective: ○ Infant does not receive nourishment at the breast for some or all of feedings ○ Maternal desire to maintain lactation and provide (or eventually provide) her breast milk for her infant's nutritional needs ○ Lack of knowledge regarding expression and storage of breast milk

Objective: ○ Separation of mother and infant

Breathing Pattern, ineffective

DEFINITION: Inspiration and/or expiration that does not provide adequate ventilation

RELATED FACTORS: ○ Neuromuscular dysfunction; SCI; neurological immaturity ○ Musculoskeletal impairment ○ Bony/chest wall deformity ○ Anxiety ○ Pain ○ Perception/cognitive impairment ○ Decreased energy/fatigue ○ Respiratory muscle fatigue ○ Body position; ○ Obesity ○ Hyperventilation; hypoventilation syndrome; [alteration of patient's normal $O_2:CO_2$ ratio (e.g., O_2 therapy in COPD)]

DEFINING CHARACTERISTICS

Subjective: ○ Shortness of breath

Objective: ○ Dyspnea; orthopnea ○ Respiratory rate: Adults (age 14 or greater) <11 or [>]24, Children 1–4 yr <20 or >30, 5–14 yr <15 or >25, Infants 0–12 mo <25 or >60 ○ Depth of breathing: Adults VT500 mL at rest, Infants 6–8 mL/kg ○ Timing ratio; prolonged expiration phases ○ Pursed-lip breathing ○ Decreased minute ventilation; vital capacity ○ Decreased inspiratory/expiratory pressure ○ Use of accessory muscles to breathe; assumption of three-point position ○ Altered chest excursion; [Paradoxical breathing patterns] ○ Nasal flaring; [grunting] ○ Increased anterior-posterior diameter

Cardiac Output, decreased

DEFINITION: Inadequate blood pumped by the heart to meet the metabolic demands of the body. [Note: In a hypermetabolic state, although cardiac output may be within normal range, it may still be inadequate to meet the needs of the body's tissues. Cardiac output and tissue perfusion are interrelated, although there are differences. When cardiac output is decreased, tissue perfusion problems will develop; however, tissue perfusion problems can exist without decreased cardiac output.]

RELATED FACTORS: ○ Altered heart rate/rhythm, [conduction] ○ *Altered stroke volume:* ○ Altered preload [e.g., decreased venous return] ○ Altered afterload [e.g., altered systemic vascular resistance] ○ Altered contractility [e.g., ventricular-septal rupture, ventricular aneurysm, papillary muscle rupture, valvular disease]

DEFINING CHARACTERISTICS

Subjective: ○ *Altered Heart Rate/Rhythm:* ○ Palpitations ○ *Altered Preload:* ○ Fatigue ○ *Altered Afterload:* ○ Shortness of breath/dyspnea ○ *Altered Contractility:* ○ Orthopnea/paroxysmal nocturnal dyspnea **[PND]** ○ *Behavioral/Emotional:* ○ Anxiety

Objective: ○ *Altered Heart Rate/Rhythm:* ○ [Dys]arrhythmias (tachycardia, bradycardia) ○ ECG changes ○ *Altered Preload:* ○ Jugular vein distention (JVD) ○ Edema ○ Weight gain ○ Increased/decreased central venous pressure (CVP ○ Increased/decreased pulmonary artery wedge pressure (PAWP) ○ Murmurs ○ *Altered Afterload:* ○ Cold, clammy skin ○ Skin [and mucous membrane] color changes [cyanosis, pallor] ○ Prolonged capillary refill ○ Decreased peripheral pulses ○ Variations in blood pressure readings ○ Increased/decreased systemic vascular resistance (SVR)/pulmonary vascular resistance (PVR) ○ Oliguria; [anuria]

NOTE: Information appearing in [ ] has been added by the authors to clarify and facilitate the use of nursing diagnoses.

○ *Altered Contractility:* ○ Crackles; cough ○ Cardiac output <4L/min ○ Cardiac index <2.5L/min; ○ Decreased ejection fraction, stroke volume index (SVI), left ventricular stroke work index (LVSWI); S₃ or S₄ sounds [gallop rhythm] ○ *Behavorial/Emotional:* ○ Restlessness

Caregiver Role Strain

DEFINITION: Difficulty in performing caregiver role

RELATED FACTORS

Care Receiver Health Status: ○ Illness severity/chronicity ○ Unpredictability of illness course ○ Instability of care receiver's health ○ Increasing care needs and/dependency ○ Problem behaviors ○ Psychological or cognitive problems ○ Addiction or codependency of care receiver

Caregiving Activities: ○ Discharge of family member to home with significant care needs [e.g., premature birth/congenital defect] ○ Unpredictability of care situation ○ 24-hour care responsibility ○ Amount/complexity of activity ○ Ongoing changes in activities; years of caregiving

Caregiver Health Status: ○ Physical problems ○ Psychological or cognitive problems ○ Inability to fulfill one's own or others' expectations ○ Unrealistic expectations of self ○ Marginal coping patterns ○ Addiction or codependency

Socioeconomic: ○ Competing role commitments ○ Alienation from family, friends, and coworkers ○ Isolation from others ○ Insufficient recreation

Caregiver–Care Receiver Relationship: ○ Unrealistic expectations of caregiver by care receiver ○ History of poor relationship ○ Mental status of elder inhibits conversation ○ Presence of abuse or violence

Family Processes: ○ History of marginal family coping/dysfunction

Resources: ○ Inadequate physical environment for providing care (e.g., housing, temperature, safety) ○ Inadequate equipment for providing care ○ Inadequate transportation ○ Insufficient finances ○ Inexperience with caregiving ○ Insufficient time; physical energy; emotional strength ○ Lack of support ○ Lack of caregiver privacy ○ Lack of knowledge about or difficulty accessing community resources ○ Inadequate community services (e.g., respite care. recreational resources) ○ Assistance and support (formal and informal) ○ Caregiver is not developmentally ready for caregiver role

[Authors' note: The presence of this problem may encompass other numerous problems/high-risk concerns such as Diversional Activity, deficient; Sleep Pattern disturbance; Fatigue; Anxiety; Coping, ineffective; Family Coping; Decisional Conflict; Denial, ineffective; Grieving, anticipatory/[actual]; Hopelessness; Powerlessness; Spiritual Distress; Health Maintenance, ineffective; Home Maintenance, impaired; Sexuality Patterns, ineffective; Family Coping: readiness for enhanced; Family Processes, interrupted; Social Isolation. Careful attention to data gathering will identify and clarify the client's specific needs, which can then be coordinated under this single diagnostic label.]

DEFINING CHARACTERISTICS

Subjective: Caregiving Activities: ○ Apprehension about possible institutionalization of care receiver, the future regarding care receiver's health and caregiver's ability to provide care, care receiver's care if caregiver becomes ill or dies

Objective: Caregiving Activities: ○ Difficulty performing/completing required tasks ○ Preoccupation with care routine ○ Dysfunctional change in caregiving activities

---

NOTE: Information appearing in [ ] has been added by the authors to clarify and facilitate the use of nursing diagnoses.

Subjective: Caregiver Health Status—physical:
○ GI upset (e.g., mild stomach cramps, vomiting, diarrhea, recurrent gastric ulcer episodes) ○ Weight change ○ Rash ○ Headaches ○ Hypertension ○ Cardiovascular disease ○ Diabetes ○ Fatigue

Objective: Caregiver Health Status—emotional:
○ Impatience ○ Increased emotional lability ○ Somatization ○ Impaired individual coping

Subjective: Emotional: ○ Feeling depressed; anger; stress; frustration; increased nervousness ○ Disturbed sleep ○ Lack of time to meet personal needs

Subjective: Socioeconomic: ○ Changes in leisure activities ○ Refuses career advancement

Objective: Socioeconomic: ○ Low work productivity; withdraws from social life

Subjective: Caregiver–Care Receiver Relationship:
○ Difficulty watching care receiver go through the illness ○ Grief/uncertainty regarding changed relationship with care receiver

Subjective: Family Processes Caregiving Activities:
○ Concern about family members

Objective: Family Processes: ○ Family conflict
[Authors' note: Although objective characteristics were not included in the NANDA diagnosis, if caregiver is in a state of denial, subjective statements may not be made by caregiver; however, statements of care receiver and observations of family members and/or other healthcare providers may indicate presence of problem.]

Caregiver Role Strain, risk for

DEFINITION: Caregiver is vulnerable for felt difficulty in performing the family caregiver role

RISK FACTORS: ○ Illness severity of the care receiver ○ Psychological or cognitive problems in care receiver ○ Addiction or codependency ○ Discharge of family member with significant home-care needs ○ Premature birth/congenital defect ○ Unpredictable illness course or instability in the care receiver's health ○ Duration of caregiving required ○ Inexperience with caregiving ○ Complexity/number of caregiving tasks ○ Caregiver's competing role commitments ○ Caregiver health impairment ○ Caregiver is female/spouse ○ Caregiver not developmentally ready for caregiver role (e.g., a young adult needing to provide care for middle-aged parent) ○ Developmental delay or retardation of the care receiver or caregiver ○ Presence of situational stressors that normally affect families (e.g., significant loss, disaster or crisis, economic vulnerability, major life events [such as birth, hospitalization, leaving home, returning home, marriage, divorce, change in employment, retirement, death]) ○ Inadequate physical environment for providing care (e.g., housing, transportation, community services, equipment) ○ Family/caregiver isolation ○ Lack of respite and recreation for caregiver ○ Marginal family adaptation or dysfunction prior to the caregiving situation ○ Marginal caregiver's coping patterns ○ Past history of poor relationship between caregiver and care receiver ○ Care receiver exhibits deviant, bizarre behavior ○ Presence of abuse or violence

Communication, impaired verbal

DEFINITION: Decreased, delayed, or absent ability to receive, process, transmit, and use a system of symbols

RELATED FACTORS: ○ Decrease in circulation to brain ○ Brain tumor ○ Anatomic deficit (e.g., cleft palate, alteration of the neurovascular visual system, auditory system, or phonatory apparatus) ○ Difference related to developmental age ○ Physical barrier (tracheostomy, intubation) ○ Physiological conditions [e.g., dyspnea]

NOTE: Information appearing in [ ] has been added by the authors to clarify and facilitate the use of nursing diagnoses.

○ Alteration of CNS ○ Weakening of the musculoskeletal system ○ Psychological barriers (e.g., psychosis, lack of stimuli) ○ Emotional conditions [depression, panic, anger]; stress ○ Environmental barriers ○ Cultural difference ○ Lack of information ○ Side effects of medication ○ Alteration of self-esteem or self-concept ○ Altered perceptions ○ Absence of SOs

DEFINING CHARACTERISTICS

Subjective: ○ [Reports of difficulty expressing self]

Objective: ○ Unable to speak dominant language ○ Speaks or verbalizes with difficulty ○ Does not or cannot speak ○ Disorientation in the three spheres of time, space, person ○ Stuttering ○ Slurring ○ Dyspnea ○ Difficulty forming words or sentences (e.g., phonia, dyslalia, dysarthria) ○ Difficulty expressing thoughts verbally (e.g., aphasia, dysphasia, apraxia, dyslexia) ○ Inappropriate verbalization, [incessant, loose association of ideas, flight of ideas] ○ Difficulty in comprehending and maintaining the usual communicating pattern ○ Absence of eye contact or difficulty in selective attending ○ Partial or total visual deficit ○ Inability or difficulty in use of facial or body expressions ○ Willful refusal to speak ○ [Inability to modulate speech] ○ [Message inappropriate to content] ○ [Use of nonverbal cues (e.g., pleading eyes, gestures, turning away)] ○ [Frustration, anger, hostility]

Conflict, decisional (specify)

DEFINITION: Uncertainty about course of action to be taken when choice among competing actions involves risk, loss, or challenge to personal life values

RELATED FACTORS: ○ Unclear personal values/ beliefs ○ Perceived threat to value system ○ Lack of experience or interference with decision making ○ Lack of relevant information, multiple or divergent sources of information ○ Support system deficit ○ [Age, developmental state] ○ [Family system, sociocultural factors] ○ [Cognitive, emotional, behavioral level of functioning]

DEFINING CHARACTERISTICS

Subjective: ○ Verbalized uncertainty about choices or of undesired consequences of alternative actions being considered ○ Verbalized feeling of distress or questioning personal values and beliefs while attempting a decision

Objective: ○ Vacillation between alternative choices ○ Delayed decision making ○ Self-focusing ○ Physical signs of distress or tension (increased heart rate; increased muscle tension; restlessness; and so on)

Confusion, acute

DEFINITION: Abrupt onset of a cluster of global, transient changes and disturbances in attention, cognition, psychomotor activity, level of consciousness, and/or sleep/wake cycle

RELATED FACTORS: ○ Over 60 years of age ○ Dementia ○ Alcohol abuse, drug abuse ○ Delirium [including febrile epilepticum (following or instead of an epileptic attack), toxic and traumatic] ○ [Medication reaction/interaction; anesthesia/surgery; metabolic imbalances] ○ [Exacerbation of a chronic illness, hypoxemia] ○ [Severe pain] ○ [Sleep deprivation]

DEFINING CHARACTERISTICS

Subjective: ○ Hallucinations [visual/auditory] ○ [Exaggerated emotional responses]

Objective: ○ Fluctuation in cognition ○ Fluctuation in sleep/wake cycle ○ Fluctuation in level of consciousness ○ Fluctuation in psychomotor activity, [tremors, body movement] ○ Increased agitation or restlessness ○ Misperceptions, [inap-

---

NOTE: Information appearing in [ ] has been added by the authors to clarify and facilitate the use of nursing diagnoses.

propriate responses] ○ Lack of motivation to initiate and/or follow through with goal-directed or purposeful behavior

Confusion, chronic

DEFINITION: Irreversible, long-standing, and/or progressive deterioration of intellect and personality characterized by decreased ability to interpret environmental stimuli; decreased capacity for intellectual thought processes; and manifested by disturbances of memory, orientation, and behavior

RELATED FACTORS: ○ Alzheimer's disease [dementia of the Alzheimer's type] ○ Korsakoff's psychosis ○ Multi-infarct dementia ○ Cerebral vascular accident ○ Head injury

DEFINING CHARACTERISTICS

Objective: ○ Clinical evidence of organic impairment ○ Altered interpretation/response to stimuli ○ Progressive/long-standing cognitive impairment ○ No change in level of consciousness ○ Impaired socialization ○ Impaired memory (short-term, long-term) ○ Altered personality

Constipation

DEFINITION: Decrease in normal frequency of defecation accompanied by difficult or incomplete passage of stool and/or passage of excessively hard, dry stool

RELATED FACTORS:

Functional: ○ Irregular defecation habits ○ Inadequate toileting (e.g., timeliness, positioning for defecation, privacy) ○ Insufficient physical activity ○ Abdominal muscle weakness ○ Recent environmental changes ○ Habitual denial/ignoring of urge to defecate

Psychological: ○ Emotional stress ○ Depression ○ Mental confusion

Pharmacological: ○ Antilipemic agents; laxative overdose; calcium carbonate; aluminum-containing antacids; nonsteroidal anti-inflammatory agents; opiates; anticholinergics; diuretics; iron salts; phenothiazides; sedatives; sympathomimetics; bismuth salts; antidepressants; calcium channel blockers

Mechanical: ○ Hemorrhoids; pregnancy ○ Obesity ○ Rectal abscess or ulcer, anal fissures, prolapse; anal strictures ○ Rectocele ○ Prostate enlargement ○ Postsurgical obstruction ○ Neurological impairment ○ Megacolon (Hirschsprung's disease) ○ Tumors ○ Electrolyte imbalance

Physiological: ○ Poor eating habits ○ Change in usual foods and eating patterns ○ Insufficient fiber intake ○ Insufficient fluid intake ○ Dehydration ○ Inadequate dentition or oral hygiene ○ Decreased motility of gastrointestinal tract

DEFINING CHARACTERISTICS

Subjective: ○ Change in bowel pattern ○ Unable to pass stool ○ Decreased volume/frequency of stool ○ Change in usual foods and eating patterns ○ Increased abdominal pressure ○ Feeling of rectal fullness or pressure ○ Abdominal pain ○ Pain with defecation ○ Nausea and/or vomiting ○ Headache ○ Indigestion ○ Generalized fatigue

Objective: ○ Dry, hard, formed stool ○ Straining with defecation ○ Hypoactive or hyperactive bowel sounds ○ Change in abdominal growling (borborygmi) ○ Distended abdomen ○ Abdominal tenderness with or without palpable muscle resistance ○ Percussed abdominal dullness ○ Presence of soft pastelike stool in rectum ○ Oozing liquid stool ○ Bright red blood with stool ○ Dark or black or tarry stool ○ Severe

---

NOTE: Information appearing in [ ] has been added by the authors to clarify and facilitate the use of nursing diagnoses.

flatus ○ Anorexia ○ Atypical presentations in older adults (e.g., change in mental status, urinary incontinence, unexplained falls, elevated body temperature)

Constipation, perceived

DEFINITION: Self-diagnosis of constipation and abuse of laxatives, enemas, and suppositories to ensure a daily bowel movement

RELATED FACTORS: ○ Cultural/family health beliefs ○ Faulty appraisal, [long-term expectations/habits] ○ Impaired thought processes

DEFINING CHARACTERISTICS

Subjective: ○ Expectation of a daily bowel movement with the resulting overuse of laxatives, enemas, and suppositories ○ Expected passage of stool at same time every day

Constipation, risk for

DEFINITION: At risk for a decrease in normal frequency of defecation accompanied by difficult or incomplete passage of stool and/or passage of excessively hard, dry stool

RISK FACTORS:

Functional: ○ Irregular defecation habits ○ Inadequate toileting (e.g., timeliness, positioning for defecation, privacy) ○ Insufficient physical activity ○ Abdominal muscle weakness ○ Recent environmental changes ○ Habitual denial/ignoring of urge to defecate

Psychological: ○ Emotional stress ○ Depression ○ Mental confusion

Physiological: ○ Change in usual foods and eating patterns ○ Insufficient fiber/ fluid intake ○ Dehydration ○ Poor eating habits ○ Inadequate dentition or oral hygiene ○ Decreased motility of gastrointestinal tract

Pharmacological: ○ Phenothiazides; nonsteroidal anti-inflammatory agents; sedatives; aluminum-containing antacids; laxative overuse; iron salts; anticholinergics; antidepressants; anticonvulsants; antilipemic agents; calcium channel blockers; calcium carbonate; diuretics; sympathomimetics; opiates; bismuth salts

Mechanical: ○ Hemorrhoids ○ Pregnancy ○ Obesity ○ Rectal abscess or ulcer ○ Rectal anal stricture; anal fissures ○ Rectal prolapse ○ Rectocele ○ Prostate enlargement ○ Postsurgical obstruction ○ Neurological impairment ○ Megacolon (Hirschsprung's disease) ○ Tumors ○ Electrolyte imbalance

Coping, community, ineffective

DEFINITION: Pattern of community activities (for adaptation and problem solving) that is unsatisfactory for meeting the demands or needs of the community

RELATED FACTORS: ○ Deficits in social support services and resources ○ Inadequate resources for problem solving ○ Ineffective or nonexistent community systems (e.g., lack of emergency medical system, transportation system, or disaster planning systems) ○ Natural or man-made disasters

DEFINING CHARACTERISTICS

Subjective: ○ Community does not meet its own expectations ○ Expressed vulnerability ○ Expressed community powerlessness ○ Stressors perceived as excessive

Objective: ○ Deficits of community participation ○ Excessive community conflicts ○ High illness rates ○ Increased social problems (e.g., homicide, vandalism, arson, terrorism, robbery, infanticide, abuse, divorce, unemployment, poverty, militance, mental illness)

NOTE: Information appearing in [ ] has been added by the authors to clarify and facilitate the use of nursing diagnoses.

Coping, community, readiness for enhanced

DEFINITION: Pattern of community activities for adaptation and problem solving that is satisfactory for meeting the demands or needs of the community but can be improved for management of current and future problems/stressors

RELATED FACTORS: ○ Social supports available ○ Resources available for problem solving ○ Community has a sense of power to manage stressors

DEFINING CHARACTERISTICS

Subjective: ○ Agreement that community is responsible for stress management

Objective: ○ Deficits in one or more characteristics that indicate effective coping ○ Active planning by community for predicted stressors ○ Active problem solving by community when faced with issues ○ Positive communication among community members ○ Positive communication between community/aggregates and larger community ○ Programs available for recreation and relaxation ○ Resources sufficient for managing stressors

Coping, defensive

DEFINITION: Repeated projection of falsely positive self-evaluation based on a self-protective pattern that defends against underlying perceived threats to positive self-regard

RELATED FACTORS: ○ To be developed by NANDA ○ [Refer to ND Coping, ineffective.]

DEFINING CHARACTERISTICS

Subjective: ○ Denial of obvious problems/weaknesses ○ Projection of blame/responsibility ○ Hypersensitive to slight/criticism ○ Grandiosity ○ Rationalizes failures ○ [Refuses or rejects assistance]

Objective: ○ Superior attitude toward others ○ Difficulty establishing/maintaining relationships, [avoidance of intimacy] ○ Hostile laughter or ridicule of others, [aggressive behavior] ○ Difficulty in reality testing perceptions ○ Lack of follow-through or participation in treatment or therapy ○ [Attention-seeking behavior]

Coping, family: compromised

DEFINITION: Usually supportive primary person (family member or close friend [significant other]) provides insufficient, ineffective, or compromised support, comfort, assistance, or encouragement that may be needed by the client to manage or master adaptive tasks related to his/her health challenge

RELATED FACTORS: ○ Inadequate or incorrect information or understanding by a primary person ○ Temporary preoccupation by a significant person who is trying to manage emotional conflicts and personal suffering and is unable to perceive or act effectively in regard to client's needs ○ Temporary family disorganization and role changes ○ Other situational or developmental crises or situations the significant person may be facing ○ Little support provided by client, in turn, for primary person ○ Prolonged disease or disability progression that exhausts the supportive capacity of significant people ○ [Unrealistic expectations of client/SOs or each other] ○ [Lack of mutual decision-making skills] ○ [Diverse coalitions of family members]

DEFINING CHARACTERISTICS

Subjective: ○ Client expresses or confirms a concern or complaint about significant other's response to his or her health problem ○ Significant person describes preoccupation with personal reaction (e.g., fear, anticipatory grief, guilt, anxiety) to client's illness/disability, or other situational or developmental crises

---

NOTE: Information appearing in [ ] has been added by the authors to clarify and facilitate the use of nursing diagnoses.

○ Significant person describes or confirms an inadequate understanding or knowledge base that interferes with effective assistive or supportive behaviors

Objective: ○ Significant person attempts assistive or supportive behaviors with less than satisfactory results ○ Significant person withdraws or enters into limited or temporary personal communication with the client at the time of need ○ Significant person displays protective behavior disproportionate (too little or too much) to the client's abilities or need for autonomy ○ [Significant person displays sudden outbursts of emotions/shows emotional lability or interferes with necessary nursing/medical interventions]

Coping, family: disabled

DEFINITION: Behavior of significant person (family member or other primary person) that disables his/her capacities and the client's capacity to effectively address tasks essential to either person's adaptation to the health challenge

RELATED FACTORS: ○ Significant person with chronically unexpressed feelings of guilt, anxiety, hostility, despair, and so forth ○ Dissonant discrepancy of coping styles for dealing with adaptive tasks by the significant person and client or among significant people ○ Highly ambivalent family relationships ○ Arbitrary handling of a family's resistance to treatment that tends to solidify defensiveness as it fails to deal adequately with underlying anxiety ○ [High-risk family situations, such as single or adolescent parent, abusive relationship, substance abuse, acute/chronic disabilities, member with terminal illness]

DEFINING CHARACTERISTICS

Subjective: ○ [Expresses despair regarding family reactions/lack of involvement]

Objective: ○ Intolerance, rejection, abandonment, desertion ○ Psychosomaticism ○ Agita-

tion, depression, aggression, hostility ○ Taking on illness signs of client ○ Neglectful relationships with other family members ○ Carrying on usual routines disregarding client's needs ○ Neglectful care of the client in regard to basic human needs and/ or illness treatment ○ Distortion of reality regarding the client's health problem, including extreme denial about its existence or severity ○ Decisions and actions by family that are detrimental to economic or social well-being ○ Impaired restructuring of a meaningful life for self, impaired individualization, prolonged overconcern for client ○ Client's development of helpless, inactive dependence

Coping, family: readiness for enhanced

DEFINITION: Effective managing of adaptive tasks by family member involved with the client's health challenge, who now exhibits desire and readiness for enhanced health and growth in regard to self and in relation to the client

RELATED FACTORS: ○ Needs sufficiently gratified and adaptive tasks effectively addressed to enable goals of self-actualization to surface ○ [Developmental stage, situational crises/ supports]

DEFINING CHARACTERISTICS

Subjective: ○ Family member attempting to describe growth impact of crisis on his or her own values, priorities, goals, or relationships ○ Individual expressing interest in making contact on a one-to-one basis or on a mutual-aid group basis with another person who has experienced a similar situation

Objective: ○ Family member moving in direction of health-promoting and enriching lifestyle that supports and monitors maturational processes, audits and negotiates treatment programs, and generally chooses experiences that optimize wellness

---

NOTE: Information appearing in [ ] has been added by the authors to clarify and facilitate the use of nursing diagnoses.

Coping, ineffective

DEFINITION: Inability to form a valid appraisal of the stressors, inadequate choices of practiced responses, and/or inability to use available resources

RELATED FACTORS: ○ Situational/maturational crises ○ High degree of threat ○ Inadequate opportunity to prepare for stressor ○ Disturbance in pattern of appraisal of threat ○ Inadequate level of confidence in ability to cope/perception of control ○ Uncertainty ○ Inadequate resources available ○ Inadequate social support created by characteristics of relationships ○ Disturbance in pattern of tension release ○ Inability to conserve adaptive energies ○ Gender differences in coping strategies ○ [Work overload, no vacations, too many deadlines; little or no exercise] ○ [Impairment of nervous system; cognitive/sensory/perceptual impairment, memory loss] ○ [Severe/chronic pain]

DEFINING CHARACTERISTICS

Subjective: ○ Verbalization of inability to cope or inability to ask for help ○ Sleep disturbance ○ Fatigue ○ Abuse of chemical agents ○ [Reports of muscular/emotional tension, lack of appetite]

Objective: ○ Lack of goal-directed behavior/resolution of problem, including inability to attend to and difficulty with organizing information ○ [Lack of assertive behavior] ○ Use of forms of coping that impede adaptive behavior [including inappropriate use of defense mechanisms, verbal manipulation] ○ Inadequate problem solving ○ Inability to meet role expectations/basic needs ○ Decreased use of social supports ○ Poor concentration ○ Change in usual communication patterns ○ High illness rate [including high blood pressure, ulcers, irritable bowel, frequent headaches/neckaches] ○ Risk taking ○ Destructive behavior toward self or others [including overeating, excessive smoking/drinking, overuse of prescribed/OTC medications, illicit drug use] ○ [Behavioral changes, e.g., impatience, frustration, irritability, discouragement]

Denial, ineffective

DEFINITION: Conscious or unconscious attempt to disavow the knowledge or meaning of an event to reduce anxiety/fear, but leading to the detriment of health

RELATED FACTORS: ○ To be developed by NANDA ○ [Personal vulnerability; unmet self-needs] ○ [Presence of overwhelming anxiety-producing feelings/situation; reality factors that are consciously intolerable] ○ [Fear of consequences, negative past experiences] ○ [Learned response patterns, e.g., avoidance] ○ [Cultural factors, personal/family value systems]

DEFINING CHARACTERISTICS

Subjective: ○ Minimizes symptoms ○ Displaces source of symptoms to other organs ○ Unable to admit impact of disease on life pattern ○ Displaces fear of impact of the condition ○ Does not admit fear of death or invalidism

Objective: ○ Delays seeking or refuses healthcare attention to the detriment of health ○ Does not perceive personal relevance of symptoms or danger ○ Makes dismissive gestures or comments when speaking of distressing events ○ Displays inappropriate affect ○ Uses home remedies (self-treatment) to relieve symptoms

Dentition, impaired

DEFINITION: Disruption in tooth development/eruption patterns or structural integrity of individual teeth

RELATED FACTORS: ○ Dietary habits ○ Nutri-

NOTE: Information appearing in [ ] has been added by the authors to clarify and facilitate the use of nursing diagnoses.

tional deficits ○ Selected prescription medications ○ Chronic use of tobacco, coffee or tea, red wine ○ Ineffective oral hygiene, sensitivity to heat or cold ○ Chronic vomiting ○ Lack of knowledge regarding dental health ○ Excessive use of abrasive cleaning agents/intake of fluorides ○ Barriers to self-care ○ Access or economic barriers to professional care ○ Genetic predisposition ○ Premature loss of primary teeth ○ Bruxism ○ [Traumatic injury/surgical intervention]

DEFINING CHARACTERISTICS

Subjective: ○ Toothache

Objective: ○ Halitosis ○ Tooth enamel discoloration ○ Erosion of enamel ○ Excessive plaque ○ Worn down or abraded teeth ○ Crown or root caries ○ Tooth fracture(s) ○ Loose teeth ○ Missing teeth or complete absence ○ Premature loss of primary teeth ○ Incomplete eruption for age (may be primary or permanent teeth) ○ Excessive calculus ○ Malocclusion or tooth misalignment ○ Asymmetrical facial expression

Development, risk for delayed

DEFINITION: At risk for delay of 25% or more in one or more of the areas of social or self-regulatory behavior, or cognitive, language, gross or fine motor skills

RISK FACTORS:

Prenatal: ○ Maternal age <15 or >35 years ○ Unplanned or unwanted pregnancy ○ Lack of, late, or poor prenatal care ○ Inadequate nutrition ○ Poverty ○ Illiteracy ○ Genetic or endocrine disorders ○ Infections ○ Substance abuse

Individual: ○ Prematurity ○ Congenital or genetic disorders ○ Vision/hearing impairment or frequent otitis media ○ Failure to thrive, inadequate nutrition ○ Chronic illness ○ Brain

damage (e.g., hemorrhage in postnatal period, shaken baby, abuse, accident) ○ Seizures ○ Positive drug screening test ○ Substance abuse ○ Lead poisoning ○ Chemotherapy ○ Radiation therapy ○ Foster or adopted child ○ Behavior disorders ○ Technology dependent ○ Natural disaster

Environmental: ○ Poverty ○ Violence

Caregiver: ○ Mental retardation or severe learning disability ○ Abuse ○ Mental illness

Diarrhea

DEFINITION: Passage of loose, unformed stools

RELATED FACTORS:

Psychological: ○ High stress levels and anxiety

Situational: ○ Laxative/alcohol abuse ○ Toxins ○ Contaminants ○ Adverse effects of medications ○ Radiation ○ Tube feedings ○ Travel

Physiological: ○ Inflammation ○ Irritation ○ Infectious processes ○ Parasites ○ Malabsorption

DEFINING CHARACTERISTICS

Subjective: ○ Abdominal pain ○ Urgency, cramping

Objective: ○ Hyperactive bowel sounds ○ At least three loose liquid stools per day

Disuse Syndrome, risk for

DEFINITION: At risk for deterioration of body systems as the result of prescribed or unavoidable musculoskeletal inactivity

(Note: Complications from immobility can include pressure ulcer, constipation, stasis of pulmonary secretions, thrombosis, urinary tract infection/retention, decreased strength/

NOTE: Information appearing in [ ] has been added by the authors to clarify and facilitate the use of nursing diagnoses.

endurance, orthostatic hypotension, decreased range of joint motion, disorientation, body image disturbance, and powerlessness.)

RISK FACTORS: ∘ Severe pain, [chronic pain] ∘ Paralysis, [other neuromuscular impairment] ∘ Mechanical or prescribed immobilization ∘ Altered level of consciousness ∘ [Chronic physical or mental illness]

Diversional Activity, deficient

DEFINITION: Decreased stimulation from (or interest or engagement in) recreational or leisure activities [Note: Internal/external factors may or may not be beyond the individual's control.]

RELATED FACTORS: ∘ Environmental lack of diversional activity as in long-term hospitalization ∘ Frequent, lengthy treatments, [homebound] ∘ [Physical limitations, bedridden, fatigue, pain] ∘ [Situational, developmental problem, lack of sources] ∘ [Psychological condition, such as depression]

DEFINING CHARACTERISTICS

Subjective: ∘ Patient's statement regarding the following: boredom, wish there were something to do, to read, etc. ∘ Usual hobbies cannot be undertaken in hospital [home or other care setting] ∘ [Changes in abilities/physical limitations]

Objective: ∘ [Flat affect; disinterest, inattentiveness] ∘ [Restlessness; crying] ∘ [Lethargy; withdrawal] ∘ [Hostility] ∘ [Overeating or lack of interest in eating; weight loss or gain]

Energy Field, disturbed

DEFINITION: Disruption of the flow of energy [aura] surrounding a person's being that results in a disharmony of the body, mind and/or spirit

RELATED FACTORS: ∘ To be developed by NANDA ∘ [Block in energy field] ∘ [Depression] ∘ [Increased state anxiety] ∘ [Impaired immune system] ∘ [Pain]

DEFINING CHARACTERISTICS

Objective: ∘ Temperature change (warmth/coolness) ∘ Visual changes (image/color) ∘ Disruption of the field (vacant/hold/spike/bulge) ∘ Movement wave/spike/tingling/dense/flowing) ∘ Sounds (tone/words)

Environmental Interpretation Syndrome, impaired

DEFINITION: Consistent lack of orientation to person, place, time, or circumstances over more than 3 to 6 months, necessitating a protective environment

RELATED FACTORS: ∘ Dementia (Alzheimer's disease, multi-infarct dementia, Pick's disease, AIDS dementia) ∘ Parkinson's disease ∘ Huntington's disease ∘ Depression ∘ Alcoholism

DEFINING CHARACTERISTICS

Subjective: ∘ [Loss of occupation or social functioning from memory decline]

Objective: ∘ Consistent disorientation in known and unknown environments ∘ Chronic confusional states ∘ Inability to follow simple directions, instructions ∘ Inability to reason; to concentrate ∘ Slow in responding to questions ∘ Loss of occupation or social functioning from memory decline

Failure to Thrive, adult

DEFINITION: Progressive functional deterioration of a physical and cognitive nature. The individual's ability to live with multisystem diseases,

NOTE: Information appearing in [ ] has been added by the authors to clarify and facilitate the use of nursing diagnoses.

cope with ensuing problems, and manage his or her care is remarkably diminished

RELATED FACTORS: ∘ Depression ∘ Apathy ∘ Fatigue ∘ [Major disease/degenerative condition] ∘ [Aging process]

DEFINING CHARACTERISTICS

Subjective: ∘ States does not have an appetite, not hungry, or "I don't want to eat" ∘ Expresses loss of interest in pleasurable outlets, such as food, sex, work, friends, family, hobbies, or entertainment ∘ Difficulty performing simple self-care tasks ∘ Altered mood state—expresses feelings of sadness, being low in spirit ∘ Verbalizes desire for death

Objective: ∘ Inadequate nutritional intake—eating less than body requirements ∘ Consumes minimal to none of food at most meals (i.e., consumes less than 75% of normal requirements at each or most meals) ∘ Anorexia—does not eat meals when offered ∘ Weight loss (decreased body mass from baseline weight)—5% unintentional weight loss in 1 month, 10% unintentional weight loss in 6 months ∘ Physical decline (decline in bodily function)—evidence of fatigue, dehydration, incontinence of bowel and bladder ∘ Cognitive decline (decline in mental processing)—as evidenced by problems with responding appropriately to environmental stimuli; demonstrates difficulty in reasoning, decision making, judgment, memory, concentration ∘ Decreased perception ∘ Apathy as evidenced by lack of observable feeling or emotion in terms of normal ADLs and environment ∘ Decreased participation in ADLs that the older person once enjoyed ∘ Self-care deficit—no longer looks after or takes charge of physical cleanliness or appearance ∘ Neglects home environment and/or financial responsibilities ∘ Decreased social skills/social withdrawal—noticeable decrease from usual past behavior in attempts to form or participate in cooperative and interdependent relationships (e.g., decreased verbal communication with staff, family, friends) ∘ Frequent exacerbations of chronic health problems such as pneumonia or urinary tract infections (UTIs)

Falls, risk for

DEFINITION: Increased susceptibility to falling that may cause physical harm

RISK FACTORS

Adults: ∘ History of falls ∘ Wheelchair use ∘ Use of assistive devices (e.g., walker, cane) ∘ Age 65 or over ∘ Female (if elderly) ∘ Lives alone ∘ Lower limb prosthesis

Physiological: ∘ Presence of acute illness ∘ Postoperative conditions ∘ Visual/hearing difficulties ∘ Arthritis ∘ Orthostatic hypotension ∘ Faintness when turning or extending neck ∘ Sleeplessness ∘ Anemias ∘ Vascular disease ∘ Endoplasms (i.e., fatigue/limited mobility) ∘ Urgency and/or incontinence ∘ Diarrhea ∘ Postprandial blood sugar changes ∘ Impaired physical mobility ∘ Foot problems ∘ Decreased lower extremity strength ∘ Impaired balance ∘ Difficulty with gait ∘ Proprioceptive deficits (e.g., unilateral neglect) ∘ Neuropathy

Cognitive: ∘ Diminished mental status (e.g., confusion, delirium, dementia, impaired reality testing)

Medications: ∘ Antihypertensive agents; ACE inhibitors; diuretics; tricyclic antidepressants; antianxiety agents; hypnotics or tranquilizers; alcohol use; narcotics

Environment: ∘ Restraints ∘ Weather conditions (e.g., wet floors/ice) ∘ Cluttered environment ∘ Throw/scatter rugs ∘ No antislip material in bath and/or shower ∘ Unfamiliar, dimly lit room

Children: ∘ <2 years of age ∘ Male gender when <1 year of age ∘ Lack of gate on stairs; window guards; auto restraints ∘ Unattended infant on

---

NOTE: Information appearing in [ ] has been added by the authors to clarify and facilitate the use of nursing diagnoses.

bed/changing table/sofa ∘ Bed located near window ∘ Lack of parental supervision

Family Processes, dysfunctional: alcoholism

DEFINITION: Psychosocial, spiritual, and physiological functions of the family unit are chronically disorganized, which leads to conflict, denial of problems, resistance to change, ineffective problem solving, and a series of self-perpetuating crises

RELATED FACTORS: ∘ Abuse of alcohol ∘ Resistance to treatment ∘ Family history of alcoholism ∘ Inadequate coping skills ∘ Addictive personality ∘ Lack of problem-solving skills ∘ Biochemical influences; genetic predisposition

DEFINING CHARACTERISTICS

Subjective: Feelings: ∘ Anxiety/tension/distress ∘ Decreased self-esteem/worthlessness ∘ Lingering resentment ∘ Anger/suppressed rage ∘ Frustration ∘ Shame/embarrassment ∘ Hurt ∘ Unhappiness ∘ Guilt ∘ Emotional isolation/loneliness ∘ Powerlessness ∘ Insecurity ∘ Hopelessness ∘ Rejection ∘ Responsibility for alcoholic's behavior ∘ Vulnerability ∘ Mistrust ∘ Depression ∘ Hostility ∘ Fear ∘ Confusion ∘ Dissatisfaction ∘ Loss ∘ Repressed emotions ∘ Being different from other people ∘ Misunderstood ∘ Emotional control by others ∘ Being unloved ∘ Lack of identity ∘ Abandonment ∘ Confused love and pity ∘ Moodiness ∘ Failure

Roles and Relationships: ∘ Family denial ∘ Deterioration in family relationships/disturbed family dynamics ∘ Ineffective spouse communication/marital problems ∘ Intimacy dysfunction ∘ Altered role function/disruption of family roles ∘ Inconsistent parenting/low perception of parental support ∘ Chronic family problems ∘ Lack of skills necessary for relationships

∘ Lack of cohesiveness ∘ Disrupted family rituals ∘ Family unable to meet security needs of its members ∘ Pattern of rejection ∘ Economic problems ∘ Neglected obligations

Objective: Roles and Relationships: ∘ Closed communication systems ∘ Triangulating family relationships ∘ Reduced ability of family members to relate to each other for mutual growth and maturation ∘ Family does not demonstrate respect for individuality and autonomy of its members

Behaviors: ∘ Expression of anger inappropriately ∘ Difficulty with intimate relationships ∘ Impaired communication ∘ Ineffective problem-solving skills ∘ Inability to meet emotional needs of its members ∘ Manipulation ∘ Dependency ∘ Criticizing ∘ Broken promises ∘ Rationalization/denial of problems ∘ Refusal to get help/inability to accept and receive help appropriately ∘ Blaming ∘ Loss of control of drinking ∘ Enabling to maintain drinking [substance use] ∘ Alcohol [substance] abuse ∘ Inadequate understanding or knowledge of alcoholism [substance abuse] ∘ Inability to meet spiritual needs of its members ∘ Inability to express or accept wide range of feelings ∘ Orientation toward tension relief rather than achievement of goals ∘ Escalating conflict ∘ Lying ∘ Contradictory, paradoxical communication ∘ Lack of dealing with conflict ∘ Harsh self-judgment ∘ Isolation ∘ Difficulty having fun ∘ Self-blaming ∘ Unresolved grief ∘ Controlling communication/power struggles ∘ Seeking approval and affirmation ∘ Lack of reliability ∘ Disturbances in academic performance in children ∘ Disturbances in concentration ∘ Chaos ∘ Failure to accomplish current or past developmental tasks/difficulty with life-cycle transitions ∘ Verbal abuse of spouse or parent ∘ Agitation ∘ Diminished physical contact ∘ Family special occasions are alcohol-centered ∘ Nicotine addiction ∘ Inability to

---

NOTE: Information appearing in [ ] has been added by the authors to clarify and facilitate the use of nursing diagnoses.

adapt to change ○ Immaturity ○ Stress-related physical illnesses ○ Inability to deal with traumatic experiences constructively ○ Substance abuse other than alcohol

Family Processes, interrupted

DEFINITION: Change in family relationships and/or functioning

RELATED FACTORS: ○ Situational transition and/or crises [e.g., economic, change in roles, illness, trauma, disabling/expensive treatments] ○ Developmental transition and/or crises [e.g., loss or gain of a family member, adolescence, leaving home for college] ○ Shift in health status of a family member ○ Family roles shift ○ Power shift of family members ○ Modification in family finances, family social status ○ Informal or formal interaction with community

DEFINING CHARACTERISTICS

Subjective: ○ *Changes in*: Power alliances ○ Satisfaction with family ○ Expressions of conflict within family ○ Effectiveness in completing assigned tasks ○ Stress-reduction behaviors ○ Expressions of conflict with and/or isolation from community resources ○ Somatic complaints ○ [Family expresses confusion about what to do; verbalizes they are having difficulty responding to change]

Objective: ○ *Changes in*: Assigned tasks ○ Participation in problem solving/decision making ○ Communication patterns ○ Mutual support ○ Availability for emotional support/affective responsiveness and intimacy ○ Patterns and rituals

Fatigue

DEFINITION: An overwhelming sustained sense of exhaustion and decreased capacity for physical and mental work at usual level

RELATED FACTORS:

Psychological: ○ Stress ○ Anxiety ○ Boring lifestyle ○ Depression

Environmental: ○ Noise ○ Lights ○ Humidity ○ Temperature

Situational: ○ Occupation ○ Negative life events

Physiological: ○ Increased physical exertion ○ Sleep deprivation ○ Pregnancy ○ Disease states ○ Malnutrition ○ Anemia ○ Poor physical condition ○ [Altered body chemistry (e.g., medications, drug withdrawal, chemotherapy)]

DEFINING CHARACTERISTICS

Subjective: ○ Verbalization of an unremitting and overwhelming lack of energy ○ Inability to maintain usual routines/level of physical activity ○ Perceived need for additional energy to accomplish routine tasks ○ Increase in rest requirements ○ Tired ○ Inability to restore energy even after sleep ○ Feelings of guilt for not keeping up with responsibilities ○ Compromised libido ○ Increase in physical complaints

Objective: ○ Lethargic or listless ○ Drowsy ○ Compromised concentration ○ Disinterest in surroundings/introspection ○ Decreased performance, [accident-prone]

Fear [specify focus]

DEFINITION: Response to perceived threat that is consciously recognized as a danger [It is a perceived threat, real or imagined.]

RELATED FACTORS: ○ Natural/innate origin (e.g., sudden noise, height, pain, loss of physical support) ○ Innate releasers (neurotransmitters) ○ Phobic stimulus ○ Learned response (e.g., conditioning, modeling from identification with others) ○ Unfamiliarity with environmental experiences ○ Separation from support

---

NOTE: Information appearing in [ ] has been added by the authors to clarify and facilitate the use of nursing diagnoses.

system in potentially stressful situation (e.g., hospitalization, hospital procedures [/treatments]) ○ Language barrier ○ Sensory impairment

DEFINING CHARACTERISTICS

Subjective: ○ *Report of:* ○ Apprehension ○ Excitement ○ Being scared ○ Alarm ○ Panic ○ Terror ○ Dread ○ Decreased self-assurance ○ Increased tension ○ Jitteriness

Cognitive: ○ Identifies object of fear ○ Stimulus believed to be a threat

Physiological: ○ Anorexia, nausea, fatigue, dry mouth, [palpitations]

Objective: Cognitive: Diminished productivity, learning ability, problem solving

Behaviors: ○ Increased alertness ○ Avoidance [/flight] or attack behaviors ○ Impulsiveness ○ Narrowed focus on "it" (i.e., the focus of the fear)

Physiological: ○ Increased pulse ○ Vomiting ○ Diarrhea ○ Muscle tightness ○ Increased respiratory rate and shortness of breath ○ Increased systolic blood pressure ○ Pallor ○ Increased perspiration ○ Pupil dilation

[Fluid Volume, deficient (hyper/hypotonic)]

[Note: NANDA has restricted Fluid Volume deficit to address only isotonic dehydration. For patient needs related to dehydration associated with alterations in sodium, the authors have provided this second diagnostic category.]

DEFINITION: [Decreased intravascular, interstitial, and/or intracellular fluid. This refers to dehydration with changes in sodium.]

RELATED FACTORS: ○ [Hypertonic dehydration: uncontrolled diabetes mellitus/ insipidus, HHNC, increased intake of hypertonic fluids/IV therapy,

inability to respond to thirst reflex/inadequate free water supplementation (high-osmolarity enteral feeding formulas), renal insufficiency/failure] ○ [Hypotonic dehydration: chronic illness/malnutrition, excessive use of hypotonic IV solutions (e.g., D_5W), renal insufficiency]

DEFINING CHARACTERISTICS

Subjective: ○ [Reports of fatigue, nervousness, exhaustion] ○ [Thirst]

Objective: ○ [Increased urine output, dilute urine (initially) and/or decreased output/oliguria] ○ [Weight loss] ○ [Decreased venous filling] ○ [Hypotension (postural)] ○ [Increased pulse rate; decreased pulse volume and pressure] ○ [Decreased skin turgor] ○ [Change in mental status (e.g., confusion)] ○ [Increased body temperature] ○ [Dry skin/mucous membranes] ○ [Hemoconcentration; altered serum sodium]

Fluid Volume, deficient [isotonic]

DEFINITION: Decreased intravascular, interstitial and/or intracellular fluid. This refers to dehydration, water loss alone without change in sodium.

RELATED FACTORS: ○ Active fluid volume loss [e.g., hemorrhage, gastric intubation, diarrhea, wounds; abdominal cancer; burns, fistulas, ascites (third spacing); use of hyperosmotic radiopaque contrast agents] ○ Failure of regulatory mechanisms [e.g., fever/thermoregulatory response, renal tubule damage]

DEFINING CHARACTERISTICS

Subjective: ○ Thirst ○ Weakness

Objective: ○ Decreased urine output ○ Increased urine concentration ○ Decreased venous filling ○ Decreased pulse volume/pressure ○ Sudden weight loss (except in third spacing) ○ Decreased BP ○ Increased pulse rate/body temper-

---

NOTE: Information appearing in [ ] has been added by the authors to clarify and facilitate the use of nursing diagnoses.

ature ○ Decreased skin/tongue turgor ○ Dry skin/mucous membranes ○ Change in mental state ○ Elevated Hct ○ Deviations affecting access, intake, or absorption of fluids (e.g., physical immobility)

Fluid Volume Excess

DEFINITION: Increased isotonic fluid retention

RELATED FACTORS: ○ Compromised regulatory mechanism [e.g., syndrome of inappropriate antidiuretic hormone—SIADH—or decreased plasma proteins as found in conditions such as malnutrition, draining fistulas, burns, organ failure] ○ Excess fluid intake ○ Excess sodium intake ○ [Drug therapies such as chlorpropamide, tolbutamide, vincristine, triptylines, carbamazepine]

DEFINING CHARACTERISTICS

Subjective: ○ Shortness of breath, orthopnea ○ Anxiety

Objective: ○ Edema, may progress to anasarca ○ Weight gain over short period of time ○ Intake exceeds output ○ Oliguria, azotemia ○ Abnormal breath sounds (rales or crackles), changes in respiratory pattern, dyspnea, pulmonary congestion, pleural effusion ○ BP changes, pulmonary artery pressure changes, increased CVP ○ jugular vein distention ○ Positive hepatojugular reflex ○ S_3 heart sound ○ Change in mental status; restlessness ○ Decreased Hb/Hct, altered electrolytes ○ Specific gravity changes

Fluid Volume, risk for deficient

DEFINITION: At risk for experiencing vascular, cellular, or intracellular dehydration

RISK FACTORS: ○ Extremes of age and weight ○ Loss of fluid through abnormal routes (e.g., indwelling tubes) ○ Knowledge deficiency

related to fluid volume ○ Factors influencing fluid needs (e.g., hypermetabolic states) ○ Medications (e.g., diuretics) ○ Excessive losses through normal routes (e.g., diarrhea)

Fluid Volume, risk for imbalanced

DEFINITION: At risk for a decrease, an increase, or a rapid shift from one to the other of intravascular, interstitial, and/or intracellular fluid. This refers to body fluid loss, gain, or both.

RISK FACTORS: ○ Scheduled for major invasive procedures ○ [Rapid/sustained loss, e.g., hemorrhage, burns, fistulas] ○ [Rapid fluid replacement] ○ Other risk factors to be determined

Gas Exchange, impaired

DEFINITION: Excess or deficit in oxygenation and/or carbon dioxide elimination at the alveoli-capillary membrane [This may be an entity of its own but also may be an end result of other pathology with an interrelatedness between airway clearance and/or breathing pattern problems.]

RELATED FACTORS: ○ Ventilation-perfusion imbalance [as in the following: altered blood flow (e.g., pulmonary embolus, increased vascular resistance), vasospasm, heart failure, hypovolemic shock] ○ Alveolar-capillary membrane changes (e.g., acute adult respiratory distress syndrome); chronic conditions such as restrictive/ obstructive lung disease, pneumoconiosis, respiratory depressant drugs, brain injury, asbestosis/silicosis ○ [Altered oxygen supply (e.g., altitude sickness)] ○ [Altered oxygen-carrying capacity of blood (e.g., sickle cell/other anemia, carbon monoxide poisoning)]

DEFINING CHARACTERISTICS

Subjective: ○ Dyspnea ○ Visual disturbances ○ Headache upon awakening ○ [Sense of impending doom]

NOTE: Information appearing in [ ] has been added by the authors to clarify and facilitate the use of nursing diagnoses.

Objective: ○ Confusion ○ [Decreased mental acuity] ○ Restlessness ○ Irritability ○ [Agitation] ○ Somnolence ○ [Lethargy] ○ Abnormal ABGs/arterial pH ○ Hypoxia/hypoxemia ○ Hypercapnia ○ Hypercarbia ○ Decreased carbon dioxide ○ Cyanosis (in neonates only) ○ Abnormal skin color (pale, dusky) ○ Abnormal rate, rhythm, depth of breathing; nasal flaring ○ Tachycardia [development of dysrhythmias] ○ Diaphoresis ○ [Polycythemia]

Grieving, anticipatory

DEFINITION: Intellectual and emotional responses and behaviors by which individuals, families, communities work through the process of modifying self-concept based on the perception of potential loss [Note: May be a healthy response requiring interventions of support and information giving.]

RELATED FACTORS: ○ To be developed by NANDA ○ [Perceived potential loss of SO, physiological/psychosocial well-being (body part/function, social role), lifestyle/personal possessions]

DEFINING CHARACTERISTICS

Subjective: ○ Sorrow, guilt, anger, [choked feelings] ○ Denial of potential loss ○ Denial of the significance of the loss ○ Expression of distress at potential loss, [ambivalence, sense of unreality] ○ Bargaining ○ Alteration in activity level, sleep/dream patterns, eating habits, ○ libido

Objective: ○ Potential loss of significant object (e.g., people, job, status, home, ideals, part and processes of the body) ○ Altered communication patterns ○ Difficulty taking on new or different roles ○ Resolution of grief prior to the reality of loss ○ [Altered affect] ○ [Crying] ○ [Social isolation, withdrawal]

Grieving, dysfunctional

DEFINITION: Extended, unsuccessful use of intellectual and emotional responses by which individuals, families, communities attempt to work through the process of modifying self-concept based upon the perception of loss

RELATED FACTORS: ○ Actual or perceived object loss (e.g., people, possessions, job, status, home, ideals, parts and processes of the body [e.g., amputation, paralysis, chronic/terminal illness] ○ [Thwarted grieving response to a loss, lack of resolution of previous grieving response] ○ [Absence of anticipatory grieving]

DEFINING CHARACTERISTICS

Subjective: ○ Expression of distress at loss; denial of loss ○ Expression of guilt; anger ○ Sadness ○ Unresolved issues ○ [Hopelessness] ○ Idealization of lost object (e.g., people, possessions, job, status, home, ideals, parts and processes of the body) ○ Reliving of past experiences with little or no reduction (diminishment) of intensity of the grief ○ Alterations in eating habits, sleep/dream patterns, activity level, libido, concentration and/or pursuit of tasks

Objective: ○ Onset or exacerbation of somatic or psychosomatic responses ○ Crying ○ Labile affect ○ Difficulty in expressing loss ○ Prolonged interference with life functioning ○ Developmental regression ○ Repetitive use of ineffectual behaviors associated with attempts to reinvest in relationships ○ [Withdrawal; isolation]

Growth, risk for disproportionate

DEFINITION: At risk for growth above the 97th percentile or below the 3rd percentile for age, crossing two percentile channels; disproportionate growth

---

NOTE: Information appearing in [ ] has been added by the authors to clarify and facilitate the use of nursing diagnoses.

RISK FACTORS:

Prenatal: ○ Maternal nutrition ○ Multiple gestation ○ Substance use/abuse ○ Teratogen exposure ○ Congenital/genetic disorders [e.g., dysfunction of endocrine gland, tumors]

Individual: ○ Organic and inorganic factors ○ Prematurity ○ Malnutrition ○ Caregiver and/ or individual maladaptive feeding behaviors ○ Insatiable appetite ○ Anorexia ○ [Impaired metabolism, greater-than-normal energy requirements] ○ Infection ○ Chronic illness [e.g., chronic inflammatory diseases] ○ Substance [use]/abuse [including anabolic steroids]

Environmental: ○ Deprivation; poverty ○ Violence ○ Natural disasters ○ Teratogen ○ Lead poisoning

Caregiver: ○ Abuse ○ Mental illness/retardation, severe learning disability

Growth and Development, delayed

DEFINITION: Deviations from age growth norms

RELATED FACTORS: ○ Inadequate caretaking, [physical/emotional neglect or abuse] ○ Indifference, inconsistent responsiveness, multiple caretakers ○ Separation from SOs ○ Environmental and stimulation deficiencies ○ Effects of physical disability [handicapping condition] ○ Prescribed dependence [insufficient expectations for self-care] ○ [Physical/emotional illness (chronic, traumatic), e.g., chronic inflammatory disease, pituitary tumors, impaired nutrition/ metabolism, greater-than-normal energy requirements; prolonged/painful treatments; prolonged/ repeated hospitalizations] ○ [Sexual abuse] ○ [Substance use/abuse, including anabolic steroids]

DEFINING CHARACTERISTICS

Subjective: ○ Inability to perform self-care or self-control activities appropriate for age

Objective: ○ Delay or difficulty in performing skills (motor, social, or expressive) typical of age group ○ [Loss of previously acquired skills, precocious or accelerated skill attainment] ○ Altered physical growth ○ Flat affect, listlessness, decreased responses ○ [Sleep disturbances, negative mood/response]

Health Maintenance, ineffective

DEFINITION: Inability to identify, manage, and/or seek out help to maintain health

RELATED FACTORS: ○ Lack of or significant alteration in communication skills (written, verbal, and/or gestural) ○ Unachieved developmental tasks ○ Lack of ability to make deliberate and thoughtful judgments ○ Perceptual or cognitive impairment (complete or partial lack of gross and/or fine motor skills) ○ Ineffective individual coping ○ Dysfunctional grieving ○ Disabling spiritual distress ○ Ineffective family coping ○ Lack of material resource, [lack of psychosocial supports]

DEFINING CHARACTERISTICS

Subjective: ○ Expressed interest in improving health behaviors ○ Reported lack of equipment, financial and/or other resources ○ Impairment of personal support systems ○ Reported inability to take the responsibility for meeting basic health practices in any or all functional pattern areas ○ [Reported compulsive behaviors]

Objective: ○ Demonstrated lack of knowledge regarding basic health practices ○ Observed inability to take the responsibility for meeting basic health practices in any or all functional pattern areas; history of lack of health-seeking behavior ○ Demonstrated lack of adaptive behaviors to internal/external environmental changes ○ Observed impairment of personal support system ○ Lack of equipment, financial

---

NOTE: Information appearing in [ ] has been added by the authors to clarify and facilitate the use of nursing diagnoses.

and/or other resources ○ [Observed compulsive behaviors]

Health-Seeking Behaviors (specify)

DEFINITION: Active seeking (by a person in stable health) of ways to alter personal health habits and/or the environment in order to move toward a higher level of health (Note: Stable health is defined as achievement of age-appropriate illness-prevention measures; client reports good or excellent health, and signs and symptoms of disease, if present, are controlled.)

RELATED FACTORS: ○ To be developed by NANDA ○ [Situational/maturational occurrence precipitating concern about current health status]

DEFINING CHARACTERISTICS

Subjective: ○ Expressed desire to seek a higher level of wellness ○ Expressed desire for increased control of health practice ○ Expression of concern about current environmental conditions on health status ○ Stated unfamiliarity with wellness community resources ○ [Expressed desire to modify codependent behaviors]

Objective: ○ Observed desire to seek a higher level of wellness ○ Observed desire for increased control of health practice

Home Maintenance, impaired

DEFINITION: Inability to independently maintain a safe growth-promoting immediate environment

RELATED FACTORS: ○ Individual/family member disease or injury ○ Insufficient family organization or planning ○ Insufficient finances ○ Impaired cognitive or emotional functioning ○ Lack of role modeling ○ Unfamiliarity

with neighborhood resources ○ Lack of knowledge ○ Inadequate support systems

DEFINING CHARACTERISTICS

Subjective: ○ Household members express difficulty in maintaining their home in a comfortable [safe] fashion ○ Household requests assistance with home maintenance ○ Household members describe outstanding debts or financial crises

Objective: ○ Accumulation of dirt, food, or hygienic wastes ○ Unwashed or unavailable cooking equipment, clothes, or linen ○ Overtaxed family members (e.g., exhausted, anxious) ○ Repeated hygienic disorders, infestations, or infections ○ Disorderly surroundings; offensive odors ○ Inappropriate household temperature ○ Lack of necessary equipment or aids ○ Presence of vermin or rodents

Hopelessness

DEFINITION: Subjective state in which an individual sees limited or no alternatives or personal choices available and is unable to mobilize energy on own behalf

RELATED FACTORS: ○ Prolonged activity restriction creating isolation ○ Failing or deteriorating physiological condition ○ Long-term stress; abandonment ○ Lost belief in transcendent values/God

DEFINING CHARACTERISTICS

Subjective: ○ Verbal cues (despondent content, "I can't," sighing); [believes things will not change/problems will always be there]

Objective: ○ Passivity, decreased verbalization ○ Decreased affect ○ Lack of initiative ○ Decreased response to stimuli, [depressed cognitive functions, problems with decisions, thought processes; regression] ○ Turning away from speaker ○ Closing eyes ○ Shrugging in response

---

NOTE: Information appearing in [ ] has been added by the authors to clarify and facilitate the use of nursing diagnoses.

to speaker ○ Decreased appetite, increased/decreased sleep ○ Lack of involvement in care/passively allowing care ○ [Withdrawal from environs] ○ [Lack of involvement/interest in SOs (children, spouse)] ○ [Angry outbursts]

Hyperthermia

DEFINITION: Body temperature elevated above normal range

RELATED FACTORS: ○ Exposure to hot environment ○ Inappropriate clothing ○ Vigorous activity ○ Dehydration ○ Inability or decreased ability to perspire ○ Medications or anesthesia ○ Increased metabolic rate; illness or trauma

DEFINING CHARACTERISTICS

Subjective: ○ [Headache]

Objective: ○ Increase in body temperature above normal range ○ Flushed skin ○ Warm to touch ○ Increased respiratory rate, tachycardia ○ [Unstable BP] ○ Seizures or convulsions ○ [Muscle rigidity/fasciculations] ○ [Confusion]

Hypothermia

DEFINITION: Body temperature below normal range

RELATED FACTORS: ○ Exposure to cool or cold environment [prolonged exposure, e.g., homeless, immersion in cold water/near drowning ○ Induced hypothermia/cardiopulmonary bypass] ○ Inadequate clothing ○ Evaporation from skin in cool environment ○ Inability or decreased ability to shiver ○ Aging [or very young] ○ [Debilitating] illness or trauma, damage to hypothalamus ○ Malnutrition ○ Decreased metabolic rate ○ Inactivity ○ Consumption of alcohol; medications [/drug overdose] causing vasodilation

DEFINING CHARACTERISTICS

Objective: ○ Reduction in body temperature below normal range ○ Shivering; piloerection ○ Cool skin ○ Pallor ○ Slow capillary refill; cyanotic nailbeds ○ Hypertension ○ Tachycardia ○ [Core temperature 95°F/35°C: increased respirations, poor judgment, shivering] ○ [Core temperature 95° to 93.2°F/35° to 34°C: bradycardia or tachycardia, myocardial irritability/dysrhythmias, muscle rigidity, shivering, lethargic/confused, decreased coordination] ○ [Core temperature 93.2° to 86°F/34° to 30°C: hypoventilation, bradycardia, generalized rigidity, metabolic acidosis, coma] ○ [Core temperature below 86°F/30°C: no apparent vital signs, heart rate unresponsive to drug therapy, comatose, cyanotic, dilated pupils, apneic, areflexic, no shivering (appears dead)]

Infant Behavior, disorganized

DEFINITION: Disintegrated physiological and neurobehavioral responses to the environment

RELATED FACTORS

Prenatal: ○ Congenital or genetic disorders, teratogenic exposure, [exposure to drugs]

Postnatal: ○ Prematurity ○ Oral/motor problems ○ Feeding intolerance ○ Malnutrition ○ Invasive/painful procedures ○ Pain

Individual: ○ Gestational/postconceptual age ○ Immature neurological system ○ Illness ○ [Infection] ○ [Hypoxia/birth asphyxia]

Environmental: ○ Physical environment inappropriateness ○ Sensory inappropriateness/overstimulation/deprivation ○ [Lack of containment/boundaries]

Caregiver: ○ Cue misreading/cue knowledge deficit ○ Environmental stimulation contribution

---

NOTE: Information appearing in [ ] has been added by the authors to clarify and facilitate the use of nursing diagnoses.

DEFINING CHARACTERISTICS

Objective: Regulatory Problems: ○ Inability to inhibit [e.g., "locking in"—inability to look away from stimulus] ○ Irritability

State-Organization System: ○ Active-awake (fussy, worried gaze) ○ Quiet-awake (staring, gaze aversion) ○ Diffuse/unclear sleep, state oscillation ○ Irritable or panicky crying

Attention-Interaction System: ○ Abnormal response to sensory stimuli (e.g., difficult to soothe, inability to sustain alert status)

Motor System: ○ Increased, decreased, or limp tone ○ Finger splay, fisting, or hands to face ○ Hyperextension of arms and legs ○ Tremors, startles, twitches; jittery, jerky, uncoordinated movement ○ Altered primitive reflexes

Physiological: ○ Bradycardia, tachycardia, or arrhythmias ○ Bradypnea, tachypnea, apnea ○ Pale, cyanotic, mottled, or flushed color ○ "Time-out signals" (e.g., gaze, grasp, hiccough, cough, sneeze, sigh, slack jaw, open mouth, tongue thrust) ○ Oximeter desaturation ○ Feeding intolerances (aspiration or emesis)

Infant Behavior, risk for disorganized

DEFINITION: Risk for alteration in integration and modulation of the physiological and behavioral systems of functioning (i.e., autonomic, motor, state, organizational, self-regulatory, and attentional-interactional systems)

RISK FACTORS: ○ Pain ○ Oral/motor problems ○ Environmental overstimulation ○ Lack of containment/boundaries ○ Invasive/painful procedures ○ Prematurity ○ [Immaturity of the CNS; genetic problems that alter neurological and/or physiological functioning conditions resulting in hypoxia and/or birth asphyxia] ○ [Malnutrition; infection; drug addiction] ○ [Environmental events or conditions such as separation from parents, exposure to loud noise, excessive handling, bright lights]

Infant Behavior, readiness for enhanced organized

DEFINITION: A pattern of modulation of the physiological and behavioral systems of functioning (i.e., autonomic, motor, state-organizational, self-regulators, and attentional-interactional systems) in an infant that is satisfactory but that can be improved resulting in higher levels of integration in response to environmental stimuli

RELATED FACTORS: ○ Prematurity ○ Pain

DEFINING CHARACTERISTICS

Objective: ○ Stable physiological measures ○ Definite sleep-wake states ○ Use of some self-regulatory behaviors ○ Response to visual/auditory stimuli

Infant Feeding Pattern, ineffective

DEFINITION: Impaired ability to suck or coordinate the suck-swallow response

RELATED FACTORS: ○ Prematurity ○ Neurological impairment/delay ○ Oral hypersensitivity ○ Prolonged NPO ○ Anatomic abnormality

DEFINING CHARACTERISTICS

Subjective: ○ [Caregiver reports infant is unable to initiate or sustain an effective suck]

Objective: ○ Inability to initiate or sustain an effective suck ○ Inability to coordinate sucking, swallowing, and breathing

---

NOTE: Information appearing in [ ] has been added by the authors to clarify and facilitate the use of nursing diagnoses.

Infection, risk for

DEFINITION: At increased risk for being invaded by pathogenic organisms

RISK FACTORS: ○ Inadequate primary defenses (broken skin, traumatized tissue, decrease in ciliary action, stasis of body fluids, change in pH secretions, altered peristalsis) ○ Inadequate secondary defenses (e.g., decreased hemoglobin, leukopenia, suppressed inflammatory response) and immunosuppression ○ Inadequate acquired immunity ○ Tissue destruction and increased environmental exposure ○ Invasive procedures ○ Chronic disease, malnutrition, trauma ○ Pharmaceutical agents [including antibiotic therapy] ○ Rupture of amniotic membranes ○ Insufficient knowledge to avoid exposure to pathogens

Injury, risk for

DEFINITION: At risk of injury as a result of environmental conditions interacting with the individual's adaptive and defensive resources

[Author's note: The potential for injury differs from individual to individual/situation to situation. It is our belief that the environment is not safe and there is no way to list everything that might present a danger to someone. Rather, we believe nurses have the responsibility to educate people throughout their life cycles to live safely in their environment.]

RISK FACTORS:

Internal: ○ Biochemical, regulatory function (e.g., sensory dysfunction) ○ Integrative or effector dysfunction; tissue hypoxia ○ Immune/autoimmune dysfunction ○ Malnutrition ○ Abnormal blood profile (e.g., leukocytosis/leukopenia, altered clotting factors, thrombocytopenia, sickle cell, thalassemia, decreased hemoglobin) ○ Physical (e.g., broken skin, altered mobility) ○ Developmental age (physiological, psychosocial) ○ Psychological (affective, orientation)

External: ○ Biological (e.g., immunization level of community, microorganism) ○ Chemical (e.g., pollutants, poisons, drugs, pharmaceutical agents, alcohol, caffeine, nicotine, preservatives, cosmetics, dyes) ○ Nutrients (e.g., vitamins, food types) ○ Physical (e.g., design, structure, and arrangement of community, building, and/or equipment), mode of transport or transportation ○ People/provider (e.g., nosocomial agent, staffing patterns; cognitive, affective, and psychomotor factors)

Injury, risk for perioperative positioning

DEFINITION: At risk for injury as a result of the environmental conditions found in the perioperative setting

RISK FACTORS: ○ Disorientation ○ Sensory/perceptual disturbances due to anesthesia ○ Immobilization, muscle weakness ○ [Preexisting musculoskeletal conditions] ○ Obesity ○ Emaciation ○ Edema ○ [Elderly]

Intracranial, adaptive capacity, decreased

DEFINITION: Intracranial fluid dynamic mechanisms that normally compensate for increases in intracranial volume are compromised, resulting in repeated disproportionate increases in intracranial pressure (ICP) in response to a variety of noxious and non-noxious stimuli

RELATED FACTORS: ○ Brain injuries ○ Sustained increase in ICP = 10 to 15 mm Hg ○ Decreased cerebral perfusion pressure = 50

NOTE: Information appearing in [ ] has been added by the authors to clarify and facilitate the use of nursing diagnoses.

to 60 mm Hg ○ Systemic hypotension with intracranial hypertension

DEFINING CHARACTERISTICS

Objective: ○ Repeated increases in ICP of >10 mm Hg for more than 5 minutes following a variety of external stimuli ○ Disproportionate increase in ICP following single environmental or nursing maneuver stimulus ○ Elevated P_2 ICP waveform ○ Volume pressure response test variation (volume-pressure ratio > 2, pressure-volume index < 10) ○ Baseline ICP equal to or greater than 10 mm Hg ○ Wide amplitude ICP waveform ○ [Altered level of consciousness—coma] ○ [Changes in vital signs, cardiac rhythm]

Knowledge, deficient [Learning Need] (specify)

DEFINITION: Absence or deficiency of cognitive information related to specific topic [Lack of specific information necessary for patients/ SO(s) to make informed choices regarding condition/treatment/lifestyle changes]

RELATED FACTORS: ○ Lack of exposure ○ Information misinterpretation ○ Unfamiliarity with information resources ○ Lack of recall ○ Cognitive limitation ○ Lack of interest in learning ○ [Patient's request for no information] ○ [Inaccurate/incomplete information presented]

DEFINING CHARACTERISTICS

SUBJECTIVE: ○ Verbalization of the problem ○ [Request for information] ○ [Statements reflecting misconceptions]

Objective: ○ Inaccurate follow-through of instruction ○ Inadequate performance of test ○ Inappropriate or exaggerated behaviors (e.g., hysterical, hostile, agitated, apathetic) ○ [Development of preventable complication]

Loneliness, risk for

DEFINITION: At risk for experiencing vague dysphoria

RISK FACTORS: ○ Affectional deprivation ○ Physical isolation ○ Cathectic deprivation ○ Social isolation

Memory, impaired

DEFINITION: Inability to remember or recall bits of information or behavioral skills (Impaired memory may be attributed to physiopathological or situational causes that are either temporary or permanent.)

RELATED FACTORS: ○ Acute or chronic hypoxia ○ Anemia ○ Decreased cardiac output ○ Fluid and electrolyte imbalance ○ Neurological disturbances [e.g., brain injury/concussion] ○ Excessive environmental disturbances ○ [Manic state, fugue, traumatic event] ○ [Substance use/abuse; effects of medications] ○ [Age]

DEFINING CHARACTERISTICS

Subjective: ○ Reported experiences of forgetting ○ Inability to recall recent or past events, factual information, [or familiar persons, places, items]

Objective: ○ Observed experiences of forgetting ○ Inability to determine if a behavior was performed ○ Inability to learn or retain new skills or information ○ Inability to perform a previously learned skill ○ Forgetting to perform a behavior at a scheduled time

Mobility, impaired bed

DEFINITION: Limitation of independent movement from one bed position to another

RELATED FACTORS: ○ To be developed by NANDA ○ [Neuromuscular impairment] ○ [Pain/ discomfort]

NOTE: Information appearing in [ ] has been added by the authors to clarify and facilitate the use of nursing diagnoses.

DEFINING CHARACTERISTICS

Subjective: ○ [Reported difficulty performing activities]

Objective: ○ *Impaired ability to:* Turn from side to side, move from supine to sitting or sitting to supine, "scoot" or reposition self in bed, move from supine to prone or prone to supine, move from supine to long-sitting or long-sitting to supine

Mobility, impaired physical [specify level]

DEFINITION: Limitation in independent, purposeful physical movement of the body or of one or more extremities

RELATED FACTORS: ○ Sedentary lifestyle, disuse or deconditioning ○ Limited cardiovascular endurance ○ Decreased muscle strength, control, and/or mass ○ Joint stiffness or contracture ○ Loss of integrity of bone structures ○ Intolerance to activity/decreased strength and endurance ○ Pain/discomfort ○ Neuromuscular/musculoskeletal impairment ○ Sensoriperceptual/cognitive impairment ○ Developmental delay ○ Depressive mood state or anxiety ○ Selective or generalized malnutrition ○ Altered cellular metabolism ○ Body mass index above 75th age-appropriate percentile ○ Lack of knowledge regarding value of physical activity ○ Cultural beliefs regarding age-appropriate activity ○ Lack of physical or social environmental supports ○ Prescribed movement restrictions ○ Medications ○ Reluctance to initiate movement

DEFINING CHARACTERISTICS

Subjective: ○ [Report of pain/discomfort on movement]

Objective: ○ Limited range of motion ○ Limited ability to perform gross fine/motor skills

○ Difficulty turning ○ Slowed movement ○ Uncoordinated or jerky movements, decreased [sic] reaction time ○ Gait changes (e.g., decreased walk, speed ○ Difficulty initiating gait, small steps, shuffling feet ○ Exaggerated lateral postural sway) ○ Postural instability during performance of routine ADLs ○ Movement-induced shortness of breath ○ Engages in substitutions for movement (e.g., increased attention to other's activity, controlling behavior, focus on preillness/ disability activity)

• *Suggested Functional Level Classification:*

    0—Completely independent
    1—Requires use of equipment or device
    2—Requires help from another person for assistance, supervision, or teaching
    3—Requires help from another person and equipment device
    4—Dependent, does not participate in activity

Mobility, impaired wheelchair

DEFINITION: Limitation of independent operation of wheelchair within environment

RELATED FACTORS: ○ To be developed by NANDA

DEFINING CHARACTERISTICS

Subjective/Objective: ○ Impaired ability to operate manual or power wheelchair on even or uneven surface, on an incline or decline, on curbs

    Note: Specify level of independence (Refer to ND Mobility , impaired physical)

Nausea

DEFINITION: Unpleasant, wavelike sensation in the back of the throat, epigastrium, or throughout the abdomen that may or may not lead to vomiting

RELATED FACTORS: ○ Postsurgical anesthesia

NOTE: Information appearing in [ ] has been added by the authors to clarify and facilitate the use of nursing diagnoses.

○ Stimulation of neuropharmacological mechanisms; chemotherapy ○ [Radiation therapy] ○ Irritation to the gastrointestinal (GI) system

DEFINING CHARACTERISTICS

Subjective: ○ Reports "nausea" or "sick to stomach"

Objective: ○ Usually precedes vomiting, but may be experienced after vomiting or when vomiting does not occur ○ Accompanied by swallowing movement affected by skeletal muscles; pallor, cold and clammy skin, increased salivation, tachycardia, gastric stasis, and diarrhea

Noncompliance [Adherence, ineffective] (specify)

DEFINITION: Behavior of person and/or caregiver that fails to coincide with a health-promoting or therapeutic plan agreed upon by the person (and/or family, and/or community) and healthcare professional. In the presence of an agreed-on health-promoting or therapeutic plan, person's or caregiver's behavior is fully or partially adherent or nonadherent and may lead to clinically ineffective, partially ineffective outcomes.

[Author's note: Noncompliance is a term that may create a negative situation for patient and caregiver fostering difficulties in resolving the causative factors. Because clients have a right to refuse therapy, we see this as a situation in which the professional needs to accept the client's point of view/behavior/choice(s) and work together with the client to find alternate means to meet original and/or revised goals.]

RELATED FACTORS:

Healthcare Plan: ○ Duration ○ SOs ○ Cost ○ Intensity ○ Complexity

Individual Factors: ○ Personal and developmental abilities ○ Knowledge and skill relevant to the regimen behavior ○ Motivational forces ○ Individual's value system ○ Health beliefs, cultural influences, spiritual values ○ [Altered thought processes such as depression, paranoia] ○ [Difficulty changing behavior, as in addictions] ○ [Issues of secondary gain]

Health System: ○ Individual health coverage ○ Financial flexibility of plan ○ Credibility of provider ○ Client-provider relationships ○ Provider continuity and regular follow-up ○ Provider reimbursement of teaching and follow-up ○ Communication and teaching skills of the provider ○ Access and convenience of care; satisfaction with care

Network: ○ Involvement of members in health plan ○ Social value regarding plan ○ Perceived beliefs of SOs' communication and teaching skills ○ [Altered thought processes such as depression, paranoia] ○ [Difficulty changing behavior, as in addictions] ○ [Issues of secondary gain]

DEFINING CHARACTERISTICS

Subjective: ○ Statements by patient or SO(s) of failure to adhere ○ [Does not perceive illness/risk to be serious, does not believe in efficacy of therapy, unwilling to follow treatment regimen or accept side effects/ limitations]

Objective: ○ Behavior indicative of failure to adhere (by direct observation) ○ Objective tests (e.g., physiological measures, detection of physiologic markers) ○ Failure to progress ○ Evidence of development of complications/exacerbation of symptoms ○ Failure to keep appointments ○ [Inability to set or attain mutual goals] ○ [Denial]

Nutrition: imbalanced, less than body requirements

DEFINITION: Intake of nutrients insufficient to meet metabolic needs

---

NOTE: Information appearing in [ ] has been added by the authors to clarify and facilitate the use of nursing diagnoses.

RELATED FACTORS: ○ Inability to ingest or digest food or absorb nutrients because of biological, psychological, or economic factors ○ [Increased metabolic demands, e.g., burns] ○ [Lack of information, misinformation, misconceptions]

DEFINING CHARACTERISTICS

Subjective: ○ Reported inadequate food intake less than recommended daily allowances (RDA) ○ Reported lack of food ○ Aversion to eating; reported altered taste sensation ○ Satiety immediately after ingesting food ○ Abdominal pain with or without pathological condition ○ Abdominal cramping ○ Lack of interest in food ○ Perceived inability to digest food ○ Lack of information, misinformation, misconceptions

Objective: ○ Body weight 20% or more under ideal [for height and frame] ○ Loss of weight with adequate food intake ○ Evidence of lack of [available] food ○ Weakness of muscles required for swallowing or mastication ○ Sore, inflamed buccal cavity ○ Poor muscle tone ○ Capillary fragility ○ Hyperactive bowel sounds; diarrhea and/or steatorrhea ○ Pale conjunctiva and mucous membranes ○ Excessive loss of hair [or increased growth of hair on body (lanugo)] ○ [Cessation of menses] ○ [Decreased subcutaneous fat/muscle mass] ○ [Abnormal laboratory studies (e.g., decreased albumin, total proteins; iron deficiency; electrolyte imbalances)]

Nutrition: imbalanced, more than body requirements

DEFINITION: Intake of nutrients that exceeds metabolic needs

RELATED FACTORS: ○ Excessive intake in relationship to metabolic need

[Note: Underlying cause is often complex and may be difficult to diagnose/treat.]

DEFINING CHARACTERISTICS

Subjective: ○ Reported dysfunctional eating patterns: ○ Pairing food with other activities ○ Eating in response to external cues such as time of day, social situation ○ Concentrating food intake at end of day ○ Eating in response to internal cues other than hunger, for example, anxiety ○ Sedentary activity level

Objective: ○ Weight 20% over ideal for height and frame [obese] ○ Triceps skinfold greater than 15 mm in men and 25 mm in women ○ Weight 10% over ideal for height and frame [overweight] ○ Observed dysfunctional eating patterns [as noted in Subjective] ○ [Percentage of body fat greater than 22% for trim women and 15% for trim men]

Nutrition: imbalanced, risk for more than body requirements

DEFINITION: At risk for intake of nutrients that exceeds metabolic needs.

RISK FACTORS: ○ Reported/observed obesity in one or both parents [/spouse; hereditary predisposition] ○ Rapid transition across growth percentiles in infants or children, [adolescents] ○ Reported use of solid food as major food source before 5 months of age ○ Reported/observed higher baseline weight at beginning of each pregnancy, [frequent, closely spaced pregnancies] ○ *Dysfunctional eating patterns:* ○ Pairing food with other activities ○ Eating in response to external cues such as time of day, social situation ○ Concentrating food intake at end of day ○ Eating in response to internal cues other than hunger (such as anxiety) ○ Observed use of food as reward or comfort measure ○ [Frequent/repeated dieting] ○ [Socially/culturally isolated; lacking other outlets] ○ [Alteration in usual activity patterns/sedentary lifestyle] ○ [Alteration in usual coping patterns] ○ [Majority of

---

NOTE: Information appearing in [ ] has been added by the authors to clarify and facilitate the use of nursing diagnoses.

foods consumed are concentrated, high-calorie/fat sources] ○ [Significant/sudden decline in financial resources, lower socioeconomic status]

Oral Mucous Membrane, impaired

DEFINITION: Disruption of the lips and soft tissue of the oral cavity

RELATED FACTORS: ○ Pathological conditions—oral cavity (radiation to head or neck) ○ Cleft lip or palate; loss of supportive structures ○ Trauma ○ Mechanical (e.g., ill-fitting dentures; braces; tubes [ET, nasogastric], surgery in oral cavity) ○ Chemical (e.g., alcohol, tobacco, acidic foods, regular use of inhalers) ○ Chemotherapy ○ Immunosuppression/compromised ○ Decreased platelets ○ Infection ○ Radiation therapy ○ Dehydration, malnutrition, or vitamin deficiency ○ NPO for longer than 24 hours ○ Lack of/impaired or decreased salivation ○ Mouth breathing ○ Ineffective oral hygiene ○ Barriers to oral self-care/professional care ○ Medication side effects ○ Stress ○ Depression ○ Diminished hormone levels (women) ○ Aging-related loss of connective, adipose, or bone tissue

DEFINING CHARACTERISTICS

Subjective: ○ Xerostomia (dry mouth) ○ Oral pain/discomfort ○ Self-report of bad/diminished or absent taste ○ Difficulty eating or swallowing

Objective: ○ Coated tongue ○ Smooth atrophic, sensitive tongue; geographic tongue ○ Gingival or mucosal pallor ○ Stomatitis ○ Hyperemia ○ Bleeding gingival hyperplasia ○ Macroplasia ○ Vesicles, nodules, or papules ○ White patches/plaques, spongy patches, or white curdlike exudate, oral lesions, or ulcers ○ Fissures ○ Chelitis ○ Desquamation ○ Mucosal denudation ○ Edema ○ Halitosis, [carious teeth] ○ Gingival recession, pockets deeper than 4 mm ○ Purulent drainage or exudates; presence of pathogens ○ Enlarged tonsils beyond what is developmentally appropriate ○ Red or bluish masses (e.g., hemangiomas) ○ Difficult speech

Pain, acute

DEFINITION: Unpleasant sensory and emotional experience arising from actual or potential tissue damage or described in terms of such damage (International Association for the Study of Pain); sudden or slow onset of any intensity from mild to severe with an anticipated or predictable end and a duration of less than 6 months

RELATED FACTORS: ○ Injuring agents (biological, chemical, physical, psychological)

DEFINING CHARACTERISTICS

Subjective: ○ Verbal or coded report [may be less from patients younger than age 40, men, and some cultural groups] ○ Changes in appetite and eating ○ [Pain unrelieved and/or increased beyond tolerance]

Objective: ○ Guarded/protective behavior; antalgic position/gestures ○ Facial mask ○ Sleep disturbance (eyes lack luster, "hecohe [beaten] look," fixed or scattered movement, grimace) ○ Expressive behavior (restlessness, moaning, crying, vigilance, irritability, sighing) ○ Distraction behavior (pacing, seeking out other people and/or activities, repetitive activities) ○ Autonomic alteration in muscle tone (may span from listless [flaccid] to rigid) ○ Autonomic responses (diaphoresis; blood pressure, respiration, pulse change; pupillary dilation) ○ Self-focusing ○ Narrowed focus (altered time perception, impaired thought process, reduced interaction with people and environment) ○ [Fear/panic]

Pain, chronic

DEFINITION: Unpleasant sensory and emotional experience arising from actual or potential tissue

---

NOTE: Information appearing in [ ] has been added by the authors to clarify and facilitate the use of nursing diagnoses.

damage or described in terms of such damage (International Association for the Study of Pain); sudden or slow onset of any intensity from mild to severe, constant or recurring without an anticipated or predictable end and a duration of greater than 6 months

[Pain is a signal that something is wrong. Chronic pain can be recurrent and periodically disabling (e.g., migraine headaches) or may be unremitting. Although chronic pain syndrome includes various learned behaviors, psychological factors become the primary contribution to impairment. It is a complex entity, combining elements from other NDs (e.g., Powerlessness; Diversional Activity deficit; Family Processes, altered; Self-Care deficit; and Disuse Syndrome).]

RELATED FACTORS: ○ Chronic physical/psychosocial disability

DEFINING CHARACTERISTICS

Subjective: ○ Verbal or coded report ○ Fear of re-injury ○ Altered ability to continue previous activities ○ Changes in sleep patterns; fatigue ○ [Changes in appetite] ○ [Preoccupation with pain] ○ [Desperately seeks alternative solutions/ therapies for relief/ control of pain]

Objective: ○ *Observed evidence of*: Protective/ guarding behavior ○ Facial mask ○ Irritability ○ Self-focusing ○ Restlessness ○ Depression ○ Reduced interaction with people ○ Anorexia, weight changes ○ Atrophy of involved muscle group ○ Sympathetic mediated responses (temperature, cold, changes of body position, hypersensitivity)

Parental Role Conflict

DEFINITION: Parent experience of role confusion and conflict in response to crisis

RELATED FACTORS: ○ Separation from child because of chronic illness [/disability] ○ Intimidation with invasive or restrictive modalities (e.g., isolation, intubation) ○ Specialized care centers, policies ○ Home care of a child with special needs (e.g., apnea monitoring, postural drainage, hyperalimentation) ○ Change in marital status ○ Interruptions of family life because of home-care regimen (treatments, caregivers, lack of respite)

DEFINING CHARACTERISTICS

Subjective: ○ Parent(s) express(es) concerns/ feeling of inadequacy to provide for child's physical and emotional needs during hospitalization or in the home ○ Parent(s) express(es) concerns about changes in parental role, family functioning, family communication, family health ○ Expresses concern about perceived loss of control over decisions relating to child ○ Verbalizes feelings of guilt, anger, fear, anxiety, and/or frustrations about effect of child's illness on family process

Objective: ○ Demonstrates disruption in caretaking routines ○ Reluctant to participate in usual caretaking activities even with encouragement and support ○ Demonstrates feelings of guilt, anger, fear, anxiety, and/or frustrations about the effect of child's illness on family process

Parenting, impaired

DEFINITION: Inability of the primary caretaker to create, maintain, or regain an environment that promotes the optimum growth and development of the child (Note: It is important to reaffirm that adjustment to parenting in general is a normal maturational process that elicits nursing behaviors to prevent potential problems and to promote health.)

NOTE: Information appearing in [ ] has been added by the authors to clarify and facilitate the use of nursing diagnoses.

RELATED FACTORS:

Social: ◦ Presence of stress (e.g., financial, legal, recent crisis, cultural move [e.g., from another country/cultural group within same country]) ◦ Unemployment or job problems ◦ Financial difficulties ◦ Relocations ◦ Poor home environments ◦ Lack of family cohesiveness ◦ Marital conflict, declining satisfaction ◦ Change in family unit ◦ Role strain or overload ◦ Single parents ◦ Father of child not involved ◦ Unplanned or unwanted pregnancy ◦ Lack of, or poor, parental role model ◦ Low self-esteem ◦ Low socioeconomic class ◦ Poverty ◦ Lack of resources, access to resources, social support networks, transportation ◦ Inadequate child-care arrangements ◦ Lack of value of parenthood ◦ Inability to put child's needs before own ◦ Poor problem-solving skills ◦ Maladaptive coping strategies ◦ Social isolation ◦ History of being abusive/being abused ◦ Legal difficulties

Knowledge: ◦ Lack of knowledge about child health maintenance, parenting skills, child development ◦ Inability to recognize and act on infant cues ◦ Unrealistic expectation for self, infant, partner ◦ Low educational level or attainment ◦ Limited cognitive functioning ◦ Lack of cognitive readiness for parenthood ◦ Poor communication skills ◦ Preference for physical punishment

Physiological: ◦ Physical illness

Infant or Child: ◦ Premature birth ◦ Multiple births ◦ Unplanned or unwanted child ◦ Not gender desired ◦ Illness ◦ Prolonged separation from parent/separation at birth ◦ Difficult temperament ◦ Lack of goodness of fit (temperament) with parental expectations ◦ Handicapping condition or developmental delay ◦ Altered perceptual abilities ◦ Attention-deficit hyperactivity disorder

Psychological: ◦ Young age, especially adolescent ◦ Lack of, or late, prenatal care ◦ Difficult labor and/or delivery ◦ Multiple births ◦ High number or closely spaced pregnancies ◦ Sleep deprivation or disruption ◦ Depression ◦ Separation from infant/child ◦ History of substance abuse or dependencies ◦ Disability ◦ History of mental illness

DEFINING CHARACTERISTICS

Subjective: Parental: ◦ Statements of inability to meet child's needs; cannot control child ◦ Negative statements about child ◦ Verbalization of role inadequacy frustration

Objective: Infant or Child: ◦ Frequent accidents/illness ◦ Failure to thrive ◦ Poor academic performance/cognitive development ◦ Poor social competence ◦ Behavioral disorders ◦ Incidence of physical and psychological trauma or abuse ◦ Lack of attachment ◦ Separation anxiety ◦ Runaway

Parental: ◦ Maternal-child interaction deficit ◦ Poor parent-child interaction ◦ Little cuddling ◦ Insecure or lack of attachment to infant ◦ Inadequate child health maintenance ◦ Unsafe home environment ◦ Inappropriate child-care arrangements ◦ Inappropriate visual, tactile, auditory stimulation ◦ Poor or inappropriate caretaking skills ◦ Inconsistent care/behavior management ◦ Inflexibility to meet needs of child, situation ◦ High punitiveness; rejection or hostility to child; child abuse; child neglect; abandonment

Parenting, risk for impaired

DEFINITION: Risk for inability of the primary caretaker to create, maintain, or regain an environment that promotes the optimum growth and development of the child (Note: It is important to reaffirm that adjustment to parenting in general is a normal maturational process that elicits nursing behaviors to prevent potential problems and to promote health.)

NOTE: Information appearing in [ ] has been added by the authors to clarify and facilitate the use of nursing diagnoses.

RISK FACTORS:

Social: ○ Stress [e.g., financial, legal, recent crisis, cultural move (e.g., from another country/cultural group within same country)] ○ Unemployment or job problems ○ Financial difficulties ○ Relocations ○ Poor home environments ○ Lack of family cohesiveness ○ Marital conflict, declining satisfaction ○ Change in family unit ○ Role strain/overload ○ Single parents ○ Father of child not involved ○ Unplanned or unwanted pregnancy ○ Lack of, or poor, parental role model ○ Low self-esteem ○ Low socioeconomic class ○ Poverty ○ *Lack of*: [Resources], access to resources, social support networks, transportation ○ Inadequate childcare arrangements ○ Lack of value of parenthood ○ Inability to put child's needs before own ○ Poor problem-solving skills ○ Maladaptive coping strategies ○ Social isolation ○ History of being abusive/being abused ○ Legal difficulties

Knowledge: ○ Lack of knowledge about child health maintenance, parenting skills, child development ○ Inability to recognize and act on infant cues ○ Unrealistic expectation of child ○ Low educational level or attainment ○ Low cognitive functioning ○ Lack of cognitive readiness for parenthood ○ Poor communication skills ○ Preference for physical punishment

Physiological: ○ Physical illness

Infant or Child: ○ Premature birth ○ Multiple births ○ Unplanned or unwanted child ○ Not gender desired ○ Illness ○ Prolonged separation from parent/separation at birth ○ Difficult temperament ○ Lack of goodness of fit (temperament) with parental expectations ○ Handicapping condition or developmental delay ○ Altered perceptual abilities ○ Attention-deficit hyperactivity disorder

Psychological: ○ Young age, especially adolescent ○ Lack of, or late, prenatal care ○ Difficult labor and/or delivery ○ Multiple births

○ High number or closely spaced pregnancies ○ Sleep deprivation or disruption ○ Depression ○ Separation from infant/child ○ History of substance abuse or dependencies ○ Disability ○ History of mental illness

Peripheral Neurovascular Dysfunction, risk for

DEFINITION: At risk for disruption in circulation, sensation, or motion of an extremity

RISK FACTORS: ○ Fractures ○ Mechanical compression (e.g., tourniquet, cast, brace, dressing, or restraint) ○ Orthopedic surgery ○ Trauma ○ Immobilization ○ Burns ○ Vascular obstruction

Personal Identity, disturbed

DEFINITION: Inability to distinguish between self and nonself

RELATED FACTORS: ○ To be developed by NANDA ○ [Organic brain syndrome] ○ [Poor ego differentiation, as in schizophrenia] ○ [Panic/dissociative states] ○ [Biochemical body change]

DEFINING CHARACTERISTICS: ○ To be developed by NANDA

Subjective: ○ [Confusion about sense of self, purpose or direction in life, sexual identification/preference]

Objective: ○ [Difficulty in making decisions] ○ [Poorly differentiated ego boundaries] ○ [See ND Anxiety, panic, for additional characteristics]

Poisoning, risk for

DEFINITION: At accentuated risk of accidental exposure to, or ingestion of, drugs or dangerous products in doses sufficient to cause poisoning [or

---

NOTE: Information appearing in [ ] has been added by the authors to clarify and facilitate the use of nursing diagnoses.

the adverse effects of prescribed medication/drug use]

RISK FACTORS:

Internal (individual): ○ Reduced vision ○ Lack of safety or drug education ○ Lack of proper precaution ○ [Unsafe habits, disregard for safety measures, lack of supervision] ○ Insufficient finances ○ Verbalization of occupational setting without adequate safeguards ○ Cognitive or emotional [/behavioral] difficulties ○ [Age, e.g., young child, elderly person] ○ [Chronic disease state, disability] ○ [Cultural or religious beliefs/practices]

External (Environmental): ○ Large supplies of drugs in house ○ Medicines stored in unlocked cabinets accessible to children or confused persons ○ Availability of illicit drugs potentially contaminated by poisonous additives ○ Flaking, peeling paint or plaster in presence of young children ○ Dangerous products placed or stored within the reach of children or confused persons ○ Unprotected contact with heavy metals or chemicals ○ Paint, lacquer, and so forth in poorly ventilated areas or without effective protection ○ Chemical contamination of food and water ○ Presence of poisonous vegetation ○ Presence of atmospheric pollutants, [proximity to industrial chemicals/pattern of prevailing winds] ○ [Therapeutic margin of safety of specific drugs (e.g., therapeutic versus toxic level, half-life, method of uptake and degradation in body, adequacy of organ function)] ○ [Use of multiple herbal supplements or megadosing]

Post-Trauma Syndrome [specify stage]

DEFINITION: Sustained maladaptive response to a traumatic, overwhelming event

RELATED FACTORS: ○ Events outside the range of usual human experience ○ Serious threat or injury to self or loved ones ○ Serious accidents; industrial and motor vehicle accidents ○ Physical and psychosocial abuse ○ Rape ○ Witnessing mutilation, violent death, or other horrors ○ Tragic occurrence involving multiple deaths ○ Natural and/or man-made disasters ○ Sudden destruction of one's home or community ○ Epidemics ○ Wars ○ Military combat ○ Being held prisoner of war or criminal victimization (torture)

DEFINING CHARACTERISTICS

Subjective: ○ Intrusive thoughts/dreams ○ Nightmares ○ Flashbacks ○ Palpitations ○ Headaches ○ [Loss of interest in usual activities, loss of feeling of intimacy/sexuality] ○ Hopelessness ○ Shame ○ [Excessive verbalization of the traumatic event, verbalization of survival guilt or guilt about behavior required for survival] ○ Gastric irritability ○ [Changes in appetite; sleep disturbance/insomnia; chronic fatigue/easy fatigability]

Objective: ○ Anxiety ○ Fear ○ Hypervigilance ○ Exaggerated startle response ○ Neurosensory irritability ○ Irritability ○ Grief ○ Guilt ○ Difficulty in concentrating ○ Depression ○ Anger and/or rage ○ Aggression ○ Avoidance; repression ○ Alienation ○ Denial ○ Detachment ○ Psychogenic amnesia ○ Numbing ○ Altered mood states ○ [Poor impulse control/irritability and explosiveness] ○ Panic attacks ○ Horror ○ Substance abuse ○ Compulsive behavior ○ Enuresis (in children) ○ [Difficulty with interpersonal relationships; dependence on others; work/school failure]

[Stages:
Acute subtype: Begins within 6 months and does not last longer than 6 months
Chronic subtype: Lasts longer than 6 months

NOTE: Information appearing in [ ] has been added by the authors to clarify and facilitate the use of nursing diagnoses.

Delayed subtype: Period of latency of 6 months or longer before onset of symptoms]

Post-trauma Syndrome, risk for

DEFINITION: At risk for sustained maladaptive response to a traumatic, overwhelming event

RISK FACTORS: ∘ Occupation (e.g., police, fire, rescue, corrections, emergency room staff, mental health worker, [and their family members]) ∘ Perception of event ∘ Exaggerated sense of responsibility ∘ Diminished ego strength ∘ Survivor's role in the event ∘ Inadequate social support ∘ Nonsupportive environment ∘ Displacement from home ∘ Duration of the event

Powerlessness [specify level]

DEFINITION: Perception that one's own action will not significantly affect an outcome; a perceived lack of control over a current situation or immediate happening

RELATED FACTORS: ∘ Health-care environment [e.g., loss of privacy, personal possessions, control over therapies] ∘ Interpersonal interaction [e.g., misuse of power, force; abusive relationships] ∘ Illness-related regimen [e.g., chronic/debilitating conditions] ∘ Lifestyle of helplessness [e.g., repeated failures, dependency]

DEFINING CHARACTERISTICS

Subjective: Severe: ∘ Verbal expressions of having no control or influence over situation, outcome, or self-care ∘ Depression over physical deterioration that occurs despite patient compliance with regimens

Moderate: ∘ Expressions of dissatisfaction and frustration over inability to perform previous tasks and/or activities ∘ Expression of doubt regarding role performance ∘ Reluctance to express true feelings; fear of alienation from caregivers

Low: ∘ Expressions of uncertainty about fluctuating energy levels

Objective: Severe: ∘ Apathy [withdrawal, resignation, crying] ∘ [Anger]

Moderate: ∘ Does not monitor progress ∘ Nonparticipation in care or decision making when opportunities are provided ∘ Dependence on others that may result in irritability, resentment, anger, and guilt ∘ Inability to seek information regarding care ∘ Does not defend self-care practices when challenged ∘ Passivity

Low: ∘ Passivity

Powerlessness, risk for

DEFINITION: At risk for perceived lack of control over a situation and/or one's ability to significantly affect an outcome

RISK FACTORS:

Physiological: ∘ Chronic or acute illness (hospitalization, intubation, ventilator, suctioning) ∘ Dying ∘ Acute injury or progressive debilitating disease process (e.g., spinal cord injury, multiple sclerosis) ∘ Aging (e.g., decreased physical strength, decreased mobility)

Psychosocial: ∘ Lack of knowledge of illness or healthcare system ∘ Lifestyle of dependency with inadequate coping patterns ∘ Absence of integrality (e.g., essence of power) ∘ Decreased self-esteem; low or unstable body image

Protection, ineffective

DEFINITION: Decrease in ability to guard self from internal or external threats such as illness or injury

RELATED FACTORS: ∘ Extremes of age ∘ Inadequate nutrition ∘ Alcohol abuse ∘ Abnormal blood profiles (e.g., leukopenia, thrombocytopenia, anemia, coagulation) ∘ Drug therapies (e.g.,

---

NOTE: Information appearing in [ ] has been added by the authors to clarify and facilitate the use of nursing diagnoses.

antineoplastic, corticosteroid, immune, anticoagulant, thrombolytic) ○ Treatments (e.g., surgery, radiation) ○ Diseases, such as cancer and immune disorders

DEFINING CHARACTERISTICS

Subjective: ○ Neurosensory alterations ○ Chilling ○ Itching ○ Insomnia ○ Fatigue ○ Weakness ○ Anorexia

Objective: ○ Deficient immunity ○ Impaired healing; altered clotting ○ Maladaptive stress response ○ Perspiring [inappropriate] ○ Dyspnea ○ Cough ○ Restlessness ○ Immobility ○ Disorientation

Rape-Trauma Syndrome

DEFINITION: Sustained maladaptive response to a forced, violent sexual penetration against the victim's will and consent. (This syndrome includes the following three subcomponents: Rape-Trauma; Rape-Trauma, compound reaction; and Rape-Trauma, silent reaction. Each appears as a separate diagnosis.) [Note: Although attacks are most often directed toward women, men also may be victims.]

RELATED FACTORS: ○ Rape [actual/attempted forced sexual penetration]

DEFINING CHARACTERISTICS

Subjective: ○ Embarrassment ○ Humiliation ○ Shame ○ Guilt ○ Self-blame ○ Loss of self-esteem ○ Helplessness ○ Powerlessness ○ Shock ○ Fear ○ Anxiety ○ Anger ○ Revenge ○ Nightmare and sleep disturbances ○ Change in relationships; sexual dysfunction

Objective: ○ Physical trauma (e.g., bruising, tissue irritation); muscle tension and/or spasms ○ Confusion ○ Disorganization ○ Inability to make decisions ○ Agitation ○ Hyperalertness ○ Aggression ○ Mood swings ○ Vulnerability ○ Dependence ○ Depression ○ Sub-

stance abuse ○ Suicide attempts ○ Denial ○ Phobias ○ Paranoia ○ Dissociative disorders

Rape-Trauma Syndrome: compound reaction

DEFINITION: Forced violent sexual penetration against the victim's will and consent. The trauma syndrome that develops from this attack or attempted attack includes an acute phase of disorganization of the victim's lifestyle and a long-term process of reorganization of lifestyle.

RELATED FACTORS: ○ To be developed by NANDA

DEFINING CHARACTERISTICS

ACUTE PHASE: ○ Emotional reactions (e.g., anger, embarrassment, fear of physical violence and death, humiliation, self-blame, revenge) ○ Multiple physical symptoms (e.g., gastrointestinal irritability, genitourinary discomfort, muscle tension, sleep pattern disturbance) ○ Reactivated symptoms of such previous conditions (i.e., physical/ psychiatric illness); reliance on alcohol and/or drugs

Long-term Phase: ○ Changes in lifestyle (e.g., changes in residence, dealing with repetitive nightmares and phobias, seeking family/social network support)

Rape-Trauma Syndrome: silent reaction

DEFINITION: Forced violent sexual penetration against the victim's will and consent. The trauma syndrome that develops from this attack or attempted attack includes an acute phase of disorganization of the victim's lifestyle and a long-term process of reorganization of lifestyle.

RELATED FACTORS: ○ To be developed by NANDA

NOTE: Information appearing in [ ] has been added by the authors to clarify and facilitate the use of nursing diagnoses.

DEFINING CHARACTERISTICS

Subjective: ○ Abrupt changes in relationships with men ○ Increase in nightmares ○ Pronounced changes in sexual behavior ○ Sudden onset of phobic reactions

Objective: ○ Increasing anxiety during interview (i.e., blocking of associations, long periods of silence; minor stuttering, physical distress) ○ No verbalization of the occurrence of rape

Relocation Stress Syndrome

DEFINITION: Physiological and/or psychosocial disturbance following transfer from one environment to another

RELATED FACTORS: ○ Past, concurrent, and recent losses ○ Feeling of powerlessness ○ Lack of adequate support system ○ Lack of pre-departure counseling ○ Unpredictability of experience ○ Isolation from family/friends ○ Language barrier ○ Impaired psychosocial health ○ Passive coping ○ Decreased health status

DEFINING CHARACTERISTICS

Subjective: ○ Anxiety (e.g., separation); anger ○ Insecurity ○ Worry ○ Fear ○ Loneliness ○ Depression ○ Unwillingness to move, or concern over relocation ○ Sleep disturbance

Objective: ○ Temporary or permanent move; voluntary/involuntary move ○ Increased [frequency of] verbalization of needs ○ Pessimism ○ Frustration ○ Increased physical symptoms/illness (e.g., gastrointestinal disturbances; weight change) ○ Withdrawal ○ Aloneness ○ Alienation ○ [Hostile behavior/outbursts] ○ Loss of identity, self-worth, or self-esteem ○ Dependency ○ [Increased confusion/cognitive impairment]

Relocation Stress Syndrome, risk for

DEFINITION: At risk for physiological and/or psychosocial disturbance following transfer from one environment to another

RISK FACTORS: ○ Moderate to high degree of environmental change (e.g., physical, ethnic, cultural) ○ Temporary and/or permanent moves; voluntary/involuntary move ○ Lack of adequate support system/group ○ Lack of pre-departure counseling ○ Passive coping ○ Feelings of powerlessness ○ Moderate mental competence (e.g., alert enough to experience changes) ○ Unpredictability of experiences ○ Decreased psychosocial or physical health status ○ Past, current, recent losses

Role Performance, ineffective

DEFINITION: Patterns of behavior and self-expression that do not match the environmental context, norms, and expectations (Note: There is a typology of roles: Sociopersonal (friendship, family, marital, parenting, community), home management, intimacy (sexuality, relationship building), leisure/exercise/recreation, self-management, socialization (developmental transitions), community contributor, and religious.

RELATED FACTORS:

Social: ○ Inadequate role socialization (e.g., role model, expectations, responsibilities) ○ Young age, developmental level ○ Lack of resources ○ Low socioeconomic status ○ Poverty ○ Stress and conflict ○ Job schedule demands ○ Family conflict ○ Domestic violence ○ Inadequate support system; lack of rewards ○ Inadequate or inappropriate linkage with the healthcare system

Knowledge: ○ Lack of knowledge about role/

NOTE: Information appearing in [ ] has been added by the authors to clarify and facilitate the use of nursing diagnoses.

role skills ○ Lack of or inadequate role model ○ Inadequate role preparation (e.g., role transition, skill, rehearsal, validation) ○ Lack of opportunity for role rehearsal ○ Education attainment level ○ Developmental transitions ○ Role transition ○ Unrealistic role expectations

Physiological: ○ Health alterations (e.g., physical health, body image, self-esteem, mental health, psychosocial health, cognition, learning style, neurological health) ○ Fatigue ○ Pain ○ Low self-esteem ○ Depression ○ Substance abuse ○ Inadequate/inappropriate linkage with healthcare system

DEFINING CHARACTERISTICS

Subjective: ○ Altered role perceptions/change in self-perception of role/usual patterns of responsibility/capacity to resume role/other's perception of role ○ Inadequate opportunities for role enactment ○ Role dissatisfaction ○ Role overload ○ Role denial ○ Discrimination [by others] ○ Powerlessness

Objective: ○ Inadequate knowledge ○ Inadequate role competency and skills ○ Inadequate adaptation to change or transition ○ Inappropriate developmental expectations ○ Inadequate confidence ○ Inadequate motivation ○ Inadequate self-management ○ Inadequate coping ○ Inadequate opportunities/external support for role enactment ○ Role strain ○ Role conflict ○ Role confusion ○ Role ambivalence ○ [Failure to assume role] ○ Uncertainty ○ Anxiety or depression ○ Pessimistic attitude ○ Domestic violence ○ Harassment ○ System conflict

Self-Care deficit [specify level] feeding, bathing/hygiene, dressing/grooming, toileting

DEFINITION: Impaired ability to perform feeding, bathing/ hygiene, dressing and grooming, or toileting activities for oneself [on a temporary, permanent, or progressing basis]

[Note: Self-care also may be expanded to include the practices used by the patient to promote health, the individual responsibility for self, a way of thinking. Refer to NDs for Home Maintenance, impaired; Health Maintenance, ineffective.]

RELATED FACTORS: ○ Weakness or tiredness ○ Decreased or lack of motivation ○ Neuromuscular/musculoskeletal impairment ○ Environmental barriers ○ Severe anxiety ○ Pain, discomfort ○ Perceptual or cognitive impairment ○ Inability to perceive body part or spatial relationship [bathing/hygiene] ○ Impaired transfer ability (self-toileting) ○ Impaired mobility status (self-toileting) ○ [Mechanical restrictions such as cast, splint, traction, ventilator]

DEFINING CHARACTERISTICS

a. Bathing/hygiene self-care deficit (levels 0–4)
   Inability to: ○ Get bath supplies ○ Wash body or body parts ○ Obtain or get to water source ○ Regulate temperature or flow of bath water ○ Get in and out of bathroom [tub] ○ Dry body
b. Dressing/grooming self-care deficit (levels 0–4)
   Inability to: ○ Choose clothing ○ Pick up clothing ○ Use assistive devices ○ Put on clothing on upper/lower body ○ Use zippers ○ Put on socks/shoes ○ Remove clothes ○ Maintain appearance at a satisfactory level ○ *Impaired ability to:* ○ Put on or take off necessary items of clothing ○ Fasten clothing ○ Obtain or replace articles of clothing
c. Feeding self-care deficit (levels 0–4)
   Inability to: ○ Prepare food for ingestion ○ Open containers ○ Handle utensils ○ Get food onto utensil ○ Bring food from a receptacle to the mouth ○ Ingest food safely ○ Manipulate food in mouth ○ Chew/swallow food ○ Pick up cup or glass ○ Use assistive

NOTE: Information appearing in [ ] has been added by the authors to clarify and facilitate the use of nursing diagnoses.

device ∘ Ingest sufficient food ∘ Complete a meal ∘ Ingest food in a socially acceptable manner

d. Toileting self-care deficit (levels 0–4)
Inability to: ∘ Get to toilet or commode ∘ Manipulate clothing ∘ Sit on or rise from toilet or commode ∘ Carry out proper toilet hygiene ∘ Flush toilet or [empty] commode

Self-Esteem, chronic low

DEFINITION: Long-standing negative self-evaluation/feelings about self or self-capabilities

RELATED FACTORS: ∘ To be developed by NANDA ∘ [Fixation in earlier level of development] ∘ [Continual negative evaluation of self/capabilities from childhood] ∘ [Personal vulnerability] ∘ [Life choices perpetuating failure; ineffective social/occupational functioning] ∘ [Feelings of abandonment by significant other; willingness to tolerate possibly life-threatening domestic violence] ∘ [Chronic physical/psychiatric conditions; antisocial behaviors]

DEFINING CHARACTERISTICS

Subjective: ∘ (*Long-standing or chronic:*) ∘ Self-negating verbalization ∘ Expressions of shame/guilt ∘ Evaluates self as unable to deal with events ∘ Rationalizes away/rejects positive feedback and exaggerates negative feedback about self

Objective: ∘ Frequent lack of success in work or other life events ∘ Overly conforming, dependent on others' opinions ∘ Lack of eye contact ∘ Nonassertive/passive ∘ Indecisive ∘ Excessively seeks reassurance ∘ Hesitant to try new things/situations (long-standing or chronic)

Self-Esteem, situational low

DEFINITION: Development of a negative perception of self-worth in response to a current situation (specify)

RELATED FACTORS: ∘ Developmental changes (specify) ∘ [Maturational transitions, adolescence, aging] ∘ Functional impairments; disturbed body image ∘ Loss (specify)[e.g., loss of health status, body part, independent functioning; memory deficit/cognitive impairment] ∘ Social role changes (specify) ∘ Failures/rejections ∘ Lack of recognition/rewards ∘ [Feelings of abandonment by SO] ∘ Behavior inconsistent with values

Self-Esteem, risk for situational low

DEFINITION: At risk for developing negative perception of self-worth in response to a current situation (specify)

Risk Factors: ∘ Developmental changes (specify) ∘ Disturbed body image; functional impairment (specify) ∘ Loss (specify) ∘ Social role changes (specify) ∘ History of learned helplessness ∘ Neglect, or abandonment ∘ Unrealistic self-expectations ∘ Behavior inconsistent with values ∘ Lack of recognition/rewards ∘ Failures/rejections ∘ Decreased power/control over environment ∘ Physical illness (specify)

Self-Mutilation

DEFINITION: Deliberate self-injurious behavior causing tissue damage with the intent of causing nonfatal injury to attain relief of tension

RELATED FACTORS: ∘ History of self-injurious behavior ∘ Family history of self-destructive behaviors ∘ Feelings of depression, rejection, self-hatred, separation anxiety, guilt, depersonalization ∘ Low or unstable self-esteem/body

---

NOTE: Information appearing in [ ] has been added by the authors to clarify and facilitate the use of nursing diagnoses.

image ∘ Labile behavior (mood swings) ∘ Feels threatened with actual or potential loss of significant relationship (e.g., loss of parent/parental relationship) ∘ Perfectionism ∘ Emotionally disturbed ∘ Battered child ∘ Substance abuse ∘ Eating disorders ∘ Sexual identity crisis ∘ Childhood illness or surgery ∘ Childhood sexual abuse ∘ Adolescence ∘ Peers who self-mutilate ∘ Isolation from peers ∘ Family divorce ∘ Family alcoholism ∘ Violence between parental figures ∘ History of inability to plan solutions or see long-term consequences ∘ Inadequate coping ∘ Mounting tension that is intolerable; needs quick reduction of stress ∘ Impulsivity ∘ Irresistible urge to cut/damage self ∘ Use of manipulation to obtain nurturing relationship with others ∘ Chaotic/disturbed interpersonal relationships ∘ Poor parent-adolescent communication ∘ Lack of family confidante ∘ Experiences dissociation or depersonalization ∘ Psychotic state (command hallucinations) ∘ Character disorders ∘ Borderline personality disorders ∘ Developmentally delayed or autistic individuals ∘ Foster, group, or institutional care ∘ Incarceration

DEFINING CHARACTERISTICS

Subjective: ∘ Self-inflicted burns (e.g., eraser, cigarette) ∘ Ingestion/inhalation of harmful substances/objects

Objective: ∘ Cuts/scratches on body ∘ Picking at wounds ∘ Biting ∘ Abrading ∘ Severing ∘ Insertion of object(s) into body orifice(s) ∘ Hitting ∘ Constricting a body part

Self-Mutilation, risk for

DEFINITION: At risk for deliberate self-injurious behavior, causing tissue damage with the intent of causing nonfatal injury to attain relief of tension

RISK FACTORS: ∘ Feelings of depression, rejection, self-hatred, separation anxiety, guilt, and

depersonalization ∘ Low or unstable self-esteem/body image ∘ Adolescence ∘ Isolation from peers ∘ Peers who self-mutilate ∘ Perfectionism ∘ Childhood illness or surgery ∘ Eating disorders ∘ Substance abuse ∘ Sexual identity crisis ∘ Emotionally disturbed and/or battered children ∘ Childhood sexual abuse ∘ Developmentally delayed or autistic individual ∘ Inadequate coping ∘ Loss of control over problem-solving situations ∘ History of inability to plan solutions or see long-term consequences ∘ Experiences mounting tension that is intolerable ∘ Inability to express tension verbally ∘ Needs quick reduction of stress ∘ Experiences irresistible urge to cut/damage self ∘ History of self-injurious behavior ∘ Chaotic/disturbed interpersonal relationships ∘ Use of manipulation to obtain nurturing relationship with others ∘ Family alcoholism ∘ Divorce ∘ History of self-destructive behaviors ∘ Violence between parental figures ∘ Loss of parent/parental relationships ∘ Feels threatened with actual or potential loss of significant relationship ∘ Character disorders ∘ Borderline personality disorders ∘ Experiences dissociation or depersonalization ∘ Psychotic state (command hallucinations) ∘ Foster, group, or institutional care ∘ Incarceration

Sensory Perception, disturbed (specify: visual, auditory, kinesthetic, gustatory, tactile, olfactory)

DEFINITION: Change in the quantity or patterning of incoming stimuli accompanied by a diminished, exaggerated, distorted, or impaired response to such stimuli

RELATED FACTORS: ∘ Altered sensory perception ∘ Psychological stress [narrowed perceptual fields caused by anxiety] ∘ Excessive/insufficient environmental stimuli ∘ [e.g., Therapeutically restricted environments (e.g., isolation, intensive

NOTE: Information appearing in [ ] has been added by the authors to clarify and facilitate the use of nursing diagnoses.

care, bedrest, traction, confining illnesses, incubator) ∘ Socially restricted environment (e.g., institutionalization, homebound, aging, chronic/terminal illness, infant deprivation); stigmatized (e.g., mentally ill/retarded/ handicapped); bereaved ∘ Excessive noise level such as work environment, patient's immediate environment (ICU with support machinery and the like)] ∘ Altered sensory reception, transmission, and/or integration: [e.g., Neurological disease, trauma, or deficit ∘ Altered status of sense organs ∘ Inability to communicate, understand, speak, or respond ∘ Sleep deprivation ∘ Pain, (phantom limb)] ∘ Biochemical imbalances ∘ Electrolyte imbalance ∘ Biochemical imbalances for sensory distortion (e.g., illusions, hallucinations) [elevated BUN, elevated ammonia, hypoxia] ∘ [Drugs, e.g., stimulants or depressants, mind-altering drugs]

DEFINING CHARACTERISTICS

Subjective: ∘ Reported change in sensory acuity [e.g., photosensitivity, hypoesthesias/hyperesthesias, diminished/altered sense of taste, inability to tell position of body parts (proprioception)] ∘ Visual/auditory distortions ∘ [Distortion of pain, e.g., exaggerated, lack of]

Objective: ∘ Measured change in sensory acuity ∘ Change in usual response to stimuli, [rapid mood swings, exaggerated emotional responses, anxiety/panic state, motor incoordination, altered sense of balance/falls (e.g., Ménière's syndrome)] ∘ Change in problem-solving abilities ∘ Poor concentration ∘ Disoriented in time, in place, or with people ∘ Altered communication patterns ∘ Change in behavior pattern ∘ Restlessness, irritability ∘ Hallucinations ∘ [Illusions] ∘ [Bizarre thinking]

Sexuality Dysfunction

DEFINITION: Change in sexual function that is viewed as unsatisfying, unrewarding, inadequate.

RELATED FACTORS: ∘ Biopsychosocial alteration of sexuality ∘ Ineffectual or absent role models ∘ Lack of significant other ∘ Vulnerability ∘ Misinformation or lack of knowledge ∘ Physical abuse ∘ Psychosocial abuse (e.g., harmful relationships) ∘ Values conflict ∘ Lack of privacy ∘ Altered body structure or function (pregnancy, recent childbirth, drugs, surgery, anomalies, disease process, trauma, [paraplegia/quadriplegia], radiation, [effects of aging])

DEFINING CHARACTERISTICS

Subjective: ∘ Verbalization of problem [e.g., loss of sexual desire, disruption of sexual response patterns such as premature ejaculation, dyspareunia, vaginismus] ∘ Actual or perceived limitation imposed by disease and/or therapy ∘ Inability to achieve desired satisfaction ∘ Alterations in achieving perceived sex role ∘ Conflicts involving values ∘ Alterations in achieving sexual satisfaction ∘ Seeking confirmation of desirability

Objective: ∘ Alteration in relationship with SO

Sexuality Patterns, ineffective

DEFINITION: Expressions of concern regarding own sexuality

RELATED FACTORS: ∘ Knowledge/skill deficit about alternative responses to health-related transitions, altered body function or structure, illness or medical treatment ∘ Lack of privacy ∘ Impaired relationship with a significant other ∘ Lack of SO ∘ Ineffective or absent role models ∘ Conflicts with sexual orientation or variant preferences ∘ Fear of pregnancy or of acquiring a sexually transmitted disease

DEFINING CHARACTERISTICS

Subjective: ∘ Reported difficulties, limitations, or changes in sexual behaviors or activities ∘ [Expressions of feeling alienated, lonely, loss, powerless, angry]

NOTE: Information appearing in [ ] has been added by the authors to clarify and facilitate the use of nursing diagnoses.

Skin Integrity, impaired

DEFINITION: Altered epidermis and/or dermis [The integumentary system is the largest multifunctional organ of the body.]

RELATED FACTORS:

External: ○ Hyperthermia or hypothermia ○ Chemical substance ○ Radiation ○ Medications ○ Physical immobilization ○ Humidity ○ Moisture ○ [Excretions/secretions] ○ Altered fluid status ○ Mechanical factors (e.g., shearing forces, pressure, restraint), [trauma: injury/surgery] ○ Extremes in age

Internal: ○ Altered nutritional state (e.g., obesity, emaciation) ○ Altered metabolic state ○ Altered fluid status ○ Skeletal prominence ○ Alterations in turgor (change in elasticity) ○ [Presence of edema] ○ Altered circulation ○ Altered sensation ○ Altered pigmentation ○ Developmental factors ○ Immunological deficit ○ [Psychogenic]

DEFINING CHARACTERISTICS

Subjective: ○ [Reports of itching, pain, numbness of affected/surrounding area]

Objective: ○ Disruption of skin surface (epidermis) ○ Destruction of skin layers (dermis) ○ Invasion of body structures

Skin Integrity, risk for impaired

DEFINITION: At risk for skin being adversely altered. Note: Risk should be determined by the use of a risk assessment tool (e.g., Braden Scale).

RISK FACTORS:

External: ○ Chemical substance ○ Radiation ○ Hypothermia or hyperthermia ○ Physical immobilization ○ Excretions and/or secretions ○ Humidity ○ Moisture ○ Mechanical factors (e.g., shearing forces, pressure, restraint) ○ Extremes of age

Internal: ○ Medication ○ Alterations in nutritional state (e.g., obesity, emaciation), metabolic state, [fluid status] ○ Skeletal prominence ○ Alterations in skin turgor (change in elasticity) ○ [Presence of edema] ○ Altered circulation, sensation, pigmentation ○ Developmental factors ○ Psychogenic ○ Immunologic

Sleep Deprivation

DEFINITION: Prolonged periods of time without sleep (sustained natural, periodic suspension of relative consciousness)

RELATED FACTORS: ○ Sustained environmental stimulation ○ Unfamiliar or uncomfortable sleep environment ○ Inadequate daytime activity ○ Sustained circadian asynchrony ○ Aging-related sleep stage shifts ○ Non–sleep-inducing parenting practices ○ Sustained inadequate sleep hygiene ○ Prolonged use of pharmacological or dietary antisoporifics ○ Prolonged physical/psychological discomfort ○ Periodic limb movement (e.g., restless leg syndrome, nocturnal myoclonus) ○ Sleep-related: enuresis/painful erections ○ Nightmares ○ Sleep-walking ○ Sleep terror ○ Sleep apnea ○ Sundowner's syndrome ○ Dementia ○ Idiopathic CNS hypersomnolence ○ Narcolepsy ○ Familial sleep paralysis

DEFINING CHARACTERISTICS

Subjective: ○ Daytime drowsiness ○ Decreased ability to function ○ Malaise ○ Tiredness ○ Lethargy ○ Anxious ○ Perceptual disorders (e.g., disturbed body sensation, delusions, feeling afloat) ○ Heightened sensitivity to pain

Objective: ○ Restlessness ○ Irritability ○ Inability to concentrate ○ Slowed reaction ○ Listlessness ○ Apathy ○ Mild, fleeting nystagmus ○ Hand tremors ○ Acute confusion ○ Transient paranoia ○ Agitated or combative ○ Hallucinations

NOTE: Information appearing in [ ] has been added by the authors to clarify and facilitate the use of nursing diagnoses.

Sleep Pattern, disturbed

DEFINITION: Time-limited disruption of sleep (natural, periodic suspension of consciousness) amount and quality

RELATED FACTORS:

Psychological: ○ Daytime activity pattern ○ Fatigue ○ Dietary ○ Body temperature ○ Social schedule inconsistent with chronotype ○ Shift work ○ Daylight/darkness exposure ○ Frequently changing sleep-wake schedule/travel across time zones ○ Circadian asynchrony ○ Childhood onset ○ Aging-related sleep shifts ○ Periodic gender-related hormonal shifts ○ Inadequate sleep hygiene ○ Maladaptive conditioned wakefulness ○ Ruminative pre-sleep thoughts ○ Anticipation ○ Thinking about home ○ Preoccupation with trying to sleep ○ Fear of insomnia ○ Biochemical agents ○ Medications ○ Sustained use of antisleep agents ○ Temperament ○ Loneliness ○ Grief ○ Anxiety ○ Fear ○ Boredom ○ Depression ○ Separation from SOs ○ Loss of sleep partner, life change ○ Delayed or advanced sleep phase syndrome

Environmental: ○ Excessive stimulation ○ Noise ○ Lighting ○ Ambient temperature, humidity ○ Noxious odors ○ Sleep partner ○ Unfamiliar sleep furnishings ○ Interruptions for therapeutics, monitoring, laboratory tests ○ Other-generated awakening ○ Physical restraint ○ Lack of sleep privacy/control

Parental: ○ Mother's sleep-wake pattern/emotional support ○ Parent-infant interaction

Physiological: ○ Position ○ Gastroesophageal reflux ○ Nausea ○ Shortness of breath ○ Stasis of secretions ○ Fever ○ Urinary urgency, incontinence

DEFINING CHARACTERISTICS

Subjective: ○ Verbal complaints [reports] of difficulty falling asleep/not feeling well rested ○ Dissatisfaction with sleep ○ Sleep onset greater than 30 minutes ○ Three or more nighttime awakenings ○ Prolonged awakenings ○ Awakening earlier or later than desired ○ Early morning insomnia ○ Decreased ability to function ○ [Falling asleep during activities]

Objective: ○ Less than age-normed total sleep time ○ Increased proportion of stage 1 sleep ○ Decreased proportion of stages 3 and 4 sleep (e.g., hyporesponsiveness, excess sleepiness, decreased motivation) ○ Decreased proportion of REM sleep (e.g., REM rebound, hyperactivity, emotional lability, agitation and impulsivity, atypical polysomnographic features) ○ Sleep maintenance insomnia ○ Self-induced impairment of normal pattern ○ [Changes in behavior and performance (increasing irritability, disorientation, listlessness, restlessness, lethargy)] ○ [Physical signs (mild fleeting nystagmus, ptosis of eyelid, slight hand tremor, expressionless face, dark circles under eyes, changes in posture, frequent yawning)]

Social Interaction, impaired

DEFINITION: Insufficient or excessive quantity or ineffective quality of social exchange

RELATED FACTORS: ○ Knowledge/skill deficit about ways to enhance mutuality ○ Communication barriers [including head injury, stroke, other neurological conditions affecting ability to communicate] ○ Self-concept disturbance ○ Absence of available significant other(s) or peers ○ Limited physical mobility [e.g., neuromuscular disease] ○ Therapeutic isolation ○ Sociocultural dissonance ○ Environmental barriers ○ Altered thought processes

DEFINING CHARACTERISTICS

Subjective: ○ Verbalized discomfort in social situations ○ Verbalized inability to receive or

---

NOTE: Information appearing in [ ] has been added by the authors to clarify and facilitate the use of nursing diagnoses.

communicate a satisfying sense of belonging, caring, interest, or shared history ○ Family report of change of style or pattern of interaction

Objective: ○ Observed discomfort in social situations ○ Observed inability to receive or communicate a satisfying sense of belonging, caring, interest, or shared history ○ Observed use of unsuccessful social interaction behaviors ○ Dysfunctional interaction with peers, family, and/or others

Social Isolation

DEFINITION: Aloneness experienced by the individual and perceived as imposed by others and as a negative or threatened state

RELATED FACTORS: ○ Factors contributing to the absence of satisfying personal relationships (e.g., delay in accomplishing developmental tasks) ○ Immature interests ○ Alterations in physical appearance/mental status ○ Altered state of wellness ○ Unaccepted social behavior/values ○ Inadequate personal resources ○ Inability to engage in satisfying personal relationships ○ [Traumatic incidents or events causing physical and/or emotional pain]

DEFINING CHARACTERISTICS

Subjective: ○ Expresses feelings of aloneness imposed by others ○ Expresses feelings of rejection ○ Expresses values acceptable to the subculture but unacceptable to the dominant cultural group ○ Inability to meet expectations of others ○ Experiences feelings of difference from others ○ Inadequacy in or absence of significant purpose in life ○ Expresses interests inappropriate to developmental age/stage ○ Insecurity in public

Objective: ○ Absence of supportive SO(s)—family, friends, group ○ Sad, dull affect ○ Inappropriate or immature interests/activities for developmental age/stage ○ Hostility projected

in voice, behavior ○ Evidence of physical/mental handicap or altered state of wellness ○ Uncommunicative ○ Withdrawn ○ No eye contact ○ Preoccupation with own thoughts ○ Repetitive meaningless actions ○ Seeking to be alone or existing in a subculture ○ Showing behavior unaccepted by dominant cultural group

Sorrow, chronic

DEFINITION: Cyclical, recurring, and potentially progressive pattern of pervasive sadness experienced (by a parent or caregiver, individual with chronic illness or disability) in response to continual loss, throughout the trajectory of an illness or disability

RELATED FACTORS: ○ Death of a loved one ○ Experiences chronic physical or mental illness or disability (e.g., mental retardation, MS, prematurity, spina bifida or other birth defects, chronic mental illness, infertility, cancer, Parkinson's disease) ○ Experiences one or more trigger events (e.g., crises in management of the illness, crises related to developmental stages, missed opportunities or milestones that bring comparisons with developmental, social, or personal norms) ○ Unending caregiving as a constant reminder of loss

DEFINING CHARACTERISTICS

Subjective: ○ Expresses one or more of the following feelings: anger, being misunderstood, confusion, depression, disappointment, emptiness, fear, frustration, guilt/self-blame, helplessness, hopelessness, loneliness, low self-esteem, recurring loss, overwhelmed ○ Client expresses periodic, recurrent feelings of sadness

Objective: ○ Feelings that vary in intensity, are periodic, may progress and intensify over time, and may interfere with the client's ability to reach his or her highest level of personal and social well-being

---

NOTE: Information appearing in [ ] has been added by the authors to clarify and facilitate the use of nursing diagnoses.

Spiritual Distress

DEFINITION: Disruption in the life principle that pervades a person's entire being and that integrates and transcends one's biological and psychosocial nature

RELATED FACTORS: ○ Separation from religious/cultural ties ○ Challenged belief and value system (e.g., due to moral/ethical implications of therapy, due to intense suffering)

DEFINING CHARACTERISTICS

Subjective: ○ Expresses concern with meaning of life/death and/or belief systems ○ Verbalizes inner conflict about beliefs ○ Verbalizes concern about relationship with deity ○ [Does not experience that God is forgiving] ○ Angry toward God [as defined by the person] ○ Displacement of anger toward religious representatives ○ Questions meaning of suffering ○ Questions meaning of own existence ○ Questions moral/ethical implications of therapeutic regimen ○ Seeks spiritual assistance ○ Unable to [or chooses not to] participate in usual religious practices ○ Description of nightmares/sleep disturbances ○ [Regards illness/situation as punishment] ○ [Unable to accept self; engages in self-blame] ○ [Describes somatic symptoms]

Objective: ○ Alteration in behavior/mood evidenced by anger, crying, withdrawal, preoccupation, anxiety, hostility, apathy, etc. ○ Gallows humor

Spiritual Distress, risk for

DEFINITION: At risk for an altered sense of harmonious connectedness with all of life and the universe in which dimensions that transcend and empower the self may be disrupted

RISK FACTORS: ○ Physical or psychological stress ○ Energy-consuming anxiety ○ Physical/mental illness ○ Situation/maturational losses ○ Loss of loved one ○ Blocks to self-love ○ Low self-esteem ○ Poor relationships ○ Inability to forgive ○ Substance abuse ○ Natural disasters

Spiritual Well-being, readiness for enhanced

DEFINITION: Process of developing/unfolding of mystery through harmonious interconnectedness that springs from inner strengths [Spiritual well-being is the ability to invest meaning, value, and purpose in one's life that gives harmony, peace, and contentment. This provides for life-affirming relationships with deity, self, community, and environment.]

RELATED FACTORS: ○ To be developed by NANDA

DEFINING CHARACTERISTICS

Subjective: ○ *Inner strengths:* ○ Sense of awareness ○ Self-consciousness ○ Sacred source ○ Unifying force ○ Inner core ○ Transcendence ○ *Unfolding mystery:* ○ One's experience about life's purpose and meaning, mystery, uncertainty, and struggles ○ *Harmonious interconnectedness:* Relatedness/connectedness/harmony with self, others, higher power/God, and the environment

Suffocation, risk for

DEFINITION: Accentuated risk of accidental suffocation (inadequate air available for inhalation)

RISK FACTORS:

Internal (Individual): ○ Reduced olfactory sensation ○ Reduced motor abilities ○ Lack of safety education, precautions ○ Cognitive or emotional difficulties [e.g., altered consciousness/mentation] ○ Disease or injury process

External (Environmental): ○ Pillow/propped bottle

NOTE: Information appearing in [ ] has been added by the authors to clarify and facilitate the use of nursing diagnoses.

placed in an infant's crib ∘ Pacifier hung around infant's head ∘ Children playing with plastic bag or inserting small objects into their mouths or noses ∘ Children left unattended in bathtubs or pools ∘ Discarded or unused refrigerators or freezers without removed doors ∘ Vehicle warming in closed garage [/faulty exhaust system] ∘ Use of fuel-burning heaters not vented to outside ∘ Household gas leaks ∘ Smoking in bed ∘ Low-strung clothesline ∘ Person who eats large mouthfuls [or pieces] of food

Suicide, risk for

DEFINITION: At risk for self-inflicted, life-threatening injury

RISK FACTORS/[INDICATORS]:

Behavioral: ∘ History of prior suicide attempt ∘ Buying a gun ∘ Stockpiling medicines ∘ Making or changing a will ∘ Giving away possessions ∘ Sudden euphoric recovery from major depression ∘ Impulsiveness ∘ Marked changes in behavior, attitude, school performance

Verbal: ∘ Threats of killing oneself ∘ States desire to die/end it all

Situational: ∘ Living alone ∘ Retired ∘ Relocation, institutionalization ∘ Economic instability ∘ Presence of gun in home ∘ Adolescents living in nontraditional settings (e.g., juvenile detention center, prison, halfway house, group home)

Psychological: ∘ Family history of suicide ∘ Abuse in childhood ∘ Alcohol and substance use/abuse ∘ Psychiatric illness/disorder (e.g., depression, schizophrenia, bipolar disorder) ∘ Guilt ∘ Gay or lesbian youth

Demographic: ∘ Age: elderly, young adult males, adolescents ∘ Race: Caucasian, Native American ∘ Gender: male ∘ Divorced, widowed

Physical: ∘ Physical/terminal illness ∘ Chronic pain

Social: ∘ Loss of important relationship ∘ Disrupted family life ∘ Poor support systems ∘ Social isolation ∘ Grief, bereavement ∘ Loneliness ∘ Hopelessness ∘ Helplessness ∘ Legal or disciplinary problem ∘ Cluster suicides

Surgical Recovery, delayed

DEFINITION: Extension of the number of postoperative days required to initiate and perform activities that maintain life, health, and well-being

RELATED FACTORS: ∘ To be developed by NANDA

DEFINING CHARACTERISTICS

Subjective: ∘ Perception more time needed to recover ∘ Report of pain/discomfort ∘ Fatigue ∘ Loss of appetite with or without nausea ∘ Postpones resumption of work/employment activities

Objective: ∘ Evidence of interrupted healing of surgical area (e.g., red, indurated, draining, immobile) ∘ Difficulty in moving about ∘ Requires help to complete self-care

Swallowing, impaired

DEFINITION: Abnormal functioning of the swallowing mechanism associated with deficits in oral, pharyngeal, or esophageal structure or function

RELATED FACTORS:

Congenital Deficits: ∘ Upper airway anomalies ∘ Mechanical obstruction (e.g., edema, tracheostomy tube, tumor) ∘ History of tube feeding ∘ Neuromuscular impairment (e.g., decreased or absent gag reflex, decreased strength or excursion of muscles involved in mastication, perceptual impairment, facial paralysis) ∘ Conditions with

---

NOTE: Information appearing in [ ] has been added by the authors to clarify and facilitate the use of nursing diagnoses.

significant hypotonia ○ Cranial nerve involvement ○ Respiratory disorders ○ Congenital heart disease ○ Behavioral feeding problems ○ Self-injurious behavior ○ Failure to thrive or protein energy malnutrition

Neurological Problems: ○ External/internal traumas ○ Acquired anatomic defects ○ Nasal or nasopharyngeal cavity defects ○ Oral cavity or oropharyngeal abnormalities ○ Upper airway/laryngeal anomalies ○ Tracheal, laryngeal, esophageal defects ○ Gastroesophageal reflux disease ○ Achalasia ○ Premature infants ○ Traumatic head injury ○ Developmental delay ○ Cerebral palsy

DEFINING CHARACTERISTICS

Subjective: ○ *Esophageal phase impairment*: ○ Complaints [reports] of "something stuck" ○ Odynophagia ○ Food refusal or volume limiting ○ Heartburn or epigastric pain ○ Nighttime coughing or awakening

Objective: ○ *Oral phase impairment*: ○ Weak suck resulting in inefficient nippling ○ Slow bolus formation ○ Lack of tongue action to form bolus ○ Premature entry of bolus ○ Incomplete lip closure ○ Food pushed out of/falls from mouth ○ Lack of chewing ○ Coughing, choking, gagging before a swallow ○ Piecemeal deglutition; abnormality in oral phase of swallow study ○ Inability to clear oral cavity ○ Pooling in lateral sulci ○ Nasal reflux ○ Sialorrhea or drooling ○ Long meals with little consumption ○ *Pharyngeal phase impairment*: ○ Food refusal ○ Altered head positions; delayed/multiple swallows ○ Inadequate laryngeal elevation ○ Abnormality in pharyngeal phase by swallow study ○ Choking, coughing, or gagging ○ Nasal reflux ○ Gurgly voice quality ○ Unexplained fevers ○ Recurrent pulmonary infections ○ *Esophageal phase impairment*: ○ Observed evidence of difficulty in swallowing (e.g., stasis of food in oral cavity, coughing/choking) ○ Abnormal-

ity in esophageal phase by swallow study ○ Hyperextension of head, arching during or after meals ○ Repetitive swallowing or ruminating; bruxism ○ Unexplained irritability surrounding mealtime ○ Acidic smelling breath ○ Regurgitation of gastric contents or wet burps ○ Vomitus on pillow ○ Vomiting ○ Hematemesis

Therapeutic Regimen: Community, ineffective management

DEFINITION: Pattern of regulating and integrating into community processes programs for treatment of illness and the sequelae of illness that are unsatisfactory for meeting health-related goals

RELATED FACTORS: ○ To be developed by NANDA ○ [Lack of safety for community members] ○ [Economic insecurity] ○ [Health care not available] ○ [Unhealthy environment] ○ [Education not available for all community members] ○ [Does not possess means to meet human needs for recognition, fellowship, security, and membership]

DEFINING CHARACTERISTICS

Subjective: ○ [Community members/agencies verbalize inability to meet therapeutic needs of all members] ○ [Community members/agencies verbalize overburdening of resources for meeting therapeutic needs of all members]

Objective: ○ Deficits in people and programs to be accountable for illness care of aggregates ○ Deficits in advocates for aggregates ○ Deficit in community activities for [primary medical care/ prevention]/secondary and tertiary prevention ○ Illness symptoms above the norm expected for the number and type of population ○ Unexpected acceleration of illness(es) ○ Number of healthcare resources insufficient [/unavailable] for the incidence or prevalence of illness(es)

NOTE: Information appearing in [ ] has been added by the authors to clarify and facilitate the use of nursing diagnoses.

○ [Deficits in community for collaboration and development of coalitions to address programs for treatment of illness and the sequelae of illness]

Therapeutic Regimen, effective management

DEFINITION: Pattern of regulating and integrating into daily living a program for treatment of illness and its sequelae that is satisfactory for meeting specific health goals

RELATED FACTORS: ○ To be developed by NANDA ○ [Complexity of healthcare management; therapeutic regimen] ○ [Added demands made on individual or family] ○ [Adequate social supports]

DEFINING CHARACTERISTICS

Subjective: ○ Verbalized desire to manage the treatment of illness and prevention of sequelae ○ Verbalized intent to reduce risk factors for progression of illness and sequelae

Objective: ○ Appropriate choices of daily activities for meeting the goals of a treatment or prevention program ○ Illness symptoms are within a normal range of expectation

Therapeutic Regimen: Family, ineffective management

DEFINITION: Pattern of regulating and integrating into family processes a program for treatment of illness and the sequelae of illness that is unsatisfactory for meeting specific health goals

RELATED FACTORS: ○ Complexity of healthcare system ○ Complexity of therapeutic regimen ○ Decisional conflicts ○ Economic difficulties ○ Excessive demands made on individual or family ○ Family conflicts

DEFINING CHARACTERISTICS

Subjective: ○ Verbalized difficulty with regula-

tion/integration of one or more effects or prevention of complication ○ [Inability to manage treatment regimen] ○ Verbalized desire to manage the treatment of illness and prevention of the sequelae ○ Verbalizes that family did not take action to reduce risk factors for progression of illness and sequelae

Objective: ○ Inappropriate family activities for meeting the goals of a treatment or prevention program ○ Acceleration (expected or unexpected) of illness symptoms of a family member ○ Lack of attention to illness and its sequelae

Therapeutic Regimen, ineffective management

DEFINITION: Pattern of regulating and integrating into daily living a program for treatment of illness and the sequelae of illness that is unsatisfactory for meeting specific health goals

RELATED FACTORS: ○ Complexity of healthcare system/therapeutic regimen ○ Decisional conflicts ○ Economic difficulties ○ Excessive demands made on individual or family ○ Family conflict ○ Family patterns of health care ○ Inadequate number and types of cues to action ○ Knowledge deficits ○ Mistrust of regimen and/or healthcare personnel ○ Perceived seriousness/susceptibility/barriers/benefits ○ Powerlessness ○ Social support deficits

DEFINING CHARACTERISTICS

Subjective: ○ Verbalized desire to manage the treatment of illness and prevention of sequelae ○ Verbalized difficulty with regulation/integration of one or more prescribed regimens for treatment of illness and its effects or prevention of complications ○ Verbalized that did not take action to include treatment regimens in daily routines/reduce risk factors for progression of illness and sequelae

---

NOTE: Information appearing in [ ] has been added by the authors to clarify and facilitate the use of nursing diagnoses.

Objective: ○ Choice of daily living ineffective for meeting the goals of a treatment or prevention program ○ Acceleration (expected or unexpected) of illness symptoms

Thermoregulation, ineffective

DEFINITION: Temperature fluctuation between hypothermia and hyperthermia

RELATED FACTORS: ○ Trauma or illness [e.g., cerebral edema, CVA, intracranial surgery, or head injury] ○ Immaturity, aging [e.g., loss/absence of brown adipose tissue] ○ Fluctuating environmental temperature ○ [Changes in hypothalamic tissue causing alterations in emission of thermosensitive cells and regulation of heat loss/production] ○ [Changes in metabolic rate/activity; changes in level/action of thyroxine and catecholamines] ○ [Chemical reactions in contracting muscles]

DEFINING CHARACTERISTICS

Objective: ○ Fluctuations in body temperature above or below the normal range ○ Tachycardia ○ Reduction in body temperature below normal range ○ Cool skin ○ Pallor (moderate) ○ Shivering (mild) ○ Piloerection ○ Cyanotic nailbeds ○ Slow capillary refill ○ Hypertension ○ Warm to touch ○ Flushed skin ○ Increased respiratory rate ○ Seizures/ convulsions

Thought Processes, disturbed

DEFINITION: Disruption in cognitive operations and activities

RELATED FACTORS: ○ To be developed by NANDA ○ [Physiological changes, aging, hypoxia, head injury, malnutrition, infections] ○ [Biochemical changes, medications, substance abuse] ○ [Sleep deprivation] ○ [Psychological conflicts, emotional changes, mental disorders]

DEFINING CHARACTERISTICS

Subjective: ○ [Ideas of reference, hallucinations, delusions]

Objective: ○ Inaccurate interpretation of environment ○ Inappropriate/nonreality-based thinking ○ Memory deficit/problems, [disorientation to time, place, person, circumstances and events, loss of short-term/remote memory] ○ Hypervigilance or hypovigilance ○ Cognitive dissonance, [decreased ability to grasp ideas, make decisions, problem-solve, use abstract reasoning or conceptualize, calculate; disordered thought sequencing] ○ Distractibility, [altered attention span] ○ Egocentricity ○ [Confabulation] ○ [Inappropriate social behavior]

Tissue Integrity, impaired

DEFINITION: Damage to mucous membrane, corneal, integumentary, or subcutaneous tissues

RELATED FACTORS: ○ Altered circulation ○ Nutritional deficit/excess ○ [Metabolic, endocrine dysfunction] ○ Fluid deficit/excess ○ Knowledge deficit ○ Impaired physical mobility ○ Irritants, chemical (including body excretions, secretions, medications); radiation (including therapeutic radiation) ○ Thermal (temperature extremes) ○ Mechanical (e.g., pressure, shear, friction), [surgery] ○ Knowledge deficit ○ [Infection]

Tissue Perfusion, ineffective (specify): renal, cerebral, cardiopulmonary, gastrointestinal, peripheral

DEFINITION: Decrease in oxygen resulting in the failure to nourish the tissues at the capillary level [Tissue perfusion problems can exist without decreased cardiac output; however, there may be

---

NOTE: Information appearing in [ ] has been added by the authors to clarify and facilitate the use of nursing diagnoses.

a relationship between cardiac output and tissue perfusion.]

RELATED FACTORS: ○ Interruption of flow—arterial, venous ○ Exchange problems ○ Hypervolemia, hypovolemia ○ Mechanical reduction of venous and/or arterial blood flow ○ Decreased Hb concentration in blood ○ Altered affinity of hemoglobin for O_2 ○ Enzyme poisoning ○ Impaired transport of the O_2 across alveolar and/or capillary membrane ○ Mismatch of ventilation with blood flow ○ Hypoventilation

DEFINING CHARACTERISTICS

Renal: Objective: ○ Altered blood pressure outside of acceptable parameters ○ Oliguria or anuria ○ Hematuria ○ Arterial pulsations, bruits ○ Elevation in BUN/Cr ratio

Cerebral: Objective: ○ Altered mental status ○ Speech abnormalities ○ Behavioral changes ○ [Restlessness] ○ Changes in motor response ○ Extremity weakness or paralysis ○ Changes in pupillary reactions ○ Difficulty in swallowing

Cardiopulmonary: Subjective: ○ Chest pain ○ Dyspnea ○ Sense of "impending doom"

Cardiopulmonary: Objective: ○ Dysrhythmias ○ Capillary refill > 3 sec ○ Altered respiratory rate outside of acceptable parameters ○ Use of accessory muscles ○ Chest retraction ○ Nasal flaring ○ Bronchospasms ○ Abnormal ABGs ○ [Hemoptysis]

Gastrointestinal: Subjective: ○ Nausea ○ Abdominal pain or tenderness

Gastrointestinal Objective: ○ Hypoactive or absent bowel sounds ○ Abdominal distention ○ [Melena]

Peripheral: Subjective: ○ Claudication

Peripheral: Objective: ○ Altered skin characteristics (hair, nails, moisture) ○ Skin temperature changes ○ Skin discolorations ○ Color diminished ○ Color pale on elevation, color does not return on lowering the leg ○ Altered sensations ○ BP changes in extremities ○ Weak or absent pulses ○ Diminished arterial pulsations ○ Bruits ○ Edema ○ Delayed healing ○ Positive Homans' sign

Transfer Ability, impaired

DEFINITION: Limitation of independent movement between two nearby surfaces

RELATED FACTORS: ○ To be developed by NANDA ○ [Conditions that result in poor muscle tone] ○ [Cognitive impairment] ○ [Fractures, trauma, spinal cord injury]

DEFINING CHARACTERISTICS

Subjective or Objective: ○ *Impaired ability to transfer:* From bed to chair and chair to bed ○ Chair to car or car to chair ○ Chair to floor or floor to chair ○ Standing to floor or floor to standing ○ On or off a toilet or commode ○ In and out of tub or shower ○ Between uneven levels

Specify level of independence—[refer to ND Mobility, impaired physical, for suggested functional level classification]

Trauma, risk for

DEFINITION: Accentuated risk of accidental tissue injury (e.g., wound, burn, fracture)

RISK FACTORS:

Internal (Individual): ○ Weakness ○ Balancing difficulties ○ Reduced large or small muscle coordination, hand/eye coordination ○ Poor vision ○ Reduced temperature and/or tactile sensation ○ Lack of safety education/precautions ○ Insufficient finances to purchase safety equipment or to effect repairs ○ Cognitive or emotional difficulties ○ History of previous trauma

---

NOTE: Information appearing in [ ] has been added by the authors to clarify and facilitate the use of nursing diagnoses.

External (Environmental) [includes but is not limited to]: ○ Slippery floors (e.g., wet or highly waxed ○ Unanchored rug ○ Litter or liquid spills on floors or stairways ○ Snow or ice collected on stairs, walkways) ○ Bathtub without handgrip or anti-slip equipment ○ Use of unsteady ladder or chairs ○ Obstructed passageways ○ Entering unlighted rooms ○ Unsturdy or absent stair rails ○ Children playing without gates at top of stairs ○ Unanchored electric wires ○ High beds ○ Inappropriate call-for-aid mechanisms for bed-resting client ○ Unsafe window protection in homes with young children ○ Pot handles facing toward front of stove ○ Bathing in very hot water (e.g., unsupervised bathing of young children) ○ Potential igniting gas leaks ○ Delayed lighting of gas burner or oven ○ Unscreened fires or heaters ○ Wearing plastic apron or flowing clothing around open flames ○ Highly flammable children's toys or clothing ○ Smoking in bed or near O_2 ○ Grease waste collected on stoves ○ Children playing with matches, candles, cigarettes ○ Playing with fireworks or gunpowder ○ Guns or ammunition stored unlocked ○ Experimenting with chemical or gasoline ○ Inadequately stored combustibles or corrosives (e.g., matches, oily rags, lye; contact with acids or alkalis) ○ Overloaded fuse boxes ○ Faulty electrical plugs, frayed wires, or defective appliances ○ Overloaded electrical outlets ○ Exposure to dangerous machinery ○ Contact with rapidly moving machinery, industrial belts, or pulleys ○ Sliding on coarse bed linen or struggling within bed [/chair] restraints ○ Contact with intense cold ○ Overexposure to sun, sunlamps, radiotherapy ○ Use of thin or worn-out pot holders [or mitts] ○ Use of cracked dishware or glasses ○ Knives stored uncovered ○ Children playing with sharp-edged toys ○ Large icicles hanging from roof ○ High-crime neighborhood and vulnerable clients ○ Driving a mechanically unsafe vehicle ○ Driving at excessive speeds ○ Driving without necessary visual aids ○ Driving after partaking of alcoholic beverages or [other] drugs ○ Children riding in the front seat of car, nonuse or misuse of seat restraints/[unrestrained infant/child riding in car] ○ Misuse [or nonuse] of necessary headgear for motorized cyclists or young children carried on adult bicycles ○ Unsafe road or road-crossing conditions ○ Playing or working near vehicle pathways (e.g., driveways, lanes, railroad tracks)

Unilateral Neglect

DEFINITION: Lack of awareness and attention to one side of the body

RELATED FACTORS: ○ Effects of disturbed perceptual abilities (e.g., [homonymous] hemianopsia, one-sided blindness; [or visual inattention]) ○ Neurological illness or trauma ○ [Impaired cerebral blood flow]

DEFINING CHARACTERISTICS

Subjective: ○ [Reports feeling that part does not belong to own self]

Objective: ○ Consistent inattention to stimuli on an affected side ○ Inadequate self-care [inability to satisfactorily perform ADLs] ○ [Lack of] positioning and/or safety precautions in regard to the affected side ○ Does not look toward affected side ○ [Does not touch affected side] ○ Leaves food on plate on the affected side ○ [Failure to use the affected side of the body without being reminded to do so]

Urinary Elimination, impaired

DEFINITION: Disturbance in urine elimination

RELATED FACTORS: ○ Multiple causality ○ Sensory motor impairment ○ Anatomical obstruction ○ UTI ○ [Mechanical trauma; fluid/volume states; psychogenic factors; surgical diversion]

NOTE: Information appearing in [ ] has been added by the authors to clarify and facilitate the use of nursing diagnoses.

DEFINING CHARACTERISTICS

Subjective: ○ Frequency ○ Urgency ○ Hesitancy ○ Dysuria ○ Nocturia, [enuresis]

Objective: ○ Incontinence ○ Retention

Urinary Incontinence, functional

DEFINITION: Inability of usually continent person to reach toilet in time to avoid unintentional loss of urine

RELATED FACTORS: ○ Altered environmental factors [e.g., poor lighting or inability to locate bathroom] ○ Neuromuscular limitations ○ Weakened supporting pelvic structures ○ Impaired vision/cognition ○ Psychological factors ○ [Reluctance to use call light or bedpan] ○ [Increased urine production]

DEFINING CHARACTERISTICS

Subjective: ○ Senses need to void ○ [Voiding in large amounts]

Objective: ○ Loss of urine before reaching toilet ○ Amount of time required to reach toilet exceeds length of time between sensing urge and uncontrolled voiding ○ Able to completely empty bladder ○ May be incontinent only in early morning

Urinary Incontinence, reflex

DEFINITION: Involuntary loss of urine at somewhat predictable intervals when a specific bladder volume is reached

RELATED FACTORS: ○ Tissue damage from radiation cystitis, inflammatory bladder conditions, or radical pelvic surgery ○ Neurological impairment above level of sacral or pontine micturition center

DEFINING CHARACTERISTICS

Subjective: ○ No sensation of bladder fullness/urge to void/voiding ○ Sensation of urgency without voluntary inhibition of bladder contraction ○ Sensations associated with full bladder such as sweating, restlessness, and abdominal discomfort

Objective: ○ Predictable pattern of voiding ○ Inability to voluntarily inhibit or initiate voiding ○ Complete emptying with [brain] lesion above pontine micturition center ○ Incomplete emptying with [spinal cord] lesion above sacral micturition center

Urinary Incontinence, stress

DEFINITION: Loss of less than 50 ml of urine occurring with increased abdominal pressure

RELATED FACTORS: ○ Degenerative changes in pelvic muscles and structural supports associated with increased age [e.g., poor closure of urethral sphincter, estrogen deficiency] ○ High intra-abdominal pressure (e.g., obesity, gravid uterus) ○ Incompetent bladder outlet ○ Overdistention between voidings ○ Weak pelvic muscles and structural supports [e.g., straining with chronic constipation] ○ [Neural degeneration, vascular deficits, surgery, radiation therapy]

DEFINING CHARACTERISTICS

Subjective: ○ Reported dribbling with increased abdominal pressure [e.g., coughing, sneezing, lifting, impact aerobics, changing position] ○ Urinary urgency ○ Frequency (more often than every 2 hours)

Objective: ○ Observed dribbling with increased abdominal pressure

Urinary Incontinence, total

DEFINITION: Continuous and unpredictable loss of urine

NOTE: Information appearing in [ ] has been added by the authors to clarify and facilitate the use of nursing diagnoses.

RELATED FACTORS: ○ Neuropathy preventing transmission of reflex [signals to the reflex arc] indicating bladder fullness ○ Neurological dysfunction [e.g., cerebral lesions] causing triggering of micturition at unpredictable times ○ Independent contraction of detrusor reflex due to surgery ○ Trauma or disease affecting spinal cord nerves [destruction of sensory or motor neurons below the injury level] ○ Anatomic (fistula)

DEFINING CHARACTERISTICS

Subjective: ○ Constant flow of urine at unpredictable times without uninhibited bladder contractions/spasm or distention ○ Nocturia ○ Lack of perineal or bladder filling awareness ○ Unawareness of incontinence

Objective: ○ Unsuccessful incontinence refractory treatments

Urinary Incontinence, urge

DEFINITION: Decreased, delayed, or absent ability to receive, process, transmit, and use a system of symbols

RELATED FACTORS: ○ Decreased bladder capacity (e.g., history of pelvic inflammatory disease—PID, abdominal surgeries, indwelling urinary catheter) ○ Irritation of bladder stretch receptors causing spasm (e.g., bladder infection, [atrophic urethritis, vaginitis]) ○ Alcohol ○ Caffeine ○ Increased fluids ○ Increased urine concentration ○ Overdistention of bladder ○ [Medication use, such as diuretics, sedatives, anticholinergic agents] ○ [Constipation/stool impaction] ○ [Restricted mobility; psychological disorder such as depression, change in mentation/confusional state (e.g., stroke, dementia, Parkinson's disease)]

DEFINING CHARACTERISTICS

Subjective: ○ Urinary urgency ○ Frequency (voiding more often than every 2 hours) ○ Bladder contracture/spasm ○ Nocturia (more than 2 times per night)

Objective: ○ Inability to reach toilet in time ○ Voiding in small amounts (<100 ml) or in large amounts (>550 ml)

Urinary Incontinence, risk for urge

DEFINITION: At risk for an involuntary loss of urine associated with a sudden, strong sensation or urinary urgency

RISK FACTORS: ○ Effects of medications, caffeine, alcohol ○ Detrusor hyperreflexia from cystitis, urethritis, tumors, renal calculi, CNS disorders above pontine micturition center ○ Detrusor muscle instability with impaired contractility ○ Involuntary sphincter relaxation ○ Ineffective toileting habits ○ Small bladder capacity

Urinary Retention [acute/chronic]

DEFINITION: Incomplete emptying of the bladder

RELATED FACTORS: ○ High urethral pressure caused by weak [/absent] detrusor ○ Inhibition of reflex arc ○ Strong sphincter ○ Blockage [e.g., benign prostatic hypertrophy—BPH, perineal swelling] ○ [Habituation of reflex arc] ○ [Infections] ○ [Neurological diseases/trauma] ○ [Use of medications with side effect of retention (e.g., atropine, belladonna, psychotropics, antihistamines, opiates)]

DEFINING CHARACTERISTICS

Subjective: ○ Sensation of bladder fullness ○ Dribbling ○ Dysuria

Objective: ○ Bladder distention ○ Small, frequent voiding or absence of urine output ○ Residual urine [150 ml or more] ○ Overflow incontinence ○ [Reduced stream]

NOTE: Information appearing in [ ] has been added by the authors to clarify and facilitate the use of nursing diagnoses.

Ventilation, impaired spontaneous

DEFINITION: Decreased energy reserves results in an individual's inability to maintain breathing adequate to support life

RELATED FACTORS: ∘ Metabolic factors [hypermetabolic state (e.g., infection), nutritional deficits/depletion of energy stores] ∘ Respiratory muscle fatigue ∘ [Airway size/resistance; problems with secretion management]

DEFINING CHARACTERISTICS

Subjective: ∘ Dyspnea ∘ Apprehension

Objective: ∘ Increased metabolic rate ∘ Increased heart rate ∘ Increased restlessness ∘ Decreased cooperation ∘ Increased use of accessory muscles ∘ Decreased tidal volume ∘ Decreased PO_2 ∘ SaO_2 ∘ Increased PCO_2

Ventilatory Weaning Response, dysfunctional

DEFINITION: Inability to adjust to lowered levels of mechanical ventilator support that interrupts and prolongs the weaning process

RELATED FACTORS:

Physical: ∘ Ineffective airway clearance ∘ Sleep pattern disturbance ∘ Inadequate nutrition ∘ Uncontrolled pain or discomfort ∘ [Muscle weakness/fatigue, inability to control respiratory muscles; immobility]

Psychological: ∘ Knowledge deficit of the weaning process, patient's role ∘ Patient's perceived inefficacy about the ability to wean ∘ Decreased motivation ∘ Decreased self-esteem ∘ Anxiety (moderate, severe) ∘ Fear ∘ Insufficient trust in the nurse ∘ Hopelessness ∘ Powerlessness ∘ [Unprepared for weaning attempt]

Situational: ∘ Uncontrolled episodic energy demands or problems ∘ Inappropriate pacing of diminished ventilator support ∘ Inadequate social support ∘ Adverse environment (noisy, active environment, negative events in the room, low nurse-patient ratio; extended nurse absence from bedside, unfamiliar nursing staff) ∘ History of ventilator dependence > 1 week ∘ History of multiple unsuccessful weaning attempts

DEFINING CHARACTERISTICS

Responds to lowered levels of mechanical ventilator support with: Mild DVWR

Subjective: ∘ Expressed feelings of increased need for O_2 ∘ Breathing discomfort ∘ Fatigue ∘ Warmth ∘ Queries about possible machine malfunction

Objective: ∘ Restlessness ∘ Slight increased respiratory rate from baseline ∘ Increased concentration on breathing

Moderate DVWR

Subjective: ∘ Apprehension

Objective: ∘ Slight increase from baseline blood pressure (<20 mm Hg) ∘ Slight increase from baseline heart rate (<20 beats/min) ∘ Baseline increase in respiratory rate (<5 breaths/min) ∘ Hypervigilance to activities ∘ Inability to respond to coaching/cooperate ∘ Diaphoresis ∘ Eye widening, "wide-eyed look" ∘ Decreased air entry on auscultation ∘ Color changes ∘ Pale, slight cyanosis ∘ Slight respiratory accessory muscle use

Severe DVWR

Objective: ∘ Agitation ∘ Deterioration in ABGs from current baseline ∘ Increase from baseline BP (>20 mm Hg) ∘ Increase from baseline heart rate (>20 beats/min) ∘ Respiratory rate increases significantly from baseline ∘ Profuse diaphoresis ∘ Full respiratory accessory muscle use ∘ Shallow, gasping breaths ∘ Paradoxical abdominal breathing ∘ Discoordinated breathing with the ventilator ∘ Decreased level of

NOTE: Information appearing in [ ] has been added by the authors to clarify and facilitate the use of nursing diagnoses.

consciousness ◦ Adventitious breath sounds, audible airway secretions ◦ Cyanosis

Violence, [actual]/risk for other-directed

DEFINITION: At risk for behaviors in which an individual demonstrates that he/she can be physically, emotionally, and/or sexually harmful to others

RISK FACTORS/[INDICATORS ◦ *History of:* ◦ Violence against others (e.g., hitting, kicking, scratching, biting or spitting, or throwing objects at someone; attempted rape, rape, sexual molestation; urinating/defecating on a person) ◦ Threats (e.g., verbal threats against property/ person, social threats, cursing, threatening notes/letters or gestures, sexual threats) ◦ Violent antisocial behavior (e.g., stealing, insistent borrowing, insistent demands for privileges, insistent interruption of meetings; refusal to eat or to take medication, ignoring instructions) ◦ Violence, indirect (e.g., tearing off clothes, urinating/defecating on floor, stamping feet, temper tantrum; running in corridors, yelling, writing on walls, ripping objects off walls, throwing objects, breaking a window, slamming doors; sexual advances) ◦ Drug/alcohol abuse ◦ Childhood abuse/witnessing family violence ◦ [Negative role modeling] Other: ◦ Body language: rigid posture, clenching of fists and jaw, hyperactivity, pacing, breathlessness, threatening stances) ◦ Neurological impairment (e.g., positive EEG, CT, or MRI; head trauma; positive neurological findings; seizure disorders, [temporal lobe epilepsy]) ◦ Cognitive impairment (e.g., learning disabilities, attention deficit disorder, decreased intellectual functioning); [organic brain syndrome] ◦ Prenatal and perinatal complications/abnormalities ◦ Psychotic symptomatology (e.g., auditory, visual, command hallucinations; paranoid delusions; loose, rambling, or illogical thought processes); [panic states; rage reactions; catatonic/manic excitement] ◦ Cruelty to animals; firesetting ◦ Motor vehicle offenses (e.g., frequent traffic violations, use of motor vehicle to release anger) ◦ Pathological intoxication, [toxic reaction to medication] ◦ Suicidal behavior; impulsivity; availability and/or possession of weapon(s) ◦ [Hormonal imbalance (e.g., premenstrual syndrome—PMS, postpartal depression/psychosis)] ◦ [Expressed intent/desire to harm others directly or indirectly] ◦ [Almost continuous thoughts of violence]

Violence, [actual]/risk for self-directed

DEFINITION: At risk for behaviors in which an individual demonstrates that he/she can be physically, emotionally, and/or sexually harmful to self

RISK FACTORS [OR INDICATORS]: ◦ Ages 15 to 19; over age 45 ◦ Marital status (single, widowed, divorced) ◦ Employment (unemployed, recent job loss/failure); occupation (executive, administrator/owner of business, professional, semiskilled worker) ◦ Conflictual interpersonal relationships ◦ Family background (chaotic or conflictual, history of suicide) ◦ Sexual orientation: bisexual (active), homosexual (inactive) ◦ Physical health (hypochondriac, chronic or terminal illness) ◦ Mental health (severe depression, psychosis, severe personality disorder, alcoholism, or drug abuse) ◦ Emotional status (hopelessness, [lifting of depressed mood], despair, increased anxiety, panic, anger, hostility) ◦ History of multiple suicide attempts ◦ Suicidal ideation (frequent, intense prolonged) ◦ Suicide plan (clear and specific; lethality: method and availability of destructive means) ◦ Personal resources (poor achievement, poor insight, affect unavailable and poorly controlled) ◦ Social resources (poor

---

NOTE: Information appearing in [ ] has been added by the authors to clarify and facilitate the use of nursing diagnoses.

rapport, socially isolated, unresponsive family) ○ Verbal clues (e.g., talking about death, "better off without me," asking questions about lethal dosages of drugs) ○ Behavioral clues (e.g., writing forlorn love notes, directing angry messages at an SO who has rejected the person, giving away personal items, taking out a large life insurance policy) ○ People who engage in autoerotic sexual acts [e.g., asphyxiation]

Walking, impaired

DEFINITION: Limitation of independent movement within the environment on foot

RELATED FACTORS: ○ To be developed by NANDA ○ [Condition affecting muscles/joints impairing ability to walk]

DEFINING CHARACTERISTICS

Subjective or Objective: ○ Impaired ability to: ○ Walk required distances ○ Walk on an incline/decline ○ Walk on uneven surfaces ○ Navigate curbs ○ Climb stairs

[Specify level of independence—refer to ND Mobility, impaired physical, for suggested functional level classification.]

Wandering

DEFINITION: Meandering, aimless or repetitive locomotion that exposes the individual to harm; frequently incongruent with boundaries, limits, or obstacles

RELATED FACTORS: ○ Cognitive impairment, specifically memory and recall deficits, disorientation, poor visuoconstructive (or visuospatial) ability, language (primarily expressive) defects ○ Cortical atrophy ○ Premorbid behavior (e.g., outgoing, sociable personality; premorbid dementia) ○ Separation from familiar people and places ○ Emotional state, especially frustration, anxiety, boredom, or depression (agitation) ○ Physiological state or need (e.g., hunger/thirst, pain, urination, constipation) ○ Over-/understimulating social or physical environment ○ Sedation ○ Time of day

DEFINING CHARACTERISTICS

Objective: ○ Frequent or continuous movement from place to place, often revisiting the same destinations ○ Persistent locomotion in search of "missing" or unattainable people or places ○ Scanning, seeking, or searching behaviors ○ Haphazard locomotion ○ Fretful locomotion or pacing ○ Long periods of locomotion without an apparent destination ○ Locomotion into unauthorized or private spaces ○ Trespassing ○ Locomotion resulting in unintended leaving of a premise ○ Inability to locate significant landmarks in a familiar setting ○ Getting lost ○ Locomotion that cannot be easily dissuaded or redirected ○ Following behind or shadowing a caregiver's locomotion ○ Hyperactivity ○ Periods of locomotion interspersed with periods of nonlocomotion (e.g., sitting, standing, sleeping)

NOTE: Information appearing in [ ] has been added by the authors to clarify and facilitate the use of nursing diagnoses.

Appendix B

NANDA Taxonomy II: Definitions of Axes

AXIS 1 DIAGNOSTIC CONCEPT: Defined as the principal element or the fundamental and essential part, the root, of the diagnostic statement.

AXIS 2 TIME: Defined as the duration of a period or interval.

> *Acute:* Less than 6 months
> *Chronic:* More than 6 months
> *Intermittent:* Stopping or starting again at intervals; periodic, cyclic
> *Continuous:* Uninterrupted, going on without stops

AXIS 3 UNIT OF CARE: Defined as the distinct population for which a nursing diagnosis is determined. Values are:

> *Individual:* a single human being distinct from others, a person.
> *Family:* two or more people having continuous or sustained relationships, perceiving reciprocal obligations, sensing common meaning, and sharing certain obligations toward others; related by blood or choice.
> *Group:* individuals gathered, classified, or acting together.
> *Community:* "'a group of people living in the same locale under the same government.' Examples include neighborhoods, cities, census tracts, and populations at risk." (Craft-Rosenberg, 1999, p 127)

When the unit of care is not explicity stated, it becomes the individual by default.

AXIS 4 AGE: Defined as the length of time or interval during which an individual has existed. Values are:

> *Fetus*   *Adolescent*
> *Neonate*   *Young adult*
> *Infant*   *Middle-aged adult*
> *Toddler*   *Young old adult*
> *Pre-school child*   *Middle old adult*
> *School-aged child*   *Old old adult*

AXIS 5 HEALTH STATUS: Defined as the position or rank on the health continuum. Values are:

> *Wellness:* the quality or state of being healthy, especially as a result of deliberate effort.
> *Risk:* vulnerability, especially as a result of exposure to factors that increase the chance of injury or loss.
> *Actual:* existing in fact or reality, existing at the present time.

AXIS 6 DESCRIPTOR: Defined as a judgment that limits or specifies the meaning of a nursing diagnosis. Values are:

> *Ability:* capacity to do or act
> *Anticipatory:* to realize beforehand, foresee
> *Balance:* in a state of equilibrium
> *Compromised:* to make vulnerable to threat

Deficient: inadequate in amount, quality, or degree; not sufficient; incomplete

Delayed: to postpone, impede, and retard

Depleted: emptied wholly or in part, exhausted of

Disproportionate: not consistent with a standard

Disabling: to make unable or unfit, to incapacitate

Disorganized: to destroy the systematic arrangement

Disturbed: agitated or interrupted, interfered with

Dysfunctional: abnormal, incomplete functioning

Effective: producing the intended or expected effect

Excessive: characterized by the amount or quantity that is greater than necessary, desirable, or useful

Functional: normal complete functioning

Imbalanced: state of disequilibrium

Impaired: made worse, weakened, damaged, reduced, deteriorated

Inability: incapacity to do or act

Increased: greater in size, amount, or degree

Ineffective: not producing the desired effect

Interrupted: to break the continuity or uniformity

Organized: to form as into a systematic arrangement

Perceived: to become aware of by means of the senses; assignment of meaning

Readiness for enhanced (for use with wellness diagnoses): to make greater, to increase in quality, to attain the more desired

AXIS 7: TOPOLOGY: Consists of parts/regions of the body—all tissues, organs, anatomical sites or structures. Values are:

auditory	*oral*
bowel	*olfactory*
cardiopulmonary	*peripheral neurovascular*
cerebral	*peripheral vascular*
gastrointestinal	*renal*
gustatory	*skin*
intracranial	*tactile*
urinary	*visual*
mucous membranes	

(NANDA: Nursing Diagnoses: Definitions & Classification 2001–2002.)

Appendix C

Assessment Tools

The following are suggested guides/tools for development by an individual/institution to create databases reflecting Diagnostic Divisions of Nursing Diagnoses in any care setting. Although the divisions are alphabetized for ease of presentation, they can be prioritized or rearranged to meet individual needs.

Adult Medical/Surgical Assessment Tool

GENERAL INFORMATION

Name : _____ Age: _____ DOB: _____ Gender: _____ Race: _____
Admission Date: _____ Time: _____ From: _____
Source of Information: _____ Reliability (1–4 with 4 = very reliable): _____

Activity/Rest

SUBJECTIVE (REPORTS)
Occupation: _____ Usual activities: _____
   Leisure time activities/hobbies: _____
   Limitations imposed by condition: _____
Sleep: Hours: _____ Naps: _____ Aids: _____
   Insomnia: _____ Related to: _____
   Rested on awakening: _____
   Excessive grogginess: _____
Feelings of boredom/dissatisfaction: _____

OBJECTIVE (EXHIBITS)
Observed response to activity:
   Cardiovascular: _____
   Respiratory: _____
Mental status (i.e., withdrawn/lethargic): _____
Neuro/muscular assessment:
   Muscle mass/tone: _____ Posture: _____
   Tremors: _____ ROM: _____
   Strength: _____ Deformity: _____

Circulation

SUBJECTIVE (REPORTS)
History of: Hypertension: _____
   Heart trouble: _____ Rheumatic fever: _____
   Ankle/leg edema: _____ Phlebitis: _____
   Slow healing: _____ Claudication: _____
   Dysreflexia: _____
   Bleeding tendencies/episodes: _____
   Palpitations: _____ Syncope: _____

OBJECTIVE (EXHIBITS)
BP: R and L: Lying: _____
   Sitting: _____ Standing: _____
Pulse pressure: _____ Auscultatory gap: _____
Pulses (palpation): Carotid: _____
   Temporal: _____
   Jugular: _____ Radial: _____ Femoral: _____
   Popliteal: _____ Post-tibial: _____
   Dorsalis pedis: _____
Cardiac (palpation): Thrill: _____

Extremities: Numbness: _____ Tingling: _____
Cough/hemoptysis: _____
Change in frequency/amount of urine: _____
Other: _____

Heaves: _____
Heart sounds: Rate: _____ Rhythm: _____
    Quality: _____
Friction rub: _____ Murmur: _____
    Vascular bruit: _____
    Jugular vein distention: _____
Breath sounds: _____
Extremities: Temperature: _____ Color: _____
    Capillary refill: _____ Homans' sign: _____
    Varicosities: _____ Nail abnormalities: _____
    Edema: _____ Distribution/quality of hair: _____
    Trophic skin changes: _____
Color: General: _____
    Mucous membranes: _____ Lips: _____
    Nailbeds: _____ Conjunctiva: _____
    Sclera: _____
Diaphoresis: _____

Ego Integrity

SUBJECTIVE (REPORTS)

Stress factors: _____
Ways of handling stress: _____
Financial concerns: _____
Relationship status: _____
Cultural factors/ethnic ties: _____
Religion: _____ Practicing: _____
Lifestyle: _____ Recent changes: _____
Sense of connectedness/harmony with self:_____
Feelings of: Helplessness _____
    Hopelessness: _____
    Powerlessness: _____

OBJECTIVE (EXHIBITS)

Emotional status (check those that apply):
    Calm: _____ Anxious: _____ Angry: _____
    Withdrawn: _____ Fearful: _____
    Irritable: _____
    Restive: _____ Euphoric: _____
Observed physiological response(s): _____
Changes in energy field:
    Temperature: _____ Color: _____
    Distribution: _____
    Movement: _____ Sounds: _____

Elimination

SUBJECTIVE (REPORTS)

Usual bowel pattern: _____
Laxative use: _____
Character of Stool: _____ Last BM: _____
    Constipation: _____ Diarrhea: _____
    History of bleeding: _____ Hemorrhoids: _____
Usual voiding pattern: _____
    Incontinence/when: _____ Urgency: _____
    Frequency: _____ Retention: _____
Character of urine: _____
Pain/burning/difficulty voiding: _____
History of kidney/bladder disease: _____
Diuretic use: _____

OBJECTIVE (EXHIBITS)

Abdomen: Tender: _____ Soft/firm: _____
    Palpable mass: _____ Size/girth: _____
    Bowel sounds: Location/type: _____
Hemorrhoids: _____ Stool guaiac: _____
Bladder palpable: _____
    Overflow voiding: _____
    CVA tenderness: _____

Food/Fluid

SUBJECTIVE (REPORTS)
Usual diet (type): _____
Carbohydrate/protein/fat intake: g/d: _____
Vitamin/food supplement use: _____
Food preferences: _____ Prohibitions: _____
No. of meals daily: _____
Dietary pattern/content: B: _____ L: _____
    D: _____
Last meal/intake: _____
Loss of appetite: _____ Nausea/vomiting: _____
Heartburn/indigestion: _____ Related to: _____
    Relieved by: _____
Allergy/food intolerance: _____
Mastication/swallowing problems: _____
    Dentures: _____
Usual weight: _____ Changes in weight: _____
Diuretic use: _____

OBJECTIVE (EXHIBITS)
Current weight: _____ Height: _____
    Body build: _____
Skin turgor: _____ Mucous membranes:
    Moist/dry: _____
Breath sounds: _____ Crackles: _____
    Wheezes: _____
Edema: General: _____ Dependent: _____
    Periorbital: _____ Ascites: _____
Jugular vein distention (JVD): _____
Thyroid enlarged: _____
Halitosis: _____ Condition of teeth/gums: _____
    Appearance of tongue: _____
    Mucous membranes: _____
Bowel sounds: _____ Hernia/masses: _____
Urine S/A or Chemstix: _____
Serum glucose (Glucometer): _____

Hygiene

SUBJECTIVE (REPORTS)
Activities of daily living: Independent/dependent
    (specify level):
    Mobility: _____ Feeding: _____ Hygiene: _____
    Dressing: _____ Toileting: _____
Preferred time of personal care/bath: _____
Equipment/prosthetic devices required: _____
Assistance provided by: _____

OBJECTIVE (EXHIBITS)
General appearance: _____
Manner of dress: _____ Personal habits: _____
    Body odor: _____ Condition of scalp: _____
    Presence of vermin: _____

Neurosensory

SUBJECTIVE (REPORTS)
Fainting spells/dizziness: _____
Headaches: Location: _____ Frequency: _____
Tingling/numbness/weakness (location): _____
Stroke/brain injury (residual effects): _____
Seizures: _____ Type: _____ Aura: _____
    Frequency: _____ Postictal state: _____
    How controlled: _____
Eyes: Vision loss: _____ Last exam: _____
    Glaucoma: _____ Cataract: _____
Ears: Hearing loss: _____ Last exam: _____
Epistaxis: _____ Sense of smell: _____
Other: _____

OBJECTIVE (EXHIBITS)
Mental status: (note duration of change)
    Oriented/disoriented: Time: _____ Place: _____
    Person: _____ Situation: _____
    Check all that apply:
    Alert: _____ Drowsy: _____ Lethargic: _____
    Stuporous: _____ Comatose: _____
    Cooperative: _____ Combative: _____
    Delusions: _____ Hallucinations: _____
    Affect (describe): _____
    Memory: Recent: _____ Remote: _____
Glasses: _____ Contacts: _____ Hearing aids: _____
Pupil shape: _____ Size/reaction: R/L: _____
Facial droop: _____ Swallowing: _____
Handgrasp/release, R/L: _____
Posturing: _____
Deep tendon reflexes: _____ Paralysis: _____

Pain/Discomfort

SUBJECTIVE (REPORTS)
Primary focus: _____ Location:
    (Intensity (0–10 with 10 most severe): _____
    Frequency: _____ Quality: _____
    Duration: _____ Radiation: _____
Precipitating factors: _____ How relieved: _____
Associated symptoms: _____
Effect on activities: _____ Relationships: _____
Additional focus: _____

OBJECTIVE (EXHIBITS)
Facial grimacing: _____ Guarding affected
    area: _____
    Posturing: _____ Behaviors: _____
Emotional response: _____ Narrowed
    focus: _____
Change in BP: _____ Pulse: _____

Respiration

SUBJECTIVE (REPORTS)
Dyspnea/related to: _____
Cough/sputum: _____
History of bronchitis: _____ Asthma: _____
    Tuberculosis: _____ Emphysema: _____
    Recurrent pneumonia: _____
    Exposure to noxious fumes: _____
Smoker: Pk/day: _____ No. of pack years: _____
Use of respiratory aids: _____ Oxygen: _____

OBJECTIVE (EXHIBITS)
Respiratory: Rate: _____ Depth: _____
    Symmetry: _____
Use of accessory muscles: _____ Nasal flaring: _____
Fremitus: _____
Breath sounds: _____ Egophony: _____
Cyanosis: _____ Clubbing of fingers: _____
Sputum characteristics: _____
Mentation/restlessness: _____

Safety

SUBJECTIVE (REPORTS)
Allergies/sensitivity: _____ Reaction: _____
Exposure to infectious diseases: _____
Previous alteration of immune system: _____
    Cause: _____
History of sexually transmitted disease
    (date/type): _____
    Testing: _____ High-risk behaviors: _____
Blood transfusion/number: _____ When: _____
    Reaction: _____ Describe: _____
Geographic areas lived in/visited: _____
Seat belt/helmet use: _____
History of accidental injuries: _____
    Fractures/dislocations: _____
Arthritis/unstable joints: _____
    Back problems: _____
Changes in moles: _____
Enlarged nodes: _____
Delayed healing: _____
Cognitive limitations: _____
Impaired vision/hearing: _____
Prosthesis: _____
Ambulatory devices: _____

OBJECTIVE (EXHIBITS)
Temperature: _____ Diaphoresis: _____
Skin integrity: Scars: _____ Rashes: _____
    Lacerations: _____ Ulcerations: _____
    Ecchymosis: _____ Blisters: _____
    Burns: (degree/percent): _____ Drainage: _____
(Mark location on diagram):

General strength: _____ Muscle tone: _____
    Gait: _____ ROM: _____
    Paresthesia/paralysis: _____
Results of cultures: _____
Immune system testing: _____
Tuberculosis testing: _____

Sexuality [Component of Social Interaction]

SUBJECTIVE (REPORTS)
Sexually active: _____
Use of condoms: _____
Birth control method: _____
Sexual concerns/difficulties: _____
Recent change in frequency/interest: _____
Female
Age at menarche: _____ Length of cycle: _____
   Duration: ___ Number of pads used/day: ___
   Last menstrual period: _____
   Pregnant now: _____
Bleeding between periods: _____
Menopause: _____ Vaginal lubrication: _____
Vaginal discharge: _____
Surgeries: _____
Hormonal therapy/calcium use: _____
Practices breast self-exam: _____
Last mammogram: _____ Last PAP smear: _____
Male
Penile discharge: _____
Prostate disorder: _____
Circumcised: _____ Vasectomy: _____
Practice self-exam: Breast: _____ Testicles: _____
Last proctoscopic/prostate exam: _____

OBJECTIVE (EXHIBITS)
Comfort level with subject matter: _____

Breast exam: _____
Genital warts/lesions: _____
Discharge: _____

Breast: _____
Penis: _____
Testicles: _____
Genital warts/lesions: _____
Discharge: _____

Social Interactions

SUBJECTIVE (REPORTS)
Marital status: _____ Years in relationship: _____

   Perception of relationship: _____
   Living with: _____
   Concerns/stresses: _____
Extended family: _____
Other support person(s): _____
Role within family structure: _____
Perception of relationship with family members: _____

Ethnic affiliation: _____
Strength of ethnic identity: _____
Lives in ethnic community (Y/N): _____
Feelings of: Mistrust: _____ Rejection: _____
   Unhappiness: ___ Loneliness/isolation: ___
Problems related to illness/condition: _____
Problems with communication: _____
   Use of communication aids: _____
Genogram: _____

OBJECTIVE (EXHIBITS)
Speech: Clear: _____ Slurred: _____
   Unintelligible: _____ Aphasic: _____
   Unusual speech pattern/impairment: _____
   Use of speech/communication aids: _____
   Laryngectomy: _____
Verbal/nonverbal communication with family/SO(s): _____
Family interaction (behavioral) pattern: _____

Teaching/Learning

SUBJECTIVE (REPORTS)

Dominant language (specify): _____ Second language: _____ Literate: _____ Education level: _____ Learning disabilities (specify): _____

Cognitive limitations: _____

Where born: _____ If immigrant, how long in this country: _____

Health and illness beliefs/practices (e.g., complementary therapies)/customs : _____

Presence of Advance Directives/Durable Medical Power of Attorney: _____

Special healthcare concerns (e.g., impact of religious/cultural practices): _____

    Health goals: _____

Familial risk factors (indicate relationship):

    Diabetes: _____ Thyroid (specify): _____

    Tuberculosis: _____ Heart disease: _____

    Strokes: _____ High BP: _____ Epilepsy: _____

    Kidney disease: _____ Cancer: _____

    Mental illness: _____ Other: _____

Prescribed medications:

    Drug: _____ Dose: _____

    Times (circle last dose): _____

    Take regularly: _____ Purpose: _____

    Side effects/problems: _____

Nonprescription drugs:

    OTC drugs: _____

    Street drugs: _____ Tobacco: _____

    Smokeless tobacco: _____

    Alcohol (amount/frequency): _____

Use of herbal supplements (specify): _____

Admitting diagnosis per provider: _____

Reason for hospitalization per client: _____

History of current complaint: _____

Client expectations of care: _____

Previous illnesses and/or hospitalizations/surgeries: _____

Evidence of failure to improve: _____

Last complete physical exam: _____

Discharge Plan Considerations

DRG projected mean length of stay: _____

Date information obtained: _____

Anticipated date of discharge: _____

Resources available: Persons: _____

    Financial: _____ Community: _____

    Support groups: _____ Socialization: _____

Areas that may require alteration/assistance:

    Food preparation: _____ Shopping: _____

    Transportation: _____ Ambulation: _____

    Medication/IV therapy: _____

    Treatments: _____ Wound care: _____

    Supplies: _____

    Self-care (specify): _____

    Homemaker/maintenance (specify): _____

Physical layout of home (specify): _____

Anticipated changes in living situation after discharge: _____

Living facility other than home (specify): _____

Referrals (date, source, services):

    Social services: _____

    Rehabilitation services: _____

    Dietary: _____

    Home care: _____

    Resp/O$_2$: _____

    Equipment: _____

    Supplies: _____

    Other: _____

EXCERPT FROM PSYCHIATRIC NURSING TOOL

Ego Integrity

SUBJECTIVE (REPORTS)

What kind of person are you (positive/negative, etc.)? _____

What do you think of your body? _____

How would you rate your self-esteem (1–10 with 10 highest)? _____

What are your problematic moods?

Depressed: _____ Guilty: _____ Sad: _____

Unreal: _____ Ups/downs: _____ Apathetic: _____

Detached: _____ Separated from the world: _____

Are you a nervous person? _____

Are your feelings easily hurt? _____

Report of stress factors: _____

Previous patterns of handling stress: _____

Financial concerns: _____

Relationship status: _____

Work history/Military service: _____

Cultural factors: _____ Religion: _____ Practicing: _____

Lifestyle: _____ Recent changes: _____

Significant losses/changes (date): _____

Stages of grief; manifestations of loss: _____

Feelings of: Helplessness: _____ Hopelessness: _____ Powerlessness: _____

Coping strategies: _____

OBJECTIVE (EXHIBITS)

Emotional status (check those that apply):

Calm: _____ Friendly: _____

Cooperative: _____ Evasive: _____

Fearful: _____ Anxious/hostile: _____

Irritable: _____ Withdrawn: _____

Restive: _____ Passive: _____

Dependent: _____ Euphoric: _____

Other (specify): _____

Defense mechanisms: Projection: _____

Denial: _____ Undoing: _____

Rationalization: _____ Passive/aggressive: _____

Repression: _____ Intellectualization: _____

Somatization: _____ Regression: _____

Identification: _____ Introjection: _____

Reaction formation: _____ Isolation: _____

Displacement: _____ Substitution: _____

Sublimation: _____

Consistency of behavior:

Verbal: _____ Nonverbal: _____

Characteristics of speech: _____

Slow/rapid/volume: _____

Pressured: _____

Impairments: _____ Aphasia: _____

Motor activity/behaviors: _____

Posturing: _____ Under/overactive: _____

Stereotypic: _____ Tics/tremors: _____

Gait patterns: _____

Observed physiological response(s): _____

Neurosensory

SUBJECTIVE (REPORTS)

Dreamlike states: _____

Walking in sleep: _____

Automatic writing: _____

Believe/feel you are another person: _____

Perception different than others: _____

Ability to follow directions: _____

Perform calculations: _____

Accomplish ADL: _____

Fainting spells/dizziness: _____

Blackouts: _____

Seizures: _____

OBJECTIVE (EXHIBITS)

Mental Status: (note duration of change)

Oriented/disoriented: Time: _____

Place: _____ Person: _____

Check all that apply:

Alert: _____ Drowsy: _____

Lethargic: _____ Stuporous: _____

Comatose: _____

Cooperative: _____ Combative: _____

Delusions: _____ Hallucinations: _____

Affect (describe): _____

Memory: Immediate: _____

Recent: _____ Remote: _____

Comprehension: _____

Thought processes (assessed through speech):

Patterns of speech (spontaneous/sudden silences): _____

Content: _____ Change in topic: _____

Delusions: _____ Hallucinations: _____

Illusions: _____

Rate or flow: _____

Clear, logical progression: _____

Expression: _____ Flight of ideas: _____

Ability to concentrate: _____

Attention span: _____

Mood: _____

Affect: _____ Appropriateness: _____

Intensity: _____ Range: _____

Insight: _____ Misperceptions: _____

Attention/calculation skills: _____

Judgment: _____

Ability to follow directions: _____

Problem solving: _____

Impulse control: _____ Aggression: _____

Hostility: _____ Affection: _____

Sexual feelings: _____

EXCERPT FROM PRENATAL ASSESSMENT TOOL

Safety

SUBJECTIVE (REPORTS)

Allergies/Sensitivity: _____

Reaction: _____

Previous alteration of immune system: _____

Cause: _____

History of sexually transmitted diseases/gynecologic infections (date/type): _____

High-risk behaviors: _____ Testing: _____

Blood transfusion/number: _____

When: _____ Reaction: _____

Describe: _____

Childhood diseases: _____

Immunization history: _____

Recent exposure to German measles: _____

Other viral infections: _____ X-ray/radiation: _____ House pets: _____

Previous obstetric problems: PIH: _____

OBJECTIVE (EXHIBITS)

Temperature: _____ Diaphoresis: _____

Skin integrity: _____ Scars: _____

Rashes: _____

Ecchymosis: _____ Vaginal warts/lesions: _____

General strength: _____ Muscle tone: _____

Gait: _____ ROM: _____

Paresthesia/paralysis: _____

Fetal status: Heart rate: _____ Location: _____

Method of auscultation: _____

Fundal height: _____ Estimated gestation: _____

Activity/movement: _____ Ballottement: _____

Results of fetal testing: _____ AFT: _____

Results of cultures, cervical/rectal: _____

Immune system testing: _____

Kidney: _____ Hemorrhage: _____
Cardiac: _____
Diabetes: _____ Infection/UTI: _____
ABO/Rh sensitivity: _____
Uterine surgery: _____ Anemia: _____
Length of time since last pregnancy: _____ Type of previous delivery: _____
History of accidental injuries:
Fractures/dislocations: _____
Physical abuse: _____ Arthritis/unstable joints: _____ Back problems: _____
Changes in moles: _____ Enlarged nodes: _____
Impaired vision: _____ Hearing: _____
Prosthesis/ambulatory devices: _____

Blood type: Maternal: _____ Paternal: _____
Screenings, i.e., Serology: _____
Syphilis: _____
Sickle cell: _____ Rubella: _____
Hepatitis: _____ HIV: _____

Sexuality (Component of Social Interactions)

SUBJECTIVE (REPORTS)

Sexual concerns: _____ Menarche: _____
Length of cycle: _____ Duration: _____
First day of last menstrual period: _____
Amount: _____
Bleeding/cramping since LMP: _____
Vaginal discharge: _____
Client's belief of when conception occurred: _____
Estimated date of delivery: _____
Practices breast self-exam (Y/N): _____
Last Pap smear: _____
Recent contraceptive method: _____
Ob history: GPTPAL: Gravida: _____
Para: _____ Term: _____
Preterm: _____ Abortions: _____
Living: _____ Multiple births: _____
Delivery History: Year: _____
Place of delivery: _____ Length of gestation: _____ Length of labor: _____ Type of delivery: _____ Born (alive or dead): _____
Weight: _____ Apgar scores: _____
Complications (maternal/fetal): _____

OBJECTIVE (EXHIBITS)

Pelvic: Vulva: _____ Perineum: _____
Vagina: _____ Cervix: _____ Uterus: _____
Adnexa: _____
Diagonal conjugate: _____ Transverse diameter: _____ Outlet (cm): _____
Shape of sacrum: _____ Arch: _____
Coccyx: _____ SS Notch: _____
Ischial spines: _____ Adequacy of inlet: _____
Mid: _____ Outlet: _____
Prognosis for delivery: _____
Breast exam: _____ Nipples: _____
Pregnancy test: _____
Serology test (date): _____
PAP smear results: _____

EXCERPT FROM INTRAPARTAL ASSESSMENT TOOL

Pain/Discomfort

SUBJECTIVE (REPORTS)

Uterine contractions began: _____
Became regular: _____ Character: _____
Frequency: _____

OBJECTIVE (EXHIBITS)

Facial expression: _____ Narrowed focus: _____
Body movement: _____
Psychological response: _____
Change in BP: _____ Pulse: _____

Duration: _____
Location of contractile pain: Front: _____
   Sacral area: _____
Degree of discomfort: Mild: _____ Moderate:
   _____ Severe: _____ How relieved: _____
   Breathing/relaxation techniques: _____
   Positioning: _____ Sacral rubs: _____
   Effleurage: _____ Other: _____

Safety

SUBJECTIVE (REPORTS)

Allergies/Sensitivity: _____
   Reaction (specify): _____
History of STD (date/type): _____
Health status of living children: _____
Month of first prenatal visit: _____
Previous/current obstetric problems/treatment:
   PIH: _____ Kidney: _____
   Hemorrhage: _____
   Cardiac: _____ Diabetes: _____
   Infection/UTI: _____ ABO/Rh sensitivity: _____
   Uterine surgery: _____ Anemia: _____
Length of time since last pregnancy: _____
Type of previous delivery: _____
Blood transfusion: _____ When: _____
   Reaction (describe): _____
Maternal stature/build: _____
Fractures/dislocations: _____
Pelvis: _____
Arthritis/Unstable joints: _____
Spinal problems/deformity:
   Kyphosis: _____ Scoliosis: _____
   Trauma: _____ Surgery: _____
   Prosthesis: _____ Ambulatory devices: _____

OBJECTIVE (EXHIBITS)

Temperature: _____
Skin integrity: _____ Rashes: _____
   Sores: _____ Bruises: _____ Scars: _____
Paresthesia/paralysis: _____
Fetal status: Heart rate: _____ Location: _____
   Method of auscultation: _____
   Fundal height: _____
   Estimated gestation: _____
   Activity/movement: _____
   Fetal assessment testing (Y/N): _____
   Date: _____ Test: _____
   Results: _____
Labor status: Cervical dilation: _____
   Effacement: _____ Fetal descent: _____
   Engagement: _____ Presentation: _____
   Lie: _____ Position: _____
Membranes: Intact: _____
   Ruptured/time: _____ Nitrazine test: _____
   Amount of drainage: _____
   Character: _____
Blood Type/Rh: Maternal: _____
Paternal: _____ Screens: Sickle cell: _____
   Rubella: _____
   Hepatitis: _____ HIV: _____
Serology: Syphilis: Pos _____ Neg _____
Cervical/Rectal culture: Pos _____ Neg _____
Vaginal warts/lesions: _____
Perineal varicosities: _____

Appendix D

NANDA Nursing Diagnoses Organized According to Maslow's Hierarchy of Needs and Nursing Framework: A Health Outcome Classification for Nursing Diagnosis

Maslow's Hierarchy of Needs

SELF-ACTUALIZATION

Coping, community, readiness for enhanced
Development, risk for delayed
Coping, family: readiness for enhanced
Growth and Development, delayed
Growth, risk for disproportionate
Health-Seeking Behaviors [specify]
Spiritual Distress
Spiritual Distress, risk for
Spiritual Well-being, readiness for enhanced
Therapeutic Regimen: effective management

SELF-ESTEEM

Adjustment, impaired
Body Image, disturbed
Conflict, decisional (specify)
Coping, defensive
Coping, ineffective
Denial, ineffective
Diversional Activity, deficient
Hopelessness
Noncompliance [Adherence, ineffective]
  (specify)

Nutrition: imbalanced, more than body requirements

Nutrition: imbalanced, risk for more than body requirements

Personal Identity, disturbed

Post-Trauma Syndrome

Post-Trauma Syndrome, risk for

Powerlessness

Powerlessness, risk for

Rape-Trauma Syndrome

Rape-Trauma Syndrome: compound reaction

Rape-Trauma Syndrome: silent reaction

Self-Esteem, chronic low

Self-Esteem, situational low

Self-Esteem, risk for situational low

Self-Mutilation

Self-Mutilation, risk for

Suicide, risk for

Violence, [actual/] risk for other-directed

Violence, [actual/] risk for self-directed

LOVE AND BELONGING

Attachment, risk for impaired parent/infant/child

Coping, family: compromised

Coping, family: disabled

Family Processes, interrupted

Family Processes, dysfunctional: alcoholism

Loneliness, risk for

Parental Role Conflict

Parenting, impaired

Parenting, risk for impaired

Relocation Stress Syndrome

Relocation Stress Syndrome, risk for

Role Performance, ineffective

Social Interaction, impaired

Social Isolation

SAFETY AND SECURITY

Autonomic Dysreflexia

Autonomic Dysreflexia, risk for

Anxiety [specify level]

Anxiety, death

Caregiver Role Strain

Caregiver Role Strain, risk for

Communication, impaired verbal

Coping, community, ineffective

Confusion, acute

Confusion, chronic

Disuse Syndrome, risk for

Environmental Interpretation Syndrome, impaired

Falls, risk for

Fear

Grieving, anticipatory

Grieving, dysfunctional

Health Maintenance, ineffective

Home Maintenance, impaired

Infant Behavior, readiness for enhanced, organized

Infection, risk for

Injury, risk for

Injury, risk for, perioperative positioning

Knowledge deficient [Learning Need] (specify)

Allergy Response, latex

Allergy Response, latex, risk for

Memory, impaired

Mobility, impaired bed

Mobility, impaired wheelchair

Peripheral Neurovascular Dysfunction, risk for

Poisoning, risk for

Protection, ineffective

Sorrow, chronic

Therapeutic Regimen: Community, ineffective management

Therapeutic Regimen: Family, ineffective management

Therapeutic Regimen: ineffective management

Transfer Ability, impaired

Trauma, risk for

Unilateral Neglect

Walking, impaired

Wandering [specify sporadic or continuous]

PHYSIOLOGICAL NEEDS

Activity Intolerance [specify level]

Activity Intolerance, risk for

Intracranial, decreased adaptive capacity

Airway Clearance, ineffective

Aspiration, risk for

Body Temperature, risk for imbalanced
Bowel Incontinence
Breastfeeding, effective
Breastfeeding, ineffective
Breastfeeding, interrupted
Breathing Pattern, ineffective
Cardiac Output, decreased
Constipation
Constipation, perceived
Constipation, risk for
Dentition, impaired
Diarrhea
Energy Field, disturbed
Failure to Thrive, adult
Fatigue
Fluid Volume, deficient
Fluid Volume, excess
Fluid Volume, risk for deficient
Fluid Volume, risk for imbalanced
Gas Exchange, impaired
Hyperthermia
Hypothermia
Infant Behavior, disorganized
Infant Behavior, risk for disorganized
Infant Feeding Pattern, ineffective
Mobility, impaired physical [specify level]
Nausea
Nutrition: imbalanced, less than body requirements
Oral Mucous Membrane, impaired
Pain, acute
Pain, chronic
Protection, ineffective
Self Care Deficit (specify): feeding, bathing/hygiene, dressing/grooming, toileting
SensoryPerception, disturbed (specify: visual, auditory, kinesthetic, gustatory, tactile, olfactory)
Sexual Dysfunction
Sexuality Patterns, ineffective
Skin Integrity, impaired
Skin Integrity, risk for impaired
Sleep Deprivation

Sleep Pattern, disturbed
Suffocation, risk for
Surgical Recovery, delayed
Swallowing, impaired
Thermoregulation, ineffective
Thought Processes, disturbed
Tissue Integrity, impaired
Tissue Perfusion, ineffective (specify type: cerebral, cardiopulmonary, renal, gastrointestinal, peripheral)
Urinary Elimination, impaired
Urinary Incontinence, functional
Urinary Incontinence, reflex
Urinary Incontinence, stress
Urinary Incontinence, total
Urinary Incontinence, urge
Urinary Incontinence, risk for urge
Urinary Retention [acute/chronic]
Ventilation, impaired spontaneous
Ventilatory Weaning Response, dysfunctional

Nursing Framework: A Health Outcome Classification for Nursing Diagnoses*

SELF-CARE OF NURSING DIAGNOSES

I. **Physiological Homeostasis**
    1.1.0. Alterations in oxygenation
        1.1.1. Impaired gas exchange
        1.1.2. Ineffective airway clearance
            1.1.2.1. Risk for aspiration
            1.1.2.2. Risk for suffocation
        1.1.3. Ineffective breathing pattern
            1.1.3.1. Inability to sustain spontaneous ventilation
            1.1.3.2. Dysfunctional ventilatory weaning response
    1.2.0. Alterations in circulation
        1.2.1. Altered tissue perfusion
        1.2.2. Altered fluid volume
            1.2.2.1. Deficit

* Modified from Jenny, J.: *Classification of Nursing Diagnoses: NANDA Proceedings from the 8th Conference.* Philadelphia: J. B. Lippincott, 1989; and Jenny, J.: Classifying nursing diagnoses: A self-care approach. *Nursing and Health Care* 10(2):1983–1988.

1.2.2.2. Excess
1.2.3. Decreased cardiac output
1.3.0. Alterations in protective mechanisms
1.3.1. Risk for infection
1.3.2. [Bleeding tendency]
1.3.3. Risk for peripheral neurovascular dysfunction
1.3.4. Dysreflexia
1.4.0. Ineffective thermoregulation
1.4.1. Risk for altered body temperature
1.4.1.1. Hypothermia
1.4.1.2. Hyperthermia
1.5.0. Sensory-perceptual alterations
1.5.1. Specific sensory deficit
1.5.1.1. Impaired vision
1.5.1.2. Impaired hearing [auditory]
1.5.1.3. Impaired touch [tactile]
1.5.1.4. Impaired taste [gustatory]
1.5.1.5. Impaired smell [olfactory]
1.5.1.6. Impaired sense of movement [kinesthetic]
1.5.1.7. [Altered proprioception]
1.5.2. [Altered consciousness]
1.5.3. Discomfort/pain
1.5.3.1. Chronic pain

II. Bodily Comfort
2.1.0. Alterations in nutrition
2.1.1. More than body requirements
2.1.2. Less than body requirements
2.1.3. Effective breastfeeding
2.1.4. Feeding difficulties
2.1.4.1. Impaired swallowing
2.1.4.2. Ineffective infant feeding pattern
2.1.4.2.1. Ineffective breastfeeding
2.1.4.2.2. Interrupted breastfeeding
2.1.5. Delayed growth
2.2.0. Alterations in elimination
2.2.1. Bowel
2.2.1.1. Constipation
2.2.1.1.1. Colonic
2.2.1.1.2. Perceived
2.2.1.2. Diarrhea
2.2.1.3. Incontinence
2.2.2. Bladder
2.2.2.1. Incontinence

2.2.2.1.1. Functional
2.2.2.1.2. Reflex
2.2.2.1.3. Stress
2.2.2.1.4. Total
2.2.2.1.5. Urge
2.2.2.2. Retention
2.2.2.3. Altered urination pattern
2.2.3. [Skin]
2.2.4. Toileting difficulties
2.3.0. Impaired tissue integrity
2.3.1. Impaired skin integrity
2.3.2. Impaired oral mucous membrane
2.4.0. Alterations in activity
2.4.1. Impaired physical mobility
2.4.1.1. [Hyperactivity]
2.4.1.2. Activity intolerance
2.4.1.3. Risk for disuse syndrome
2.4.2. Sleep pattern disturbance
2.4.3. Fatigue
2.4.4. Diversional activity/recreation deficit
2.5.0. Altered grooming pattern
2.5.1. Specific grooming difficulties
2.5.1.1. Bathing/perineal care
2.5.1.2. [Mouth care]
2.5.1.3. Dressing
2.5.2. [Self neglect]
2.5.2.1. Neglect, unilateral

III. Ego Integrity
3.1.0. Altered self concept
3.1.1. Disturbance in body image
3.1.2. Disturbance in self esteem
3.1.2.1. Chronic low
3.1.2.2. Situational low
3.1.3. Disturbance in personal identity
3.2.0. Altered thought processes
3.2.1. [Impaired information processing]
3.2.2. [Memory loss]
3.2.3. [Confusion]
3.2.4. [Impaired learning]
3.2.5. [Impaired self-orientation]
3.3.0. [Diminished feelings of personal control]
3.3.1. Anxiety
3.3.2. Fear
3.3.3. Grieving
3.3.3.1. Anticipatory

3.3.3.2. Dysfunctional
3.3.4. Risk for violence
   3.3.4.1. Risk for self mutilation
3.3.5. Post-trauma response
   3.3.5.1. Rape-trauma syndrome
      3.3.5.1.1. Compound reaction
      3.3.5.1.2. Silent reaction
3.3.6. Powerlessness
3.3.7. Hopelessness
3.4.0. Spiritual distress

IV. **Social Interaction**
4.1.0. [Alterations in communication]
   4.1.1. Verbal, impaired
   4.1.2. [Nonverbal, impaired]
4.2.0. [Alterations in relationships]
   4.2.1. Social isolation
   4.2.2. [Social withdrawal]
   4.2.3. Altered sexuality pattern
      4.2.3.1. Sexual dysfunction
4.3.0. Alterations in role
   4.3.1. Impaired parenting
      4.3.1.1. Parental role conflict
   4.3.2. [Impaired work functioning]
      4.3.2.1. Caregiver role strain
4.4.0. Alterations in family process
   4.4.1. Family coping, potential for growth
   4.4.2. Ineffective family coping
      4.4.2.1. Compromised
      4.4.2.2. Disabling
4.5.0. [Risk for abuse]
4.6.0. Developmental delay

V. **Health Protection**
5.1.0. Health-seeking behaviors
5.2.0. Altered health maintenance
   5.2.1. [Inadequate self monitoring]
   5.2.2. [Inadequate self protection]
   5.2.3. [Reduced use of health services]
5.3.0. [Ineffective stress management]
   5.3.1. Ineffective individual coping
      5.3.1.1. Decisional conflict
      5.3.1.2. Ineffective denial
      5.3.1.3. Coping, defensive
5.4.0. Risk for injury
   5.4.1. Risk for trauma
   5.4.2. [Risk for abuse]

VI. **Health Restoration**
6.1.0. Ineffective management of therapeutic regimen
   6.1.1. Noncompliance [specify]
   6.1.2. Impaired adjustment
   6.1.3. [Risk for transmitting infection]

VII. **Environmental Management**
7.1.0. Impaired home maintenance management
   7.1.1. [Coping with dysfunctional facilities]
   7.1.2. [Inability to perform household tasks]
7.2.0. [Exposure to hazards]
7.3.0. [Separation from community services/resources]
7.4.0. Relocation stress syndrome

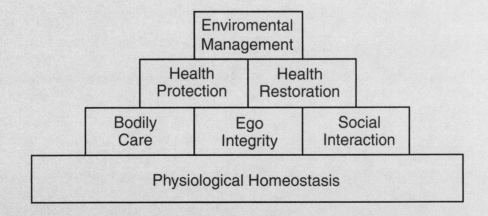

Appendix E

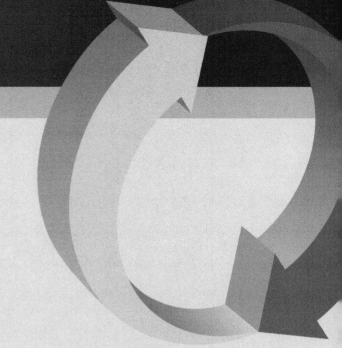

Code for Nurses

1. The nurse, in all professional relationships, practices with compassion and respect for the inherent dignity, worth, and uniqueness of every individual, unrestricted by considerations of social or economic status, personal attributes, or the nature of health problems.
2. The nurse's primary commitment is to the patient, whether an individual, family, group, or community.
3. The nurse promotes, advocates for, and strives to protect the health, safety, and rights of the patient.
4. The nurse is responsible and accountable for individual nursing practice and determines the appropriate delegation of tasks consistent with the nurse's obligation to provide optimum patient care.
5. The nurse owes the same duties to self as to others, including the responsibility to preserve integrity and safety, to maintain competence, and to continue personal and professional growth.
6. The nurse participates in establishing, maintaining, and improving health care environments and conditions of employment conducive to the provision of quality health care and consistent with the values of the profession through individual and collective action.
7. The nurse participates in the advancement of the profession through contributions to practice, education, administration, and knowledge development.
8. The nurse collaborates with other health professionals and the public in promoting community, national, and international efforts to meet health needs.
9. The profession of nursing, as represented by associations and their members, is responsible for articulating nursing values, for maintaining the integrity of the profession and its practice, and for shaping social policy.

Reprinted with permission from Code of Ethics for Nurses, 2001, American Nurses Association, Washington, DC.

Appendix F

Lunney's Ordinal Scale for Degrees of Accuracy of a Nursing Diagnosis

Value	Criteria
+5	Diagnosis is consistent with all of the cues, supported by highly relevant cues, and precise.
+4	Diagnosis is consistent with most or all of the cues and supported by relevant cues but fails to reflect one or a few highly relevant cues.
+3	Diagnosis is consistent with many of the cues but fails to reflect the specificity of available cues.
+2	Diagnosis is indicated by some of the cues but there are insufficient cues relevant to the diagnosis, and/or the diagnosis is lower priority than other diagnoses.
+1	Diagnosis is suggested by only one or a few cues.
0	Diagnosis is not indicated by any of the cues. No diagnosis is stated when there are sufficient cues to state a diagnosis. The diagnosis cannot be rated.
–1	Diagnosis is indicated by more than one cue but should be rejected based on the presence of at least two disconfirming cues.

Reprinted with permission from Lunney, M. (1990). Accuracy of nursing diagnosis: Concepts and developments. *Nursing Diagnosis* 1:12–17.

Self-Monitoring of Accuracy Using the Integrated Model: A Guide

1. Pre-encounter data
   a. What data did I collect before seeing the patient? Did I collect enough (or too much) information at this point?
   b. How did I interpret the data before seeing the patient (e.g., relevance of data, priority of data, nursing responsibilities related to data, health status of patient)? What were my biases?
   c. Did I cluster two or more cues, before contact with the patient, as having specific meaning when occurring together?
   d. Was I naming hypotheses before I saw the patient? Should I have connected the data with hypotheses?
2. Entering the data search field and shaping the direction of data gathering
   a. In what ways did seeing the patient affect my initial assessment?
   b. How did I interpret the data that I initially collected in relation to other data, previous expectations, priorities, my responsibilities,

or specific hypotheses? How did the patient interpret my behavior?
   c. Did I rearrange any clusters that existed (in my mind) before seeing the patient?
   d. For which hypotheses was I collecting data? Did I consider hypotheses related to the individuality of the patient? Did the patient express diagnostic hypotheses? Were the diagnoses the same as those that were generated by pre-encounter data, or did seeing the patient revise the names that I was considering?
3. Coalescing the cues into clusters or chunks
   a. To what extent did the clustering of cues make me aware of the need for further data collection?
   b. Did I assign validity and reliability estimates to the data while coalescing them into clusters or chunks?
   c. Did the clusters or chunks of data have meanings that can be validated through the literature?

d. To what extent would other nurses agree with the names that I was considering for the clusters or chunks?

4. **Activating possible diagnostic explanations**
   a. What data did I collect to support hypotheses? If the answer is none, did I close data collection prematurely? Did limitations in my knowledge prevent me from collecting data for certain diagnoses?
   b. How did I judge the relevance of the data that activated diagnostic hypotheses, for example, were they relevant enough to validate the diagnosis or just predictive? Was my judgment consistent with the judgment of the patient?
   c. Considering the literature on diagnostic concepts, how well did the clusters support the activation of diagnostic hypotheses? Did I consider the unique aspects of this patient when clustering the data for hypotheses?
   d. Did I consider the names of the important hypotheses?

5. **Hypothesis- and data-directed searching of the data field**
   a. Was my data collection efficient enough to produce highly relevant data for high-priority diagnoses as well as to rule out competitive diagnoses? Was I able to obtain the greatest quantity of relevant data with the least amount of cost to the patient and myself (cost equals time spent, time lost, and effort expended)?
   b. Was I able to interpret the data in relation to many conflicting hypotheses? Was my interpretation specific enough to direct me to precise diagnoses? Was I able to identify the need for further data?
   c. Were previous clusters used, or were they rearranged to produce new clusters?
   d. What diagnostic concepts were considered relevant and valid for testing the goodness of fit after a search of the data field? Were there concepts that I considered briefly during the previous steps but did not pursue?

6. **Testing diagnostic hypotheses for goodness of fit**
   a. What cues were used to test the goodness of fit?
   b. Were my interpretations of these cues derived from legitimate sources of information: theory, research, norms, and the unique patterns of the patient?
   c. Were the clusters of cues sufficiently well developed for testing the goodness of fit?
   d. Did the diagnostic label fulfill the criteria for goodness of fit?

Appendix H

Clinical (Critical) Pathways: A Sample

Clinical pathways may be used as a standardized plan of care or as a guideline for developing an individualized plan for a specific patient. Pathways are best used for acute problems for which there are predictable outcomes that must be achieved within a specific time frame. For example, Donald may be admitted initially to a medical, or step-down unit, during the acute phase of alcohol withdrawal. Following is a sample clinical pathway for his 5-day length of stay. After completing this phase, he would be transferred to the Behavioral Unit for the rehabilitation program, and a new clinical pathway would be implemented.

CLINICAL PATHWAY: ALCOHOL WITHDRAWAL—LOS: 5 DAYS

ND and Categories of Care	Time Dimension	Goals/Actions	Time Dimension	Goals/Actions	Time Dimension	Goals/Actions
Risk for injury R/T CNS agitation	Day 1	Verbalize understanding of unit policies, procedures, and safety concerns relative to individual needs Cooperate with therapeutic regimen	Day 3 Day 4	Vital signs stable I&O balanced Display marked decrease in objective symptoms	Day 5	Be free of injury resulting from ETOH withdrawal Display no objective symptoms of withdrawal
Referrals	Day 1	CNS/Psychiatrist If indicated: Internist, Cardiologist, Neurologist				
Diagnostic studies	Day 1	BA level Drug screen (urine and blood) If indicated: CXR, ECG Pulse oximetry	Day 2	SMA 20 Serum Mg, amylase RPR UA	Day 4	Repeat of selected studies as indicated
Additional assessments	Day 1 Day 1–4 Ongoing Stage I Stage II	VS, temp, respiratory status/breath sounds q4h I&O q8h Motor activity, body language, verbalizations, need for/type of restraint Withdrawal symptoms: Tremors, N/V, hypertension, tachycardia, diaphoresis, sleeplessness Increased hyperactivity, hallucinations, seizure activity	Day 2–3	VS q8h if stable	Day 4–5	VS qd

ND and Categories of Care	Time Dimension	Goals/Actions	Time Dimension	Goals/Actions	Time Dimension	Goals/Actions
	Stage III	Extreme autonomic hyperactivity, profound confusion, anxiety, fever				
Medications Allergies:	Day 1–4	Thiamine 100 mg IM				
	Day 1–5	Serax 15mg PO tid				
Patient education	Day 1	Orient to room/unit, schedule, procedures	Day 3	Need for ongoing therapy	Day 5	Schedule of follow-up visits if indicated
			Day 3–4	Goals/availability of AA program		
Additional nursing actions	Day 1	Bed rest 12 hr if in withdrawal	Day 3–5	Activity as tolerated		
		Position change, HOB elevated; C, DB exercises if on bedrest				
		Assist with ambulation, self-care as needed				
	Day 1–2	Encourage fluids if free of N/V				
	Ongoing	Provide environmental safety measures, seizure precautions as indicated				
		Reorient as needed				
Ineffective coping R/T personal vulnerability, situational crisis, inadequate coping methods	Day 1–5	Participate in development/evaluation of treatment plan	Day 3	Verbalize understanding of relationship of ETOH abuse to current situation	Day 5	Plan in place to meet needs post-discharge
	Day 2–5	Interact in group sessions				

ND and Categories of Care	Time Dimension	Goals/Actions	Time Dimension	Goals/Actions	Time Dimension	Goals/Actions
Referrals	Day 1 Day 2–5	Psychiatrist Group sessions	Day 4	Identify/make contact with potential resources, support groups		
Additional assessments	Day 1	Understanding of current situation Drinking pattern, previous withdrawal, other drug use, attitudes toward substance use History of violence	Day 4	Community classes: Assertiveness training Stress management		
	Day 1–2	Relationships with others: personal, work/school Readiness for group activities	Day 2–3	Previous coping strategies/consequences Perception of drug use on life, employment, legal issues		
			Day 3–5	Congruency of actions based on insight		
Medications			Day 5	Naltrexone 50 mg qd if indicated		
Patient education	Day 1	Physical effects of ETOH abuse	Day 3–5	Human behavior and interactions with others/ transactional analysis (TA)	Day 5	Medication dose, frequency, side effects Written instructions for therapeutic program
	Day 1–2	Types/use of relaxation techniques	Day 4–5	Community resources for self/family Identify goals for change		
	Day 2	Consequences of ETOH abuse				

ND and Categories of Care	Time/Dimension	Goals/Actions	Time/Dimension	Goals/Actions	Time/Dimension	Goals/Actions
Additional nursing actions	Day 1–5	Support patient's taking responsibility for own recovery Provide consistent approach/expectations for behavior Set limits/confront inappropriate behaviors	Day 2–5	Discuss alternative solutions Provide positive feedback for efforts Support during confrontation by peer group Encourage verbalization of feelings, personal reflection		
Imbalanced nutrition: less than body requirements R/T poor intake, effects of ETOH on digestive system, and hypermetabolic response to withdrawal	Day 2–5	Select foods appropriately to meet individual dietary needs	Day 4	Verbalize understanding of effects of ETOH abuse and reduced dietary intake on nutritional status	Day 5	Display stable weight or initial weight gain as appropriate, and laboratory results WNL
Referrals Diagnostic studies	Day 1 and prn Day 1	Dietitian CBC, liver function studies Serum albumin, transferrin	Day 2–5	Fingerstick glucose prn		
Additional assessments	Day 1 Day 1–2 Day 1–5	Weight, skin turgor, condition of mucous membranes, muscle tone Bowel sounds, characteristics of stools Appetite, dietary intake Antacid ac and hs			Day 5	Weight

ND and Categories of Care	Time Dimension	Goals/Actions	Time Dimension	Goals/Actions	Time Dimension	Goals/Actions
Medications	Day 1–5	Imodium 2 mg prn	Day 2–5	Multivitamin tab qd		
Patient education	Day 1–2	Individual nutritional needs	Day 4	Principles of nutrition, foods for maintenance of wellness		
Additional nursing actions	Day 1	Liquid/bland diet as tolerated	Day 2–5	Advance diet as tolerated		
	Day 1–5	Encourage small, frequent, nutritious meals/snacks Encourage good oral hygiene pc and hs				

Appendix I

Common Medical Abbreviations

Abbreviations are used as a time and space saver for those writing notes. In order to assure that everyone in the hospital/agency can understand what has been written by others, most facilities have a list of abbreviations approved by the medical record department for use in that particular facility. Therefore, the list of acceptable abbreviations varies from one facility to the next. The following is a representation of common abbreviations used by nurses. Note: The context of use determines the appropriate choice when more than one definition is provided.

A	assessment	bid	twice a day
ABD	abdomen	bilat.	bilateral
ac	before meals	BK	below knee
ACTH	adrenocorticotrophic hormone	BM	bowel movement
ad lib	at discretion	BP	blood pressure
ADL	activities of daily living	bpm	beats per minute
adm	admission	BR	bedrest
AFO	ankle-foot orthosis	BRP	bathroom privileges
AK	above knee	BS	blood sugar
AM	morning	B/S	bedside
AMA	against medical advice	BUN	blood urea nitrogen (blood test)
Amb	ambulate, ambulatory	C	Centigrade
AP	anteroposterior	C & S	culture and sensitivity
APN	advanced practice nurse	CA	carcinoma, cancer; cardiac arrest
AROM	active range of motion	CABG	coronary artery bypass graft
ASA	aspirin	CAD	coronary artery disease
ASAP	as soon as possible	cal	calories
ASHD	arteriosclerotic heart disease	CBC	complete blood count
assist.	assistance	CBS	chronic brain syndrome
as tol	as tolerated	CC, C/C	chief complaint
AV	atrioventricular; arteriovenous	cc	cubic centimeter

CCU	coronary care unit	I&O	intake and output
CHF	congestive heart failure	ICU	intensive care unit
cm	centimeter	IDDM	insulin-dependent diabetes mellitus
CNA	certified nursing assistant		
CNS	central nervous system; clinical nurse specialist	IM	intramuscular
		imp.	impression
c/o	complains of	in	inches
CO_2	carbon dioxide	IPPB	intermittent positive-pressure breathing
COLD	chronic obstructive lung disease		
cont.	continue	IV	intravenous
COPD	chronic obstructive pulmonary disease	JVP	jugular venous pressure
		kcal	kilocalories
CP	cerebral palsy	kg	kilogram
CSF	cerebrospinal fluid	KUB	kidney, ureter, bladder
CVA	cerebrovascular accident; costovertebral angle	L, l	liter
		lb	pound
CVP	central venous pressure	LBP	low back pain
DAR	data, action, response (charting)	LE	lower extremity
D&C	dilation & curettage	LOC	loss of consciousness; locus of control
DO	doctor of osteopathy; osteopath		
DOB	date of birth	LP	lumbar puncture
Dx	diagnosis	LPN/LVN	licensed practical/vocational nurse
ECG	electrocardiogram	L&W	living and well
EDD	expected date of delivery	m	meter
EEG	electroencephalogram	MD	medical doctor; doctor of medicine
ER/D	emergency room/department		
FBS	fasting blood sugar	Meds	medications
FHT	fetal heart tones	mEq	milliequivalent
Fx	fracture	mg	milligram
GU	genitourinary	MI	myocardial infarction
HA, H/A	headache	mL	milliliter
Hb, Hgb	hemoglobin	mm	millimeter
HCVD	hypertensive cardiovascular disease	Mn	midnight
		MRI	magnetic resonance imaging
HEENT	head, ear, eyes, nose, throat	MSW	medical social worker
HHA	home health agency	NA	nurse's aide
HIV	human immunodeficiency virus	ND	nursing diagnosis; nursing doctorate
HNP	herniated nucleus pulposus		
HOB	head of bed	neg	negative
HR	heart rate	NG	nasogastric
hr	hour	NIDDM	non–insulin-dependent diabetes mellitus
hs	at bedtime		
ht	height	NP	nurse practitioner
Ht	hematocrit	O_2	oxygen
Htn	hypertension	occ	occasional
Hx, hx	history	OOB	out of bed

OR	operating room	SOAP	subjective, objective, assessment, plan (charting)
OTC	over-the-counter		
PEEP	positive end-expiratory pressure	S/P	status post
PERRLA	pupils equal, round, and reactive to light and accommodation	spec	specimen
		STD	sexually transmitted disease
PO	per os (by mouth)	stat	immediately, at once
POMR	problem-oriented medical record	Sx	symptoms
pos	positive	T	temperature
poss	possible	T&A	tonsillectomy and adenoidectomy
post op	after surgery (operation)	tab	tablet
pre op	before surgery (operation)	TB	tuberculosis
PROM	passive range of motion; premature rupture of membranes	tbsp	tablespoon
		TENS, TNS	transcutaneous electrical nerve stimulator
prn	whenever necessary		
PT	physical therapy, physical therapist	THR	total hip replacement
		TIA	transient ischemic attack
Pt., pt.	patient	tid	three times daily
PVD	peripheral vascular disease	TKR	total knee replacement
PWB	partial weight bearing	TMJ	temporomandibular joint
q	every	t.o.	telephone order
qd	every day	TPR	temperature, pulse, and respiration
qh	every hour	tsp	teaspoon
qid	four times a day	TUR	transurethral resection
qn	every night	UA	urine analysis
qod	every other day	UE	upper extremity
qs	sufficient quantity	UMN	upper motor neuron
qt	quart	URI	upper respiratory infection
RA	rheumatoid arthritis	US	ultrasound
RBC	red blood cell count	UTI	urinary tract infection
RD	registered dietitian	UV	ultraviolet
re:	regarding	VD	venereal disease
resp	respiratory, respiration	vo	verbal orders
RN	registered nurse	vol	volume
R/O	rule out	vs	vital signs
ROM	range of motion	WBC	white blood cell count
ROS	review of systems	w/c	wheelchair
RT	respiratory therapist	WIC	women, infants, and children (nutritional program)
Rx	treatment, prescription, therapy		
sec	seconds	wk	week
sc	subcutaneous	WNL	within normal limits
sig	directions for use, give as follows, let it be labeled	wt	weight
		X	number of times performed ($\times 2$ = twice)
SLE	systemic lupus erythematosus		
SLR	straight leg raise	y/o	years old
SNF	skilled nursing facility	yd	yard
SO(s)	significant other(s)	yr	year

Appendix J

Glossary

Analysis: The process of examining and categorizing information to reach a conclusion about a client's needs.

Assessment: The first step of the nursing process, during which data are collected.

Baseline Assessment: Initial data collection done at the time of admission/beginning of shift, and so on, with which future assessments are compared.

Charting: The written record of relevant details of the care given to a client and the client's response, including observations and changes in the patient's condition.

Client Database: The compilation of data collected about a client; it consists of the nursing history, physical examination, and results of the diagnostic studies.

Client Diagnostic Statement: The outcome of the diagnostic reasoning process; a three-part statement identifying the client's problem/need, etiology of the problem/need, and the associated signs/symptoms.

Collaborative Problem: A need identified by another discipline that will contain a nursing component requiring nursing intervention and/or monitoring.

Concept-mapping: Diagrams of important ideas (client problems and treatments) that are linked together.

Cue(s): A signal that indicates a possible need/direction for care.

DAR: Format for charting—data, actions, response (called FOCUS CHARTING™).

Defining Characteristics: Clinical criteria that represent the presence of a diagnostic category; cluster of signs and symptoms indicating a specific nursing diagnosis.

Diagnosis: Identification of a disease/condition or human response by a scientific evaluation of signs/symptoms, history, and diagnostic studies.

Diagnostic Error: A mistaken assumption leading to a wrong conclusion.

Diagnostic Reasoning: Process of problem/need identification used during the second step of the nursing process: problem-sensing, rule-out process, synthesizing the data, evaluation or confirming the hypothesis, listing patient problems/needs.

Etiology: Identified causes and/or contributing factors responsible for the presence of a specific client problem/need.

Evaluation: The fifth step of the nursing process during which the client's movement toward specified outcomes is determined and the plan of care is modified or care is terminated depending on the findings.

Focus Assessment: Gathering of data narrowed to a specific area/topic.

Goal: Broad guidelines indicating the overall direction for movement as a result of the interventions of the healthcare team; divided into long-term and short-term goals.

Implement/Implementation: The fourth step of the nursing process in which the plan of care is put into action; performing identified interventions/activities.

Inference: To conclude/deduce from evidence presented.

Intuition: A sense of something that is not clearly evidenced by known facts.

JCAHO (Joint Commission on Accreditation of Healthcare Organizations): Surveying body that certifies clinical and organizational performance of an institution according to established guidelines.

Long-term Goals: May not be achieved before discharge from care.

Measurable Verb: An action/behavior that can be quantified by specific amounts of time and can be seen or heard.

Medical Diagnosis: Illness/condition for which treatment is directed by a licensed physician; medical diagnosis focuses on correction/prevention of pathology of specific organs/body systems.

Mind-mapping: A graphic representation of the connections between concepts and ideas that are related to a central subject. Used to plan nursing care.

NANDA International (Formerly North American Nursing Diagnosis Association): A group responsible for the development of nursing diagnoses.

Need Identification: The second step of the nursing process in which the data collected are analyzed and, through the process of diagnostic reasoning, specific client diagnostic statements are created.

Nurse-Patient Relationship: A therapeutic relationship built on a series of interactions, developing over time, and meeting the needs of the patient.

Nursing Audit: Procedure to evaluate the quality of nursing care provided, using established criteria/standards. Concurrent audit is done while nursing care is being performed. Retrospective audit is done after the client is discharged from care.

Nursing Diagnosis: Noun: a label approved by NANDA identifying specific client problems/needs. The means of describing health problems amenable to treatment by nurses; may be physical, sociologic, or psychological. Verb: process of identifying specific client problems/needs; used by some as the title of the second step of the nursing process.

Nursing Interventions: Prescriptions for specific behaviors expected for the client, and/or actions to be carried out by nurses to promote, maintain, or restore health.

Nursing Process: An orderly, logical five-step problem-solving approach to administering nursing care. Composed of assessment, diagnosis/need identification, planning, implementation, and evaluation.

Nursing Standard: Identified criterion against which nursing care is compared and evaluated; generally reflects the minimum level for nursing care.

Objective Data: What can be observed; for example, vital signs, behaviors, diagnostic studies.

Outcome: The result of actions undertaken to achieve a broader goal; measurable steps to achieve the goals of treatment and to meet discharge criteria.

PES: Format for combining a client problem label, etiology, and signs/symptoms to create an individualized diagnostic statement.

Planning: The third step of the nursing process during which goals/outcomes are determined and interventions chosen.

Plan of Care: Written evidence of the second and third steps of the nursing process that identifies the client's problems/needs, goals/outcomes of care, and interventions to treat the problems/needs.

POMR or PORS (Problem-Oriented Medical Record): A method of recording data about the health status of the client relative to specific problems.

Protocol: Written guidelines of steps to be taken for providing client care in a particular situation/condition.

Related Factor: The conditions/circumstances

that contribute to the development/maintenance of a nursing diagnosis; related to components of the client diagnostic statement.

Risk Factor: The environmental factors and physiological, psychological, genetic, or chemical elements that increase the vulnerability of an individual, family, or community to an unhealthful event.

Risk Nursing Diagnosis: A problem that may occur/recur, particularly if intervention is not undertaken. Because it has not yet occurred, there are no signs/symptoms when the client diagnostic statement is written; instead, risk factors are identified.

Short-term Goals: Those goals that usually must be met before discharge or movement to a less acute level of care.

Sign: Objective or observable evidence or manifestation of a health problem.

SOAP: Format for documentation—subjective, objective, analysis, plan.

SOAPIER: Format for documentation—subjective, objective, analysis, plan, implementation, evaluation, revision.

Subjective Data: What the client reports, believes, or feels.

Symptom: Subjectively perceptible change in the body or its functions that indicates disease or the kind or phase of disease.

Synthesize: Viewing all data as a whole to provide a comprehensive picture of the client.

Validating: The process of assuring that data are factual.

Wellness: A state of optimal health, physical and psychosocial.

Appendix K

Nursing Outcomes Classification

The Nursing Outcomes Classification (NOC) uses the following 16 different Likert scales to measure variability in the patient state, behavior, or perception depicted in the outcome:

Scale No. 1: 1—Extremely compromised; 2—Substantially compromised; 3—Moderately compromised; 4—Mildly compromised; 5—Not compromised—used to measure outcomes such as Bowel Elimination, Cognitive Ability, Well-being

Scale No. 2: 1—Extreme deviation from expected range to 5—No deviation from expected range, to measure Growth, Physical Aging Status, or Vital Signs Status

Scale No. 3: 1—Dependent, does not participate to 5—Completely independent, for outcomes such as Balance, Self Care, and Transfer Performance

Scale No. 4: 1—No motion to 5—Full motion for Joint Movement outcomes

Scale No. 5: 1—Not at all to 5—To a very great extent, for outcomes such as Dignified Dying, Energy Conservation, Immune Hypersensitivity Control

Scale No. 6: 1—Not adequate to 5—Totally adequate, measuring Abuse Protection, Breastfeeding, Role Performance

Scale No. 7: 1—Over 9 to 5—None, for Safety Status: Falls Occurrence

Scale No. 8: 1—Extensive to 5—None, for Caregiver Stressors and Loneliness

Scale No. 9: 1—None to 5—Extensive, for outcomes such as Abuse Recovery, Knowledge, and Social Support

Scale No. 10: 1—None to 5—Complete, for Bone Healing and Wound Healing

Scale No. 11: 1—Never positive to 5—Consistently positive, measuring Body Image and Self Esteem

Scale No. 12: 1—Very weak to 5—Very strong, for Health Beliefs and Health Orientation

Scale No. 13: 1—Never demonstrated to 5—Consistently demonstrated, for outcomes such as Aggression Control, Memory, Suicide Self Restraint

Scale No. 14: 1—Severe to 5—None, to measure Infection Status, Pain Level, Substance Addiction Consequences

Scale No. 15: 1—No evidence to 5—

Extensive evidence, for Abuse Cessation and Neglect Cessation

Scale No. 16: 1—Extreme delay from expected range to 5—No delay from expected range, to measure Child Development outcomes

Scale No. 17: 1—Poor to 5—Excellent, to measure Community Health Status, Physical Fitness outcomes

SAMPLE OF NOC OUTCOME MEASUREMENT:

PAIN CONTROL BEHAVIOR

	Never 1	Rarely 2	Sometimes 3	Often 4	Consistently Demonstrated 5
Indicators:					
Reports symptoms to healthcare professional				✓	
Uses preventive measures			✓		
Uses nonanalgesic relief measures				✓	
Reports pain controlled					✓

Appendix L

Keys to Practice Activities

Key for Practice Activity 2–1: Determining Types of Data

1. Identify subjective (S) versus objective (O) data:

O Skin cool/damp	O Pitting edema of feet and ankles
S or O Sputum pale yellow	S Usually voids three times per day
S Allergic to eggs and sulfa	S Chest pain lasting 15 minutes

2. Match the technique in column A to the statements in column B:

Column A	Column B
a. Open-ended question	A What would you like to talk about?
b. Hypothetical question	B The next time this comes up, what would you do to handle it?
c. Reflection	C That feeling in your chest, can you describe it more fully?
d. Closed-ended question	D Do you use alcohol regularly?
e. Leading question	E You're feeling better today aren't you?

Rewrite the following using effective data collection techniques (see Box 2–3):

a. You felt like crying, didn't you? *You're sad about what happened and are concerned about what you can do.*

b. You're in pain again? *I notice you seem to be in pain, tell me about it.*

c. Do you want to change occupations? *I'd like to hear more about your interests, what you would enjoy doing.*

d. Since your doctor has talked with you, you don't have any questions, do you? *What is your understanding of what the doctor told you?*

e. Did you eat lunch? *Tell me what you ate for lunch.*

Key to Practice Activity 2–2: Organizing Data: Diagnostic Divisions and Functional Health Patterns

Donald has been admitted to the psychiatric hospital acute substance abuse unit for treatment of depression and withdrawal from alcohol.

Organize the data below according to diagnostic divisions and functional health patterns. Place the number of the listed data next to the category where you believe it fits (see Table 2–1).

1. 46-year-old male

2. Divorced, not currently involved in a relationship

3. Loan banker, laid off 7 months ago

4. Unsteady gait

5. Clothes rumpled, has not shaved for 2 days, dry skin

6. Eats one or two meals a day—donuts, sandwiches, meat and potatoes, no vegetables or fruits; coffee 4+ cups/day

7. Stools have been loose, 3–4/day

8. BP 136/82, right arm/sitting; radial pulse 92

9. Alert and oriented

10. Catholic, not practicing

11. Sleeps usually 3–4 hours a night, awakens around 5:00 AM

12. "I've been drinking a lot lately." Bourbon one fifth/day

13. Worries about financial situation, unable to make child support payments

14. Congested nonproductive cough

15. Reports constant throbbing pain, left knee—old sports injury

Genogram:

Diagnostic Divisions	Functional Health Patterns
Activity/Rest: 3, 11	Health Perception/Health
Circulation: 8	Management: 4, 12, 15
Ego Integrity: 2, 10, 13	Nutritional/Metabolic: 6, 8, 14
Elimination: 7	Elimination: 7
Food/Fluid: 6	Activity/Exercise: 4, 5
Hygiene: 5	Cognitive/Perceptual: 9
Neurosensory: 9	Sleep/Rest: 11
Pain/Discomfort: 15	Self Perception/Self Concept: 13
Respiration: 14	Role/Relationship: 1, 2, 3, 16
Safety: 4, 15	Sexuality/Reproductive: 2
Sexuality: 1, 2	Coping/Stress Tolerance: 12, 13
Social Interaction: 2, 16	Value/Belief: 10
Teaching/Learning: 12	

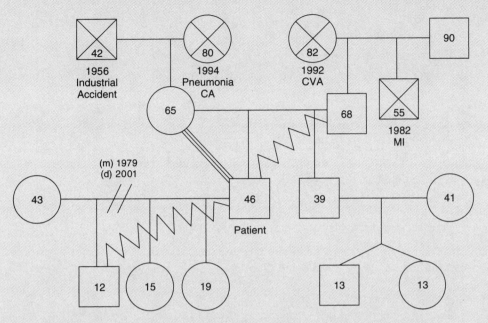

GENOGRAM: Graphic representation of a family (may include several generations), reflecting medical data and relationships/roles.

Key to Practice Activity 3–1: Activity Intolerance (Level II)

Client's medical diagnosis: *Pneumonia, recurrent*

ASSESSMENT

Subjective Data Entry:

Reports being weak most of the time. Stays at home; activity limited to short walks and watching baseball on TV. Shortness of breath has contributed to activity limitations. History of smoking 49 pack/years. Dyspnea when walking too long and in closed places.

Objective Data Entry:

BP 178/102, P 100 after short walk on unit. Leans forward to help himself breathe while in a sitting position. Respirations at rest are 28 and shallow. AP chest diameter is increased.

Key to Practice Activity 3–2: Identifying the PES Components of the Client Diagnostic Statement

Instructions (questions 1 through 5): Identify the "PES" components of each of these diagnostic statements:

1. Anxiety, severe, related to changes in health status of fetus/self and threat of death as evidenced by restlessness, tremors, focus on self/fetus.

P = Anxiety, *severe*
E = *Changes in health status of fetus/self and threat of death*
S = *Restlessness, tremors, focus on self/fetus*

2. Thought Processes, altered, related to pharmacological stimulation of the nervous system as evidenced by altered attention span, disorientation, and hallucinations.
P = *Thought processes, altered*
E = *Pharmacological stimulation of the nervous system*
S = *Altered attention span, disorientation, and hallucinations*

3. Coping, ineffective, related to maturational crisis as evidenced by inability to meet role expectations and alcohol abuse.
P = *Coping, ineffective*
E = *Maturational crisis*
S = *Inability to meet role expectations and alcohol abuse*

4. Hyperthermia related to increased metabolic rate and dehydration as evidenced by elevated temperature, flushed skin, tachycardia, and tachypnea.
P = *Hyperthermia*
E = *Increased metabolic rate and dehydration*
S = *Elevated temperature, flushed skin, tachycardia, and tachypnea*

5. Pain, acute related to tissue distention and edema as evidenced by verbal reports, guarding behavior, and changes in vital signs.
P = *Pain, acute*
E = *Tissue distention and edema*
S = *Verbal reports, guarding behavior, and changes in vital signs*

6. Explain the difference between actual and risk diagnoses: *An actual diagnosis is one that is currently present and manifested by signs and symptoms. In recording the need/concern, you would use a three-part diagnostic statement. A risk diagnosis is one that you believe could develop, but because it has not occurred yet, there are no signs or symptoms, only "risk factors." Therefore the need would be written as a two-part statement.*

7. Give an example of an actual and a risk problem for a client with second-degree burns of the hand.

   Actual: impaired Skin Integrity; acute Pain; Self- Care deficit; deficient Knowledge: treatment needs
   Risk: risk for Infection; risk for impaired Adjustment; risk for disturbed Body Image

Practice Activity 3–3: Identifying Correct and Incorrect Client Diagnostic Statements

Label each client diagnostic statement as correct or incorrect. Identify why a statement is incorrect:

correct   1. Ineffective Airway Clearance related to increased pulmonary secretions and bronchospasm as evidenced by wheezing, tachypnea, and ineffective cough.

correct   2. Impaired Thought Processes related to delusional thinking or reality base as evidenced by persecutory thoughts of "I am victim," and interference with ability to think clearly and logically.

incorrect   3. Impaired Gas Exchange related to bronchitis as evidenced by rhonchi, dyspnea, and cyanosis. Related to medical diagnosis. In considering the pathophysiology of bronchitis, the underlying problem may actually be Airway Clearance, ineffective, related to excessive, thickened mucous secretions as evidenced by rhonchi, dyspnea, and cyanosis.

incorrect   4. Deficient Knowledge diabetic care, related to inaccurate follow-through of instructions as evidenced by information misinterpretation and lack of recall. "Related to" and "evidenced by" statements are reversed.

correct   5. Acute Pain related to tissue distention and edema as evidenced by reports of severe colicky pain in right flank, elevated pulse and respirations, and restlessness.

Key to Practice Activity 4–1: Prioritizing Nursing Diagnoses

Instructions: Prioritize the nursing diagnoses listed in each separate set by using the Maslow and Kalish models. Rank the four diagnoses by using 1 to designate the most basic or more immediate client need and continuing to 4, which designates the highest-level need (but least in priority). Review Appendix A as needed to compare definitions of these nursing diagnoses.

a.   2   Urinary Incontinence, stress

      4   Sexuality Patterns, ineffective

      1   Airway Clearance, ineffective

      3   Skin Integrity, risk for impaired

b.   1   Gas Exchange, impaired

      4   Knowledge, deficient

      2   Hypothermia

      3   Infection, risk for

c.   1   Pain, acute

      4   Self Esteem, chronic low

      2   Mobility, impaired physical

      3   Social Isolation

Practice Activity 4–2: Identifying Correctly Stated Outcomes

Instructions: Identify which of the following outcome statements are written correctly, or state why it is not correct. Modify those statements that are not correct.

1. Client will: List individual risk factors and appropriate interventions. *Incorrect—RATIONALE: There is no time frame indicated. Corrected example: Client will: List individual risk factors and appropriate interventions within 72 hours.*

2. Client will: Identify four adaptive/protective measures for individual situation by discharge. *Correct—RATIONALE: All elements of a measurable outcome are present.*

3. Client will: Understand behaviors, lifestyle changes necessary to promote physical safety within 72 hours. *Incorrect—RATIONALE: "Understands" is not a measurable verb. Corrected example: Client will: Verbalize understanding of behaviors, lifestyle changes necessary to promote physical safety within 72 hours.*

4. Airway patent, aspiration prevented, ongoing. *Incorrect—RATIONALE: There is no active verb, no subject, and this may represent two separate outcomes. Corrected example: Client will: maintain patent airway, ongoing. OR Client will: demonstrate techniques to prevent aspiration, within 24 hours.*

5. Client will: Assume responsibility for own learning by participating in group discussions twice a day no later than 10/29/02. *Correct—RATIONALE: All elements of a measurable outcome are present.*

Practice Activity 4–3: Identifying Correctly Stated Interventions

Instructions: Identify which of the following interventions are correctly stated, and rewrite those that are not.

1. Walk length of hall 2 to 3×/day with assistance from two staff members. *Correct.*

2. Force fluids. *Incorrect—RATIONALE: The quantity of fluid is not indicated. Corrected example: Force fluid to a minimum of 2000 ml/day.*

3. Pericare after each BM. *Incorrect—RATIONALE: No verb and no indication of who is responsible for the activity. Corrected example: Provide [nurse], OR Assist with [nurse and client] OR Encourage [client] pericare after each BM.*

4. Encourage deep-breathing exercises and cough q2h. *Correct.*

5. Reduce environmental stimuli. *Incorrect—RATIONALE: How/what? Corrected example: Maintain low lighting in room, OR Keep hallway door closed.*

6. Provide written handout for side effects of medications before discharge. *Correct.*

Practice Activity 4–4

Does not require a key because student is simply copying information from Box 4–3 into a 5-column form.

Practice Activity 4–5

PLANNING

Desired Outcome and Client Criteria: The Client will: *Report measurable increase in activity level. Demonstrate a decrease in physiological signs of intolerance.*

TIME OUT! The desired outcome must meet criteria to be accurate. The outcome must be specific, realistic, and measurable, and include a time frame for completion. Does the action verb describe the client's behavior to be evaluated? Can the outcome be used in the evaluation step of the nursing process to measure the client's response to the nursing interventions listed below?

Interventions	Rationale for Selected Intervention and References
Measure vital signs before/during/after activity.	*Determines pt's response to physical activity & appropriateness of activity.*
Adjust activities to pt. tolerance.	*Prevents overexertion.*
Teach energy conserving methods.	*May enhance pt's ability to perform ADLs.*
Plan care with rest periods between activities.	*Reduces fatigue, enhances sense of well-being*
Encourage participation in social activities.	*Provides stimulation, opportunities to form new relationships, and maximizes cognitive function.*

EVALUATION

TIME OUT! Do your interventions assist the client in achieving outcome? Do your interventions address further monitoring of the client's response to your interventions and to the achievement of the desired outcome? Are qualifiers **when, how, amount, time,** and **frequency** used? Is the focus of the action's verb on the nurse's actions and not on the client? Do your rationales provide sufficient reason and directions?

What was your client's response to the interventions?

Was the desired outcome achieved? ☐ Yes ☐ No   If no, what revisions to either the desired outcome or interventions would you make?

Documentation Focus: Now that you have completed the evaluation, the next step is to document your care and the client's response. Use the areas below to enter your progress note information.

DOCUMENTATION

Reassessment Data:

Interventions Implemented:

Patient's Response:

INSTRUCTOR'S COMMENTS:

Key to Practice Activity 5–1: Setting Your Work Schedule for Implementing the Plan of Care

Vignette: Michelle incurred compound fractures of the right lower leg 3 days ago. In reviewing the plan of care, you note the following:

○ Assist with bed bath ○ Calculate I&O every 8 hours (2 PM) ○ Change dressing twice a day and prn (9 AM) ○ Assess vital signs every 4 hours (8 AM, 12 noon) ○ Monitor circulation/nerve function R lower leg every hour × 24 hr, then every 4 hr and prn ○ IV medications (8 AM, 2 PM) ○ Up in chair with meals (7:30 AM, 12 noon) ○ Walk in halls 3 times a day after instructed in crutch walking.

1. Organize the above interventions and activities on the following worksheet:

Worksheet

Pt.	7	8	9	10	11	12	1	2	3	Comments
Michelle	Chair	VS Circ ✔ Med	Bath Dress	Walk	VS Circ ✔ Chair			I&O Med Walk		

2. During nursing rounds, just after the change-of-shift report on 6/13, you find Michelle is crying and she reports sudden throbbing pain in her R lower leg. How will this affect your work plan?

The plan needs to be reordered because after you assess Michelle's pain and administer medication, she requires time to relax and for the medication to take effect. For example: You may choose to leave Michelle in bed for her breakfast and have her up in the chair after her bath or following her walk.

Key to Practice Activity 5–2: Legal and Ethical Concerns of Care

As noted, Robert had completed a form directing healthcare providers to withhold advanced life support measures, including the use of a mechanical ventilator.

1. Have you and your family members completed advance directives stating specific healthcare desires? <u>Self-answer</u>

   If not, why: <u>Self-answer</u>

2. As a nurse, how do you feel about adhering to advance directives as stipulated by an elderly client? <u>Self-answer</u>

   For a premature infant as stipulated by the parents? <u>Self-answer</u>

3. Review the Code for Nurses (see Appendix D) and choose two principles you believe may address your responsibility to clients/guardians in regard to their decisions to limit care.

a. *No. 1—A client has the moral right to determine his or her own care by accepting, rejecting, or terminating treatment based on personal value system and lifestyle. Nurses have an obligation to be knowledgeable about the moral and legal rights of the client and to protect and support those rights.*

b. *No. 3—Denying or negating the client's rights (moral and/or legal) results in unethical or illegal practice. The nurse has a duty to be knowledgeable regarding agency policies and procedures, nursing standards of practice, the Code for Nurses, and laws governing nursing and healthcare practices to protect and advocate for the client.*

c. *No. 4—The professional nurse bears the primary responsibility for nursing care provided (or not provided) and neither physicians' orders nor agency policies relieve the nurse of accountability for actions taken and judgments made.*

Key to Practice Activity 5–3: Communicating Nursing Information to Other Caregivers

Work through the questions below.

1. Two methods of communicating your observations about client care and activities to other nurses are by:

a. *Written record*   b. *Verbal report*

2. Discuss the benefits of nursing rounds: *Aids in verifying the status of invasive treatments, appearance of wounds/dressings, and the current condition of the client.*

3. Underline the information listed below that you would include in your change-of-shift report:
   <u>Sally Ate well Age 30 Dr. Jefferson</u>
   <u>Weak and unsteady while up in hall</u>
   <u>*Episiotomy reddened, slight edema*</u>, no drainage second day postpartum
   <u>Scheduled for discharge tomorrow</u>
   <u>*Received oral pain medication at 11 AM*</u> with reported relief
   Does not want to go home
   Sister in to visit at lunchtime
   <u>Coordination for home care services in progress with the discharge planner</u>
   Spent afternoon talking on phone
   <u>Has not named Baby B and at times has ignored infant cues</u>

4. The wife of a prominent local politician is admitted for treatment of alcoholism. You could discuss her admission and course of therapy with which of the following people? (check any answers that seem appropriate)
   x   attending/primary physician
   x   nursing supervisor
          pediatric nurse (her best friend)
          your husband
          client's son
          interested newspaper reporter
   x   other nurses on your unit
Note: Client permission is required for release of information even to family members.

Key to Practice Activity 6–1: Evaluating Client Outcomes

Read over the case study information below. It has been used to develop a plan of care for Michelle.

When Michelle was admitted to the hospital the evening of 6/11, a physiological (Maslow's) or survival (Kalish's) need of pain avoidance was identified (i.e., Acute Pain). A higher-level problem of safety or stimulation was noted (i.e., impaired physical Mobility), as was a safety need of protection (i.e., risk for Infection).

The following morning (6/12) during the 8 AM assessment, Michelle indicates she was successful in obtaining relief of pain following periodic injection of analgesics. Michelle also found that deep-breathing exercises and focusing her attention on the scenic picture at the foot of her bed helped to minimize the severity of recurrent muscle spasms in her right leg. In addition, frequent weight shifts using the overhead trapeze and range-of-motion exercises reduced general aches and joint stiffness and meditation enhanced general relaxation.

The nurse noticed that most of Michelle's breakfast tray was untouched. Michelle reported she was not very hungry but did want fruit juice and other fluids. Following the morning bed bath, the dressings were changed and the right leg wound was evaluated. Skin edges were pink and serous drainage was odorless. Pin sites were also cleaned and no signs of inflammation noted. At lunch, Michelle's intake was poor. She indicated she was having difficulty opening her mouth and chewing and had an aching sensation located in the right temple and ear.

During the afternoon assessment at 4:30 PM, Michelle's nurse verified that Michelle understood and was using infection control techniques of proper handwashing and avoidance of contact with wound and pin sites.

When Michelle was set up on the side of the bed before her dinner, she reported dizziness and sharp pain in her right leg, and she became pale and diaphoretic. She was returned to the supine position and a focused assessment was performed, revealing a BP of 92/60. Within 20 minutes, Michelle's color had improved, the dizziness was gone, and the pain was relieved with medication.

In reviewing the excerpts from Michelle's plan of care, complete the status column denoting whether the outcomes have been met (m), partially met (pm), or not met (nm) appropriately for the timeframes indicated.

ACUTE PAIN

Although Michelle is reporting relief of pain following administration of medication, this is an ongoing outcome and will remain active. Michelle has identified methods that enhance pain relief and is successfully using relaxation techniques; thus the second and third outcomes have been met.

RISK FOR INFECTION

Michelle is able to identify and is practicing interventions to reduce risk of infection, meeting the first outcome.

IMPAIRED PHYSICAL MOBILITY

Michelle is participating in activities to maintain muscle strength, meeting the first outcome. However, the initial attempt to get Michelle out of bed was unsuccessful, and the second outcome has not been met.

Practice Activity 6–1 Plan of Care: Michelle

Patient: Michelle   Age: 14—03/2/88   Sex: F   Admitted: 6/11/02 5:30 PM   Dx: Compound   Fx R Tibia/Fibula, closed head injury/ mild concussion

Date	Patient Diagnostic Statement	Goal	Interventions	Outcomes	Status
6/11/02	Acute Pain, related to movement of bone fragments, soft tissue injury/edema, evidenced by verbal reports, guarding, muscle tension, narrowed focus, and tachycardia	Pain-free or controlled by discharge	1. Maintain limb rest R leg × 24 hr to 5 PM 6/12. 2. Elevate lower leg with folded blanket. 3. Apply ice to area as tolerated × 48 hr to 5 PM 6/13. 4. Place cradle over foot of bed. 5. Document reports and characteristics of pain. 6. Medicate with Demerol 75 mg and Phenergan 25 mg IM q4h prn, or Vicodin 5 mg PO q4h prn. 7. Demonstrate/encourage use of progressive relaxation techniques, deep-breathing exercises, visualization. 8. Provide alternate comfort measures, position change, backrub. 9. Encourage use of diversional activities.	Verbalizes relief of pain within 30–60 minutes of administration of medication Identifies methods that provide relief by 9 AM, 6/12 Uses relaxation skills to reduce level of pain by 9 AM, 6/12	 M/6/12 M/6/12
6/11/02	Risk for Infection: risk factors of broken skin, traumatized tissues, decreased hemoglobin levels, invasive procedures, environmental exposure	Free of infection	1. Monitor temp, VS, q4h. 2. Aseptic dressing change bid 9 AM, 9 PM, and prn. 3. Pin care per protocol bid 9 AM, 9 PM. 4. Routine IV site care daily. 5. Document condition of wound, IV, and pin sites q4h. 6. Review ways client can reduce risk of infection. 7. Cefoxitin 2 g IV piggyback q8h (8 AM, 4 PM, 12 AM).	Identifies and practices interventions to reduce risk of infection by 5 PM 6/12. Identifies signs/ symptoms requiring medical evaluation by 9 AM, 6/13 Displays initial wound healing free of purulent drainage/signs of infection by discharge	M/6/12

(Continued)

Practice Activity 6–1 Plan of Care: Michelle (Continued)

Patient: Michelle   **Age:** 14—03/2/88   **Sex:** F   **Admitted:** 6/11/02 5:30 PM   **Dx:** Compound   Fx R Tibia/Fibula, closed head injury/mild concussion

Date	Patient Diagnostic Statement	Goal	Interventions	Outcomes	Status
6/11/02	Impaired Physical Mobility: related to musculoskeletal impairment and pain, evidenced by reluctance to attempt movement and imposed restrictions	Ambulates safely with assistive device	1. Monitor circulation/nerve function R leg q1h × 24 hr, then q4h and prn. 2. Support R leg fixator during movement. 3. Support feet with footboard. 4. Encourage use of side rails/overhead trapeze for position change. 5. Demonstrate/assist with ROM exercises to unaffected limbs q2h. 6. Assist out of bed, non-weight-bearing 6 PM, 6/12. 7. Instruct in/monitor use of crutches 6/13.	Participates in activities to maintain muscle strength by 9 AM, 6/12 Increases level of activity beginning 6 PM, 6/12 and ongoing Demonstrates techniques/behaviors that enable resumption of activities by 6 PM, 6/13 Maintains position of function R leg, free of foot drop—ongoing	M/6/12 M/6/12

294

Key to Practice Activity 6–2: Modification of the Plan of Care

Based on your evaluation, how would you alter Michelle's plan of care from Practice Activity 6–1?

Michelle has learned ways to control her pain, and she seeks pharmacological relief appropriately. The need will remain active for the duration of this admission, although at a lesser level of concern. Intervention 1 can be deleted.

At this time, Michelle's wounds show no signs of infection, and Michelle is aware of ways to help reduce the risk of infection. Components of this problem will remain active for the duration of this hospitalization. Intervention 6 can be deleted.

Michelle is able to reposition herself and participates in activities/behaviors to maintain function. Michelle's initial attempt to be out of bed was not successful. The timeframe will need to be extended while Michelle is evaluated for adequacy of circulation and appropriateness of premedication before activity is initiated again.

A concern regarding nutrition has also been identified. Assessing the integrity of Michelle's jaws/teeth and TM joint and providing a semisoft diet may help improve her intake. In addition, Michelle's knowledge of her nutritional needs will require assessment because a proper diet is necessary to promote healing and reduce risk of infection. Obtain a baseline weight for future comparison.

Key for Practice Activity 7–1: Elements of Progress Notes

Give a brief explanation of how progress notes provide for the following elements of the nurse/client relationship.

1. Staff communication: *Recorded information can be reviewed by other staff members/healthcare providers at any time.*

2. Evaluation: *Tracks the client's responses to treatment, progress toward outcomes, and interventions used to obtain these outcomes to determine quality of care provided.*

3. Relationship monitoring: *Documents client's interactions with others, which may have an impact on well-being, recovery, and independence.*

4. Reimbursement: *Proof of services necessary for payment.*

5. Legal documentation: *Verifies implementation of the plan of treatment, events, activities, and progress toward outcomes.*

6. Accreditation: *Meets standards necessary to gain accreditation.*

7. Training/Supervision: *A model for coworkers; gives an impression of abilities and identifies areas for additional training or supervision.*

Practice Activity 7–2: Writing Nonjudgmental Statements

Circle either the J or O/B for each of the following statements to identify either judgmental (J) or observational/behavioral (O/B) documented statements. If the statement is judgmental, rewrite to reflect observation/behavioral language:

1. Mrs. Jewel has a poor body image since undergoing a mastectomy. <u>J</u> Example of behavioral language: *Mrs. Jewel says she thinks her husband will not want to look at her body, and she doesn't feel like a woman anymore.*

2. Mr. Dunn needs to be evaluated regarding his competence to manage his household affairs because of his left-sided weakness since his stroke. <u>O/B</u>

3. Miss Janus does a good job of breast self-examination. <u>J</u> Example of behavioral language: *Miss Janus performs her breast examination 10 or more times a year.*

4. Mary Bird does not eat enough for her current level of activity. <u>J</u> Example of behavioral language: *Mary Bird's caloric intake is 1000 calories, which represents maintenance level and is not sufficient to maintain her weight at her current level of activity.*

5. Mr. Lambert stops taking his medication; then when he has a seizure, he presents at the doctor's office for treatment. <u>O/B</u>

6. It has been a long time since Mr. Babbitt has had his medications evaluated. <u>J</u> Example of behavioral language: *Mr. Babbitt has not had his medications evaluated since last November.*

Appendix M

Keys to Chapter Work Pages

Key to Work Page: Chapter 1

1. The ANA has defined nursing as:
   The diagnosis and treatment of human responses to actual or potential health problems.
2. My own definition of nursing is: *Self-answer*
3. How has the information in this chapter affected your definition? *Self-answer*
4. The ANA Social Policy Statement defines the phenomena of concern for nurses as: *human responses to health and illness.*
5. The definition of nursing process is: *an orderly, logical five-step problem-solving approach for administering nursing care.*
6. Name and define the five steps of the nursing process and provide an example of each step:

Steps	Definition	Example
a. *Assessment*	*Systematic collection of data.*	*Low BP, thirst, dry mouth, dark urine.*
b. *Diagnosis/Need Identification*	*Analysis of data to identify client's needs/problems.*	*Fluid volume deficit.*
c. *Planning*	*Setting goals/outcomes and choosing interventions.*	*Increase circulating volume. Encourage oral fluids*
d. *Implementation*	*Putting the plan into action.*	*Place water and juice of choice at bedside.*
e. *Evaluation*	*Assessing the effectiveness of the plan and changing the plan if indicated.*	*Monitor BP, urine output, and mucous membranes to note improvement.*

7. List the three advantages of using nursing process:
   a. *Provides framework for meeting individual needs of the client, family, and community.*
   b. *Focuses attention on individual human responses to provide holistic care.*
   c. *Provides an organized, systematic method of problem solving.*
   d. *Promotes active involvement of the client.*
   e. *Enables the nurse to exert greater control over own practice.*
   f. *Provides a common language for practice.*
   g. *Provides a means for assessing nursing's economic contribution to client care.*

8. List two of the fundamental philosophical beliefs that you believe are basic to decision making within the nursing process:

Client is a human being who has worth and dignity.

If basic human needs are not met, intervention is required until individual can resume responsibility for self.

Clients have a right to quality health and nursing care with a focus on wellness and prevention.

Therapeutic nurse-client relationship is important to this process.

9. Identify the steps of the nursing process by placing the appropriate number of the activity in the space following the data presented in the following vignette: 1 = Assessment; 2 = Diagnosis/Need Identification; 3 = Planning; 4 = Implementation; 5 = Evaluation

VIGNETTE:

Robert, a 72-year-old African-American male, is admitted with recurrent bilateral lower lobe pneumonia. 1

He reports this is his second episode in 6 months. 1

Temperature is 101°F; skin hot and flushed. 1

He reports frequent, hacking cough with moderate amount of thick greenish mucus. 1

Auscultation of the chest reveals scattered rhonchi throughout. 1

His mucous membranes are pale, and his lips are dry and cracked. 1

He says when he was sick last month, the doctor prescribed an antibiotic, which he discontinued after 6 days because he was feeling better. 1

You determine Robert has an airway clearance problem, a fluid volume deficit, and is not managing his therapeutic regimen effectively, which will require teaching to promote adequate self-care and to prevent recurrence. 2

You establish the following outcomes:

Expectorates secretions completely with breath sounds clear and respirations noiseless. 3

Demonstrates adequate fluid balance with moist mucous membranes and loose respiratory secretions. 3

Verbalizes understanding of cause of condition and therapeutic regimen. 3

You decide to set up a regular schedule for respiratory activities and fluid replacement. 3

In addition, you formulate a teaching plan to cover the identified concerns for self-care and illness prevention. 3

You provide a tube of petroleum jelly for Robert to use on his lips. 4

Every 2 hours, you visit Robert to encourage him to deep-breathe, cough, change his position, and drink a glass of fluid of his choice. 4

You use this time to discuss avoidance of crowds and individuals with upper respiratory infections and the necessity of continuing the treatment plan after discharge. 4

The following day, Robert's skin is no longer hot and flushed, temperature is 99°F, secretions are loose and readily expectorated, and breath sounds are clearing. 5

Robert's lips and oral mucous membranes are moist. He is able to explain in his own words how to care for himself and ways to prevent pneumonia. 5

You decide that the current treatment plan is achieving the identified outcomes and to continue the plan as written. 5

Key to Work Page: Chapter 2

1. Rewrite the following questions so that they are open-ended:
   a. You're feeling better after the respiratory treatment, aren't you? *How are you feeling after your respiratory treatment?*
   b. Have you taken your medicine today? *Tell me about your medication schedule. How is that working for you?*
   c. Do you understand these directions? *Explain your understanding of these directions.*
2. Using the technique of reflection, write a response to clarify these client statements:
   a. Do you think I should tell my doctor about my concern?
   What do you think you need to do?
   b. What do you want to talk about today?
   I'm interested in what your concerns are.
   c. I don't think I can go on without my husband.
   It seems difficult without him.
   d. Do you think it is important to get married?
   I'd be interested in your thoughts about that.
3. When might a closed-ended question be helpful?
   In an emergency.
4. Describe the three components of the client database:
   a. *Client history*
   b. *Physical examination*
   c. *Diagnostic studies*
5. The four activities involved in the physical assessment are:
   a. *Inspection*
   b. *Percussion*
   c. *Auscultation*
   d. *Palpation*
6. The client database is important to the provision of client care because *it provides a profile of the client's health status on which need identification is based.*
7. For assessment purposes, the difference between subjective data and objective data is: *Subjective data are what the client/significant other(s) say that reflects their thoughts, feelings, perceptions. Objective data are observable and measurable and include data gathered from other sources.*
8. Underline the subjective data, and circle the objective data in the following vignette:

VIGNETTE:

Sally comes to the obstetric department for evaluation of her stage of labor. Back pains began about 3 hours ago (8 PM) while she was on her job as a respiratory therapist. Contractions are 5 minutes apart, lasting 30 seconds for the last 45 minutes. BP 146/84, left arm/lying; P 110; respirations 24. Weight 155 pounds (up 4 pounds this week). Cervix dilated 4 cm, membranes intact. Fetal head engaged, heart tones slightly muffled in right lower quadrant, rate 132. Nauseated since a dinner of fried chicken 4 hours ago. Appears anxious and seems irritated that her physician is not here. Voided 1 hour ago, has not had a bowel movement for 2 days. Stopped smoking 8 months ago. Lungs clear. No allergies. Married, husband plans to attend the birth. Two children are in the care of their grandmother tonight. Appearance is well groomed with a well-fitting maternity uniform and low-heeled shoes. Requests to leave contacts in to observe the birth. Last physical examination 1 week ago. Gestation 37 weeks, with due date 3 weeks off—3/11/02.

9. An important benefit of doing "research" or reviewing available information before an interview *is to gather information and generate questions*.
10. An interview should be "requested" because *it promotes a more positive interaction*.
11. Check those information resources that can be useful in helping the nurse to prepare for the interview:

    x Family/significant other   x Physician notes
    x Old medical records   x Textbooks/reference journals
    x Diagnostic studies   x Other nurse/healthcare providers

12. Sensitivity of the nurse is important during the interview process to *respect the client's right to privacy and enhance trust*.
13. List three abilities of the nurse that are necessary in order to collect a relevant client database.
    a. *Knowledge base*
    b. *Choice of questions to be asked*
    c. *Method of asking questions*
    d. *Ability to give meaning to response*
14. In the following vignette, cluster and record the assessed data (following the numbers) into the appropriate diagnostic divisions listed below. Refer to Table 2–1 as needed for the type of data included in the specific divisions to assist you in clustering the data.

VIGNETTE:

Robert, a 72-year-old (1) African-American (2) male admitted to the medical unit at 1 PM for (3) bilateral lower lobe pneumonia. (4) Has had liquids only by mouth for several days. (5) Last BM—2 days ago, brown/formed stool, (6) voided at 1:20 PM—clear, dark amber. He reports (7) "My chest hurts," as he splints chest while coughing. (8) Small amount thick, green sputum expectorated with cough. (9) Appears anxious, fidgeting with sheets, face tense, watching nurse intently. (10) Tympanic temperature (TMT) 101°F, (11) BP 178/102 (left arm/lying), P 100/regular, (12) respirations 28/shallow. (13) Skin warm, moist, color pale. (14) Has difficulty hearing questions, left hearing aid (R ear) at home. (15) Reports "This is the second episode in a month." (16) Doctor did prescribe antibiotic (drug unknown) a month ago, client did not complete treatment. (17) States he lives alone (widower), and (18) is responsible for meeting own needs. In reviewing diagnostic studies, you note the (19) chest x-ray reveals infiltrates both lower lobes, and a (20) Gram stain of the sputum reveals Gram-negative bacteria.

Diagnostic Divisions

Activity/Rest: <u>none</u> Hygiene: <u>18</u> Safety: <u>10, 14, 20</u>
Circulation: <u>8, 11, 13</u> Neurosensory: <u>14</u> Sexuality: <u>2</u>

Ego Integrity: <u>9</u> Pain/Discomfort: <u>7</u>
Social Interaction: <u>1, 17</u> Elimination: <u>5, 6</u>
Respiration: <u>8, 12, 19</u> Teaching/Learning: <u>3, 15, 16</u>
Food/Fluid: <u>4</u>

Key to Work Page: Chapter 3

1. What is the definition of Need Identification? *The process of data analysis using diagnostic reasoning to determine if nursing intervention is indicated.*
2. What two factors influenced the development and acceptance of nursing diagnosis as the language of nursing? *ANA Social Policy Statement and ANA Standards of Practice.*
3. List three reasons for using nursing diagnosis:
   a. *Provides a common language for improved communication.*
   b. *Promotes identification of appropriate goals and interventions and provides guidance for evaluation.*
   c. *Provides framework for client classification system for staffing needs and third-party reimbursement.*
   d. *Can be a standard for nursing practice.*
   e. *Provides opportunity for documentation and validation of process.*
4. List the six steps of diagnostic reasoning:
   a. *Problem-sensing*
   b. *Rule-out process*
   c. *Synthesizing data*
   d. *Evaluating/confirming the hypothesis*
   e. *List client's needs/concerns*
   f. *Re-evaluate the problem list*
5. Name the components of the Client Diagnostic Statement:
   a. *Problem (or need)*
   b. *Etiology*
   c. *Signs/Symptoms*
6. If a risk diagnosis is identified, how is the client diagnostic statement altered? *Etiology and signs/symptoms are replaced by risk factors.*
7. What is the difference between a medical and a nursing diagnosis? *Medical diagnoses are illnesses/conditions; nursing diagnoses are human responses to actual or potential health problems/life processes that are amenable to treatment by nurses.*
8. Which of these client diagnostic statements are stated correctly? Indicate by placing a C before correct, or an I before incorrect statements. Then, differentiate actual (A) from risk (R) problems by placing an A or R by each statement.
   C/A a. Deficient Knowledge drug therapy related to misinterpretation and unfamiliarity with resources as evidenced by request for information and statement of misconception.
   C/R b. Risk for Infection, risk factors of altered lung expansion, decreased ciliary action, decreased hemoglobin, and invasive procedures.
   I/A c. Impaired Urinary Elimination related to indwelling catheter as evidenced by inability to void.
   C/A d. Anxiety [moderate] related to change in health status, role functioning, and socioeconomic status as evidenced by apprehension, insomnia, and feelings of inadequacy.
9. Underline the cues in the client database below that indicate that a problem may exist, and write a client diagnostic statement based on your findings:

VIGNETTE:

Sally is 2 days post delivery. She reports her bowels have not moved but says she has been drinking plenty of fluids, including fruit juices, and has been eating a balanced diet.

ELIMINATION (EXCERPT FROM THE CLIENT DATABASE)

Subjective

Usual bowel patterns: Every morning
Laxative use: Rare/MOM PM
Character of stool: Brown, formed   Last BM: <u>4 days ago</u>
History of bleeding: No   Hemorrhoids: <u>Last 5 weeks</u>
Constipation: <u>Since delivery</u>   Diarrhea: No
Usual voiding pattern: 3–4 ×/day   Incontinence: No   Urgency: No
Character of urine: Yellow   Pain/burning/difficulty voiding: No
History of kidney/bladder disease: Several bladder infections, last one 6 years ago
Associated complaints: <u>Pain with stool, nausea, "I just can't go no matter what I do."</u>

Objective

Abdomen tender: Yes   Soft/firm: <u>Somewhat firm</u>
Palpable mass: No   Size/girth: <u>Enlarged/postpartal</u>
Bowel sounds: Present all four quadrants, <u>hypoactive, every 1 to 2 minutes</u>
Hemorrhoids: Visual examination not done

Now, write the Client Diagnostic Statement. (Refer to the listing of nursing diagnoses in Appendix A to compare diagnostic labels addressing bowel elimination.) *Constipation related to weak abdominal musculature and pain on defecation evidenced by decreased frequency of stool, abdominal fullness, nausea, and hypoactive bowel sounds.*

Key to Work Page: Chapter 4

1. List three reasons why the plan of care is important:
   a. *Provides continuity of care*
   b. *Enhances communication*
   c. *Assists with determining unit priorities*
   d. *Supports documentation of the nursing process*
   e. *Serves as a teaching tool*
2. Briefly explain why setting priorities is necessary:
   Helps ensure that basic needs are met first, then other needs in order of importance.
3. What is the difference between a goal and an outcome?
   A goal is stated broadly, reflecting the general direction in which the client is expected to progress.
   An outcome is a specific measurable step taken toward achieving the goal.
4. Identify five important components of client outcomes:
   a. *Specific*

    b. *Realistic*
    c. *Consider the client's circumstances and desires*
    d. *Indicate a time frame*
    e. *Provide measurable evaluation criteria*

5. List four types of information that nursing interventions need to contain:
    a. *Date intervention is written*
    b. *Action verb reflecting activity to be performed*
    c. *Qualifiers of how, when, where, time/frequency, and amount*
    d. *Signature and/or initials of the nurse*

6. Explain the difference between a measurable and a nonmeasurable verb and give an example of each: *Measurable verbs describe an action that can be observed and/or quantified, for example, "verbalizes," "ambulates"; nonmeasurable verbs cannot be observed, for example, "understands."*

7. When does discharge planning begin? *When the client is admitted.*

8. How is the plan of care documented? *On a single or multipage form that is kept in a Kardex, the client's chart, or at the bedside.*

9. Identify two additional problems facing Michelle; then set a goal with one outcome and two interventions for each problem.

VIGNETTE:

> Michelle, the 14-year-old female with compound fractures of the right lower leg and a mild concussion, has other problems in addition to Acute Pain, as was previously discussed.
>
>   Her wound was contaminated by dirt and she had significant blood loss before paramedics arrived. Although the wound was flushed with sterile saline and antibiotic solution before being packed and dressed, a cast was not applied because of tissue swelling and concerns about the wound and bone. Instead, an external fixation device (a metal frame with pins extending through the skin and bone) is currently being used for immobilization of the tibia and fibula. The device is heavy and awkward for Michelle to move without causing increased pain, and she is to remain on bedrest for 24 hours. In addition, IV antibiotics are to be administered q4h.

    a. Problem: *risk for infection, risk factors of broken skin, traumatized tissues, decreased hemoglobin, invasive procedures, increased environmental exposure.*
    Goal: *Free of infection.*
    Outcome: *Client will achieve timely wound healing free of purulent drainage and will be afebrile by discharge.*
    OR
    Outcome: *Client will identify behaviors to reduce risk of infection within 24 hours.*

INTERVENTIONS

> ◦ Monitor temperature/vital signs ◦ Maintain aseptic technique with dressing change ◦ Assess/document wound condition and pin sites ◦ Administer antibiotic—monitor response ◦ Instruct client in ways to reduce risk of infection.

b. Problem/Need: *impaired physical mobility related to musculoskeletal impairment and pain as evidenced by reluctance to attempt movement, imposed restrictions of movement.*
Goal: *Ambulates safely with assistive device.*
Outcome: *Client will maintain position of function R leg, free of footdrop—ongoing.*
OR
Outcome: *Client will increase level of activity within 24 hours.*

INTERVENTIONS:

> ○ Monitor circulation/nerve function of R leg ○ Support foot in upright position with bed board/blanket roll ○ Assist out of bed ○ Instruct in/monitor use of crutches.

c. Problem/Need: *deficient knowledge: self-care/treatment needs related to lack of exposure to resources evidenced by request for information.*
Goal: *Managing own care effectively.*
Outcome: *Client will verbalize understanding of condition and treatment needs within 3 days.*
OR
Outcome: *Client will list signs/symptoms requiring medical evaluation/intervention, within 36 hours.*

INTERVENTIONS:

> ○ Review appropriate pathophysiology of injury in lay terms ○ Demonstrate proper wound and pin care ○ Identify signs/symptoms suggestive of complications ○ Discuss actions, side-effects, and possible adverse reactions of medications.

Key to Work Page: Chapter 5

1. Identify three activities involved in implementing the plan of care:
   a. *Identifying priorities*
   b. *Providing client care*
   c. *Ongoing data collection*
   d. *Documentation*
   e. *Communication*
2. Discuss the importance of understanding the expected effect and potential hazards of the interventions you will implement:
   It is important to understand the expected effect and potential hazards of the interventions you will implement to be sure the intervention will be beneficial, that you are achieving the desired effects, or that you have allowed for changes necessary to provide for specific needs/safety.
3. Explain the purpose for ongoing data collection throughout the implementation step of the nursing process:
   Provides information that will be used to determine appropriateness of care; need to alter interventions, and/or refer to other resources; necessity of shifting priorities, development of new client problems/needs.

4. List two reasons why documentation of the care provided is important:
   a. *Legal requirement for all healthcare settings*
   b. *Communication tool*
   c. *Resource to aid in determining effectiveness of care*
   d. *Assisting in setting priorities for ongoing care*
5. Name three activities you might use to carry out interventions for planned client care:
   a. *"Hands-on" care*
   b. *Assisting the client with care*
   c. *Instructing*
   d. *Counseling*
   e. *Monitoring*
6. What is the advantage of reporting "by exception"? *Provides for giving important information in a brief, concise manner that saves time.*
7. When and where is client confidentiality important? *When discussing the client in any area/situation where the conversation can be overheard by others who are not involved in the client's care.*
8. Flexibility in providing client care is important because: *it allows the nurse to respond to changed circumstances, interruptions, and so on, in a timely manner.*

VIGNETTE:

> Robert signed advance directives asking that no extraordinary means (e.g., intubation and mechanical ventilation) be used to prolong his life. When his condition changed, his daughter was notified as required. While visiting with her father, she is surprised to learn of his decision. She is very upset and a confrontation develops. Robert tells her "it is none of your business" and refuses to enter into further conversation.

9. What can you do now? *Ask the daughter to step out of the room with you, making sure that the client is "settled" before leaving the room. Find a quiet, private area, offer something to drink and sit down facing the daughter. Acknowledge her feelings of distress and encourage her to talk about the situation. Answer questions and provide information, as indicated, in verbal and written form regarding advance directives. Review what will be done for her father under advance directives. Facilitate a conference between father and daughter if both are agreeable, helping with clarification of terms and promoting understanding. If necessary, refer to a clinical nurse specialist or social worker for additional conflict resolution.*

Key to Work Page: Chapter 6

1. What is the difference between assessment and evaluation? *Assessment identifies the client's current status, and evaluation determines the client's movement toward specified outcomes.*
2. What is the primary purpose of the evaluation process? *Determines effectiveness of the plan of care.*
3. The evaluation process provides what three opportunities for the client and nurse?

  a. *Provides positive feedback to client and caregivers for efforts to date.*
  b. *Provides encouragement to continue to strive for higher level of functioning.*
  c. *Provides for problem solving.*
  d. *Provides for personal growth.*
4. List the three methods by which client outcomes may be evaluated, and give an example for each:
  a. *Direct observation.   Ambulated the length of the hall without difficulty.*
  b. *Client interview.   Reports decreased level of pain.*
  c. *Review of records.   Temperature has remained within normal range.*
5. Because it is advisable to deal with only three to five nursing diagnoses at a time, how are needs prioritized? *According to the hierarchy of needs, meeting basic/life threatening needs first.*
6. When is consideration of discharge planning begun? *On admission.*

VIGNETTE:

> Today is Donald's fifth hospital day. At the start of the shift, you have completed a focused assessment to evaluate progress/changes in status of the identified client problems. Donald's initial nausea has resolved and his intake yesterday was approximately 3000 calories. During rounds, you notice he has eaten all of the food on his breakfast tray. He fills out the next day's menu, neglecting to include any vegetables and selecting only one fruit.
>
> Later, during group, Donald talks about his options for employment and says he knows an employment agency and a business where he can check about possible jobs. He also mentions a friend who he believes might be willing to help him. He says he is realizing that he is really OK, even though the loss of his job was a devastating event for him following so soon after his divorce. He acknowledges that his feelings of anxiety led to an increase in his drinking. He further says he still has feelings of sadness and occasionally feels a sense of despair but believes he will feel better as he begins to get his life back together again. He seems tentative in accepting his need to be involved in AA, saying he doesn't know "where they meet, or anyone who attends the meetings."

  a. **Evaluation:** Based on the above information, evaluate Donald's progress regarding his problems of imbalanced Nutrition: less than body requirements, ineffective Coping, and ineffective Role Performance as outlined in the Plan of Care.
    Problem 4: Donald's intake is meeting daily caloric requirements, achieving the second outcome. However, his menu choices do not include all appropriate food groups; therefore, the first outcome is only partially met.
    Problem 5: Donald recognizes the impact that his loss of employment and recent divorce have had on his current feelings of anxiety and helplessness, meeting the first outcome.
    Problem 6: Donald is expressing awareness of feelings related to his situation and has some optimism for the future. This meets the first outcome. In addition, Donald has developed a realistic plan with two job-hunting strategies, meeting the second outcome.
  b. **Modification:** How would you change Donald's plan of care? *Investigate Donald's menu choices and how he plans to meet dietary needs without adequate intake of fruits and vegetables.*
  c. **Termination:** How might new concerns regarding the client affect your discharge plans? *Identify a contact person from AA to provide support for Donald to promote continued involvement in the treatment plan.*

Key to Work Page: Chapter 7

1. You are writing a paper regarding documentation. Identify three goals of the documentation process you will include:
   a. *Facilitate the quality of client care.*
   b. *Ensure documentation of progress with regards to client-focused outcomes.*
   c. *Facilitate interdisciplinary consistency and communication of treatment goals and progress.*

2. Steps of the Nursing Process are documented on which form:

Steps	Form
c Assessment	a. Plan of care
a Diagnosis/Need identification	b. Progress notes
a Planning	c. Client database
b, d Implementation	d. Flow sheets
a, b Evaluation	

3. List five functions of progress notes:
   a. *Staff communication*
   b. *Legal documentation*
   c. *Evaluation*
   d. *Accreditation*
   e. *Training and supervision*
   f. *Reimbursement*
   g. *Relationship monitoring*

4. Complete the following statements describing the JCAHO's standards for documentation.
   a. A medical record is **initiated** and **maintained** for every individual assessed or treated. The medical record incorporates information from subsequent contacts between the **client** and the **organization**.
   b. The medical record contains **sufficient information** to identify the client, support the **diagnosis**, justify the **treatment**, document the course and results accurately, and facilitate **continuity** of care among healthcare providers.

5. When documenting for reimbursement, five factors need to be included: *These are the when, where, how, what, and who of services.*

6. Two ways in which the plan of care can be used for supervision are: *the identification of employees' abilities identifying the need for further supervision, training, or education.*

7. The best way to ensure clarity of the progress notes is: *to use descriptive/observational statements.*

8. Rewrite the following judgmental statements to make them nonjudgmental:
   a. He is uncooperative today.
   Mr. Jones refused his bath and did not want to get out of bed this morning.
   b. He is a manipulative client.
   Mr. Smith told me I was the only nurse who listened to him and wanted me to let him skip his medication and not tell the doctor.
   c. She had a bad attitude about taking her medication this morning.
   Mrs. Wharton stated she was tired of taking her medicine and threw the cup across the room this morning.
   d. The new client is really difficult.
   Mr. Bemish did not want to go to bed and cursed when I went in to obtain his admitting information.

9. List three types of judgmental statements:
   a. *Contain undefined periods of time*
   b. *Contain undefined quantities*
   c. *Contain undefined qualities*
   d. *Fail to specify any objective basis for the judgment made*
10. Name three types of data that are important to record in the progress note:
   a. *Unsettled or unclear problems that need to be dealt with*
   b. *Noteworthy incidents or interview*
   c. *Significant phone calls, home visits, and family interactions; additional critical incident data*
   d *Care or observations not recorded elsewhere*
11. List five additional factors that can enhance accurate communication:
   a. *Correct grammar and spelling*
   b. *Legible writing, use of nonerasable ink*
   c. *Avoidance of repetition of data*
   d. *Avoidance of abbreviations*
   e. *Brevity*
12. What actions can be taken to correct an error in charting? *Draw a line through the error, write "error," and initial.*
13. Name three charting formats:
   a. *Block*
   b. *POMR/SOAP*
   c. *FOCUS™ CHARTING/DAR*
   d. *Narrative—time.*
14. Read the following vignette and record the client data using the SOAP and DAR formats, and the format used in your facility/agency, if different.

VIGNETTE:

Sally was discharged home with the twins on the evening of her third postpartal day. On the morning of day 5, she is visited by the public health nurse specializing in maternal/newborn care.

Sally is dressed in a robe and slippers, her hair is uncombed, her color is pale, and she has dark circles under her eyes. She is sitting in a recliner, bottle feeding Baby A. The grandmother is sitting on the couch feeding Baby B. The living area is noted to be clean and neat with comfortable ambient temperature. The two older children are reported to be at preschool from 9 AM to 2:30 PM daily.

Postpartal assessment form is completed with physical findings within normal limits. Sally reports her bowels are working "slowly" (small firm BM this AM) with fluid intake approximately 2 L/day and moderate appetite—"just too tired to really eat or do anything else." Sally's mother indicates she is providing household assistance—cooking, cleaning, and child care. Sally and her mother agree fatigue is a major concern for Sally. Both Sally and her mother are up twice during the night to feed the twins. Sally does take short naps during the day. Sally is observed to display usual attachment behaviors toward Baby A (Laura); however, her interaction with Baby B (unnamed) is of short duration, appears to lack warmth, and is restricted to caretaking activities.

You provide Sally with a teaching sheet describing postpartal fatigue and discussing dietary needs/supplements, energy conservation techniques, and the importance of balanced activity/exercise and rest. You suggest Sally's husband might get up for one feeding during the night to allow her a longer period of uninterrupted sleep and to provide him additional opportunity for interaction with his daughters.

Next, you ask Sally how she feels about being the mother of twins. Sally becomes tearful and states "I just don't know what I'm going to do when Mom goes home." You ask if she would like to have a visit from a member of the Mothers of Multiples group. You also suggest having a family meeting to problem-solve her concerns. You then discuss your observation that Sally appears more comfortable with Laura than with her twin, asking Sally to describe her perceptions of and feelings for Baby B. After reflecting on the question, Sally says she has felt so overwhelmed that she has not truly accepted the reality of having twins. She is visibly upset, berating herself for being a "poor mother." You tell her that it is not unusual to be overwhelmed by the reality of a multiple birth, even when planned for in advance of delivery.

You ask Sally to think about what she needs to help her resolve this situation. Sally decides she needs to spend more time getting to know Baby B, allowing other family members to care for and interact with Laura. After a discussion about the individual characteristics of her other children, Sally says Baby B is unique in her level of alertness and "her acceptance" of anyone who cares for her. "She deserves a name reflecting family ties and thanksgiving for the special gift of twins." You encourage Sally to read the literature about twins provided before her discharge and to apply techniques she has found successful in dealing with previous stressful situations. You schedule a follow-up visit for 1 week and leave a contact number if Sally has any questions or needs assistance before your next visit. When you depart, Sally appears focused on ways to improve her current situation, displaying a lighter mood, smiling, and giving a firm handshake.

The SOAP format requires that chart entries be tied to a problem. In reviewing this vignette, you might choose to address the problem of constipation as follows:

SOAP: PROBLEM #4 (CONSTIPATION)

S: Bowels working slowly.

O: Small firm BM this AM.

A: Constipation beginning to resolve.

P: Continue oral fluid intake of 2+ L/day and monitor diet for adequate bulk and roughage.

I: Verified Sally has reviewed teaching sheet.

E: States she understands interventions.

R: Reassess on next visit.
Or you might choose to address the problem of fatigue:

SOAP: PROBLEM #6 (FATIGUE)

S: "Too tired to eat or do anything else." Concern expressed about coping once her mother leaves.

O: Tearful. Color pale with dark circles under her eyes.

A: Postpartum fatigue.

P: Provide information, review activity schedule, identify possible role model.

I: Teaching sheet regarding postpartal fatigue provided. Discussed dietary needs/supplements, energy conservation techniques, and activity/rest program. Suggested family meeting to problem-solve concerns and to involve husband more in provision of care for infants. Referral made to Mothers of Multiples group.

E: Sally appears receptive to plan and with mother's assistance will likely follow through. Will reassess at next visit in 1 week.

> The DAR format provides for chart entries to be tied to a problem sign/symptom, event, or specific standard of care. Therefore, an initial entry addressing the home visit is acceptable, or you could choose to address the problem of fatigue.

DAR: HOME VISIT

D: See Postpartal Assessment form attached. Reports constipation slowly resolving. Primary concern is fatigue and whether she will be able to cope once mother leaves. Bonding with Baby B appears weak, interaction is of short duration and restricted to caretaking activities, appears uncomfortable and lacks warmth. Tearful, berated self for being a "poor" mother.

A: Provided teaching sheet re Postpartal Fatigue. Discussed dietary needs/supplements, energy conservation techniques, activity/rest program. Suggested family meeting to problem-solve concerns and to have husband increase infant care activities. Encouraged Sally to identify special/individual characteristics of Baby B and review discharge literature re twins. Noted successful coping skills previously used and referral to Mothers of Multiples group provided. Follow-up visit scheduled for 1 week.

R: Sally has clarified current needs. She is focused on problem-solving activities and has identified actions to improve interactions and relationship with Baby B. Mood lighter, smiling, and handshake firm.

Key to Work Page: Chapter 8—Now is the time for you to put your knowledge "to the test" and show what you have learned.

Index

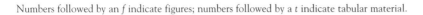

Numbers followed by an *f* indicate figures; numbers followed by a *t* indicate tabular material.